Cambridge History of Medicine
EDITORS: CHARLES WEBSTER
AND CHARLES ROSENBERG

Madness, Morality and Medicine

Other books in this series

Charles Webster, ed. *Health, medicine and mortality in the sixteenth century*
Ian Maclean *The Renaissance notion of woman*
Michael MacDonald *Mystical bedlam*
Robert E. Kohler *From medical chemistry to biochemistry*
Walter Pagel *Joan Baptista Van Helmont*
Nancy Tomes *A generous confidence*
Roger Cooter *The cultural meaning of popular science*

Madness, Morality and Medicine
A STUDY OF THE YORK RETREAT, 1796–1914

Anne Digby
Institute for Research in the Social Sciences
University of York

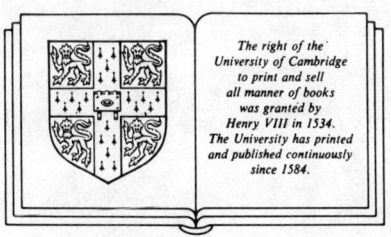

CAMBRIDGE UNIVERSITY PRESS
CAMBRIDGE
LONDON   NEW YORK   NEW ROCHELLE
MELBOURNE   SYDNEY

Published by the Press Syndicate of the University of Cambridge
The Pitt Building, Trumpington Street, Cambridge CB2 1RP
32 East 57th Street, New York, NY 10022, USA
10 Stamford Road, Oakleigh, Melbourne 3166, Australia

© Cambridge University Press 1985

First published 1985

Printed in the United States of America

Library of Congress Cataloging in Publication Data
Digby, Anne.
Madness, morality and medicine.
(Cambridge history of medicine)
Bibliography: p.
Includes index.
1. York Retreat. 2. Psychiatric hospitals – England –
History. 3. Mentally ill – Care and treatment – England –
History. I. Title. II. Series. [DNLM: 1. Hospitals,
Psychiatric – history – England.   WM 28 FE5 D5m]
RC450.G72Y673   1985   362.2'1'0942843   84 – 21486
ISBN 0 521 26067 1

For my parents

Contents

	List of illustrations and tables	*page* ix
	Preface	xiii
	A note on terminology	xvii
1	The birth of the asylum	1
2	The Retreat: a distinctive concept	14
	Founding the Retreat	14
	A distinctive lay therapy	25
3	Moral treatment	33
	A therapeutic environment	37
	Occupational therapy	42
	A domestic milieu	49
4	Moral management	57
	Patients as children	57
	Educating the insane	61
	Rewards and punishments	66
	Moral management and moral treatment	85
5	A Quaker institution	88
6	The ascendancy of medicine	105
	From lay therapist to medical practitioner	105
	Medical treatment	122
	The classification of insanity	135
	Old and new ideas	137
7	A hidden dimension: the asylum attendant	140
	Recruitment and wages	141
	Duties	144
	Performance	150
	William Waller	156
	From attendant to mental nurse	165

8	Patients	171
	The changing social character of patients	173
	The patients' world	186
9	The Retreat's record	202
	Admissions	202
	Alleged causes of insanity	207
	Short- and long-stay patients	213
	Outcome of treatment	221
	Readmissions	233
10	The Retreat's influence	237
	Appendix: selected case-notes of patients	259
	Notes	295
	Index	319

Illustrations and tables

FIGURES

5.1	Quaker and non-Quaker populations within the Retreat, 1820–1914	page 103
6.1	Drug costs and patients under medication	125
9.1	Patient numbers, 1796–1914	203
9.2	Annual admissions of patients, 1796–1909	204
9.3	Moral and physical causes of mental disorders among first admissions	211
9.4	Deaths as a percentage of average numbers of residents, 1798–1913	226
9.5	Recoveries as a percentage of annual admissions: five-year averages, 1801–1910	232
10.1	Visitors to the Retreat 1815–61	246

PLATES

1	Pencil sketch of three generations of Tukes: William, Henry and Samuel (1826)	19
2	Silhouettes of George and Catherine Jepson	22
3	The Sixth Gallery in 1900	41
4	New dining-room for ladies, 1899	41
5	Perspective view of north front of the Retreat	44
6	The Appendage (shown on right)	44
7	Cricket team, 1901	47
8	The Lodge (rebuilt in 1875) with cricket match	47
9	Plan of the Retreat in 1827	68
10	Patients taking the air at Scarborough	70
11	Throxenby Hall, 1904	70
12	Early bill showing purchase of means of mechanical restraint	80

x   *Illustrations and Tables*

13	Thomas and Mary Allis	109
14	Hannah Ponsonby	110
15	Dr Thurnam	110
16	Dr Kitching	116
17	Dr Baker	116
18	Drs Pierce, McKenzie (Assistant Medical Officer) and Kemp	117
19	West Villa	118
20	East Villa	118
21	Belle Vue House	119
22	William Waller	163
23	Elizabeth Slee	163
24	Nurses in c.1900. E. Rowntree is on the left.	167
25	Thomas W.	188
26	Robert H.	190
27	Barnard R.	190
28	Notice of escape	198
29	A patient's view of his treatment (1899)	201
30	Signatures in the Visitors Book of six Senecan Indians and their chief who visited the Retreat in 1818	257

TABLES

5.1	Characteristics of Quaker moral insanity cases	95
6.1	Average cost of drugs per patient, 1800–1914	126
6.2	Diagnoses of first admissions, June 1796–June 1843	136
7.1	Ratio of attendants to patients	146
7.2	Length of attendants' service in 1896	166
7.3	Timetables of nurses in 1902	168
8.1	Religious affiliation of first admissions (in %)	174
8.2	Gender of first admissions (in %)	174
8.3	Marital status of first admissions (in %)	175
8.4	Ages of first admissions (in %)	177
8.5	Geographical origins of first admissions (in %)	179
8.6	Geographical origins of Quaker and non-Quaker first admissions, 1796–1910 (in %)	180
8.7	Class of first admissions (in %)	183

8.8	Class of Quaker and non-Quaker first admissions, 1796–1910 (in %)	184
8.9	Class of Quaker first admissions in Retreat and in the Quaker community (in %)	185
9.1	Alleged causes of mental disorder of first admissions (in %)	209
9.2	Duration of stay of first admissions (in %)	219
9.3	Duration of stay of first admissions in relation to religious affiliation, 1796–1910 (in %)	220
9.4	Duration of mental illness prior to admission in relation to outcome, 1796–1840 (in %)	227
9.5	Outcome of treatment of first admissions in relation to duration of stay, 1796–1910 (in %)	227
9.6	Duration of stay in relation to outcome of first admissions, 1796–1910 (in %)	228
9.7	Gender in relation to outcome of treatment in first admissions, 1796–1910 (in %)	228
9.8	Marital status in relation to outcome of treatment of first admissions, 1796–1910 (in %)	229
9.9	Age in relation to outcome of treatment of first admissions, 1796–1910 (in %)	230
9.10	Religious affiliation in relation to outcome of treatment of first admissions, 1796–1910 (in %)	230
9.11	Outcome of treatment of first admissions under different superintendents between 1796 and 1910 (in %)	231
9.12	Total number of stays of patients (in %)	236

Preface

Most studies of the history of mental illness pay tribute to the past work of the Retreat in York in promoting mild methods of treatment. Yet although there is consensus on its historical significance the image of the institution that is presented is to some extent a misleading one. It is derived from Samuel Tuke's *Description of the Retreat,* written in 1813 as the first full-length account of any asylum and enormously influential in the early nineteenth century because of this. But the fact that this book was written from a reformist standpoint has usually been overlooked, and so its ahistorical nature in neglecting the Retreat's antecedents, its selectivity in describing its therapy and its optimism as to the outcome of treatment have been accepted as a reflection of a static historical reality. In the past Tuke's view of the Retreat has been serviceable in helping to construct a Whiggish identification of the rise of the asylum with psychiatric progress. More recently the limitations of such an interpretation have become apparent, with general studies that have questioned whether the asylum was a progressive reform and that have emphasised the extent to which its creation was a response to wider social, economic and intellectual changes. Yet modern hypotheses, like their Whiggish predecessors, have had to erect large models on fragmentary foundations since histories of individual asylums are few in number. In this context, a detailed study of the Retreat seemed to be particularly needed because of its historical and historiographical importance.

The Retreat was not a typical asylum. Its distinctive features naturally contributed to its historical significance but, less obviously perhaps, added to both the interest and the feasibility of research on its past. The Quaker character of its founders, managers and therapists gave a special moral and religious dimension to life within the institution and to the treatment there, since it contrasted with more secular preoccupations in other establishments for the care of the mentally ill. Contemporaries frequently referred to it as the Quaker Retreat, and in its early days it was in many respects a microcosm of the wider Society of Friends. Close relationships between Friends at the Retreat and those elsewhere produced abundant correspondence, so that the historian is fortunately placed to try to evaluate such intangible features of asylum life as relatives' attitudes to mental illness. The permanent smallness of this private, charitable hospital differed markedly from the increasing size of large numbers of public asylums created during the nineteenth century. This enabled the Retreat's therapists to give greater importance to patients as individuals and to develop original ideas on their treatment. The quality of case-records that they kept on their relatively small number of patients gave an added attraction to the Retreat as a subject for enquiry by a social historian.

These extensive archives made possible the first large-scale study of all the patients in an English asylum that has yet been undertaken. This quantitative, computerised examination of patients highlighted the way in which an original Quaker clientele was gradually outnumbered by non-Quakers, and analysis of case-records indicated an interesting differentiation in their medical histories. Continuity in the hospital's records, and open access to them until an unusually late date, enabled the investigation to be extended into the underresearched era of the late-Victorian and Edwardian era. This dynamic, long-term view revealed a fascinating change in the balance between curative and custodial aspects of treatment, the deterioration of the Retreat's well-publicised moral treatment into a more repressive moral management and the growing ascendancy of medical therapy. The fortunate discovery of the private papers of William Waller, who worked as a Retreat attendant during the 1840s and 1850s, gave a unique insight into an important but usually concealed area of an asylum: the relationship between patients and those who looked after them. And extensive use of a rich but neglected source in the case histories of patients has given a clearer view of individuals usually hidden from, and forgotten by, history.

Yet much remains elusive. The opaqueness of the language used to categorise mental illness and to denote progress by patients leaves vital topics of interest highly problematical. Even apparently more

Preface

accessible, administrative records pose difficulties since they were intended to articulate the viewpoint of asylum managers and doctors, and only inadvertently do they reveal the feelings of patients. The attempt to try to penetrate beyond this official facade and to reconstruct a more complex reality than the one-sidedness of the "official" record has proved both challenging and rewarding.

I have been particularly fortunate in this task because of the help given me by individuals and institutions.

For permission to use the Retreat's library I should like to thank the Committee of Management, and for making me welcome on visits there I am grateful to Miss Eileen Cope and Mr Leonard Barnard. I owe a special debt to the Retreat's medical director, Dr Alistair Gordon, and his colleague, Dr Michael Bearpark, for sharing their expertise with me. And at the Borthwick Institute of Historical Research David Smith, Bill Sheils and Chris Webb have made the Retreat's archives available to me with exemplary efficiency.

Many librarians and archivists have furthered my researches and I should like to acknowledge the help given by the staffs of the libraries of the Universities of York, Leeds, Cambridge and Manchester; the Wellcome Library for the History of Medicine; the Library of the Society of Friends; the British Library; York City Reference Library; York City Archives; the West Riding Record Office; the Public Record Office; the Royal Bethlem Archives; the Stanley Royd Hospital, Wakefield; and Bootham Park Hospital, York.

My ideas have been clarified and my focus of enquiry sharpened during enjoyable conversations with Bill Bynum, Anne Crowther, Nicholas Hervey, Kay Jones, Mike Jones, Bill Luckin, Charlotte McKenzie, Alan Peacock, John Pickstone, Roger Smith and John Walton. I hope they feel that I have developed shared ideas fruitfully. In addition I have profited from many interesting suggestions made in discussion following papers given at conferences, seminars and meetings in Cambridge, Lancaster, London, Manchester and York.

I am very appreciative of the assistance given me by Bill and Margot Sessions, who enlightened a non-Quaker through their insight into the history and beliefs of the Society of Friends; Brian Walster, who altruistically gave me access to his private archive on William Waller; David Whiteley, who skilfully produced clear photographs from faded antique prints; Dr Arthur Bowen, who first showed me the potentialities of research in this field; Dr Peter Kennedy and his colleagues at Bootham Park Hospital, whose comments expanded my field of vision; Jessica Feinstein, who was an exemplary and ever-willing research assistant; Roy Porter, who provided scholarly and stimulating comment on the text of this book; and Charles Webster, who brought both acumen and forbearance to the task of editing this volume. And I have derived incalculable benefit from Charles Feinstein's sustained encouragement, intellectual companionship and constructive advice and criticism.

I would like to acknowledge the generosity of the Retreat's Committee of Management for permission to use many of the photographs in this book and to Brian Walster for the use of the photographs of William Waller and Elizabeth Slee.

Finally, I am grateful both to the Social Science Research Council for funding this research, and to the Institute for Research in the Social Sciences in the University of York for the facilities it placed at my disposal. My obligation to my IRISS colleague, Eileen Sutcliffe, for her help in computerising my data is substantial. My thanks are due to Michael Doe and Helen Humphreys who drew the figures meticulously. Only the IRISS secretaries – Sally Baker, Sally Cuthbert and Barbara Olive – who jointly converted my manuscript palimpsest into a model typescript, possess the secret of how many times I find it necessary to rewrite drafts.

Anne Digby

A note on terminology

The language contemporaries used to refer to mental illness has been retained since the social nuances it embodied provide us with rich insights. It is helpful to appreciate, however, that there was considerable plasticity in the general terms used so that lunacy, madness or mental disorder were deployed interchangeably. This diffuseness was also found in the more specialist vocabulary developed by "professionals" working in the field of mental illness, whose vocabulary was neither static nor precise, but was often merely speculative.

1

The birth of the asylum

Perceptions of madness are culturally responsive: definitions of what constitutes insanity are a reflection of ideas and values current at a particular time in contemporary society. Amongst these are the prevailing notions regarding sanity: in characterising individuals as mad emphases on uncontrollable passions, an undisciplined will or an irrational mind provide an implicit contrast with the ideal attributes of the sane. As views of humanity change so the interface between sanity and madness alters. And the treatment of the mad reflects the extent to which this fluid boundary between sanity and insanity is seen as permeable. If those deemed insane are believed in some degree to partake of the attributes of the rest of humanity then resocialisation or rehabilitation is more likely to be prominent in their therapy. If they are seen as animal, or as having lost their spiritual element, discipline and coercion will probably be the dominant or sole methods of treatment.

Georgian England is extraordinarily interesting for a study of changing perspectives on insanity. By the end of the eighteenth century the lunatic was beginning to be seen less as brute than as human, heroic therapeutics inherited from classical times were being challenged by milder methods and the growth of specialist treatment in asylums and madhouses provided an increasing therapeutic optimism. It was within this context of transitional theory and practice that the Retreat opened its doors in 1796.

Although there was a range of attitudes towards madness, the dominant conception within this spectrum was beginning to change in the early modern period. Madness was seen less as a spiritual disease, in which the mad, possessed by the devil, were sinful or immoral, and more as a secular condition. Metaphor and allusion in literature and art give us a useful insight into the extent of this transition. In 1615 Thomas Adams's famous sermon, *Mystical Bed-*

lam, or the World of Mad Men, retained the traditional idea that spiritual and mental afflictions were identical: 'every wilfull sinne is Madness'. The oldest lunatic establishment in England – Bethlem Hospital popularly known as Bedlam – was depicted metaphorically as a theological establishment that housed twenty different kinds of moral madness. But by the late seventeenth century Bedlam was being demystified and secularised: it could now be regarded as a kind of zoo and its mad inmates as akin to animals. Their degradation was depicted poetically, with excremental vividness, in Pope's 'Dunciad' of 1726; a few years later Hogarth's artistry emphasised the brutish degeneration of Tom Rakewell, chained up in the squalor of Bedlam, during the final phase of his 'Rake's Progress'.[1] These images both reflected changes in attitudes towards madness and acted as a catalyst in transforming social sensibility.

The shift in attitudes that was making madness into more of a secular condition was complex: profuse and sometimes contradictory evidence is not amenable to the imposition of simple analytical patterns. In this context it is worth noting that within the mental world of laymen, contemporaries could hold very varied perceptions of insanity, and that even specialists in the treatment of madness frequently maintained a breath-taking eclecticism in both theory and practice. Old stereotypes frequently coexisted with new ideas whereas fresh philosophical, psychological or medical insights into the nature of insanity did not necessarily overturn conventional practices. Within this complicated, and often confusing, intellectual terrain it is helpful to isolate a strategic change in opinion that placed an increased emphasis on the fundamental rationality of human beings and, associated with it, a much greater concern to control the passions of the individual.

'I cannot conceive of a man without thought, that would be a stone or a brute', wrote Pascal. In seeing reason as the essential attribute of humanity and thus the touchstone of sanity, this statement reflected a general secularisation in outlook that had occurred during the seventeenth century. Madness was no longer perceived primarily as a moral state, its religious undertones were less dominant and the connection with another world had lessened. Instead, the individual madman was seen as responsible for his own misfortune to some extent; irrationality might even be viewed as the product of individual choice rather than external agency.² In this identification of madness as a denial of reason related states also tended to partake of the undesirability of madness: an antipathy to 'fancy' was part of a pervasive distrust of subjectivity; dreams were seen as a form of temporary madness; unrestrained imagination and excessive enthusiasm were felt to be dangerous in their denial of rationality. By the eighteenth century religious enthusiasm was itself increasingly seen as a form of madness, thus denying both the independence of spiritual authority and the validity of the 'voice of the spirit'.³ Such irrationality came to be feared precisely because it was now internalised within the individual: the mad were in some sense authors of their own misfortunes since their control over their passions was inadequate. External discipline should therefore be applied to correct them.

In an age of reason the forces of irrationality – represented by the mad – needed to be excluded. Their conditions while confined were to be appropriate to their ambiguous state. Having lost their reason, which constituted their badge of humanity, the mad were seen as animals. This brutish view of the lunatic was reinforced by a much older intellectual tradition that regarded the universe as a great Chain of Being. Man, the middle link within this chain, was located where the transition occurred from lower sentient beings to higher intellectual ones. But the mad, having lost their rationality, slipped off the lowest rung of humanity and thus took on an animal character.⁴ In functional, as well as intellectual, terms the mad might be seen as the dregs of society as was evident in a contemporary association of madness with poverty. The insane were poor because they were idle: with other antisocial groups antagonistic to the work ethic they needed the corrective of institutionalisation.⁵ But the custodialism of early institutions also contained the potential for a more therapeutic function and this emerged later with the development of the specialised asylum.

The earliest institutional provision for the insane was more for the protection of the public than for the care of the inmates. Bethlem Hospital, founded in 1247 as the priory of St Mary of Bethlehem, was between the early fifteenth and eighteenth centuries the only English institution to provide 'specialist facilities' for the mad. In Augustan England about 100,000 people a year were willing to pay a penny entrance fee for the entertainment provided by the antics of the mad in this human zoo – Bedlam. Yet this brutish existence was probably preferable to the alternatives facing the majority of deranged individuals. Some were found in overtly custodial institutions such as prisons, houses of correction or workhouses. Others, less troublesome, might be looked after or restrained in the home of a householder who was compensated for his trouble by payment from the rates. From the mid-seventeenth century onwards, certain individuals began to make a living from this through their organisation of private madhouses.[6] But it was not until the middle of the eighteenth century, when there was an appreciation that the mad could be managed, rather than brutalised, that a different kind of provision for the insane could develop.

Madness is, contrary to the opinion of some unthinking persons, as manageable as many other distempers, which are equally dreadful and obstinate, and yet are not looked upon as incurable: and that such unhappy objects ought by no means to be abandoned, much less shut up in loathsome prisons as criminals or nuisances to society.[7]

This statement by Dr Battie, first physician to St Luke's Hospital, indicated the therapeutic optimism that had stimulated its foundation in 1751. Other specialist asylums followed: Manchester opened its doors in 1766; Newcastle in 1767; York in 1777; Liverpool in 1792; and Leicester in 1794. In these asylums lunatics were secluded from other 'problem populations' and specialist treatment was made possible. At Liverpool the objective of the new asylum was defined explicitly as being distinct from the custodialism of the workhouse, house of correction or gaol. Lunatics should be freed from the workhouse, which aimed to 'extirpate vice, disorder, guilty idleness from this great family of the lowest and most ignorant class of society', and should not be consigned to 'a prison-house for the insane', but to an asylum, which had 'the greater object of restoring reason itself'.[8] The therapeutic function of these early asylums was confirmed by their location when, as at Liverpool and Manchester, the lunatic establishment was administered as part of a larger hospital: the infirmary treated diseases of the body and the asylum those of the mind.

The humanity of the asylum's professed objectives was not necessarily matched by its medical therapy. Heroic therapeutics, based on a tradition that had originated with the classical practices of Hippocrates and Galen, still dominated mad-doctors' treatments during the early eighteenth century. These were based on the convention that mental health depended on a balance of the four humours in the body: blood, choler, phlegm and bile. Bold actions were justified in order to eliminate an excess of one or more of these elements, and so vigorous purgatives, emetics and bleedings were periodically used. These were intended to correct the humoral imbalance and restore the individual's appropriate temperament or character. Vigorous measures were directed particularly at the maniac whose violent behaviour must have appeared implicitly to sanction such extremity. Amongst these, a concern over the consistency of the blood led to much depletion through cupping and leeching. A similar desire to counteract morbid processes in the brain led to the use of counter-irritants: scarifications (surgical incisions in the skin), setons (threads through the skin) and artificially induced blisters were designed to give relief through the suppurations of the body.[9] The impact of such strenuous measures must have been as much to subdue as to treat those disordered in mind.

In the more scientific ethos of Georgian England, custom no longer seemed an entirely adequate sanction for medical treatment. The anecdotalism that had characterised earlier references to case histories in psychiatric literature was gradually replaced by an empiricism based on careful observations of individual patients. From the mid-eighteenth century books by mad-doctors showed a certain amount of scepticism towards traditional methods. A concern to test them experimentally and to justify their use or discontinuance on the basis of medical trials was evident.[10] Dr Battie, physician at St Luke's Hospital, suggested in 1758 that general bleedings, emetics, blisters and cathartics were inappropriate and that medical remedies should be used with caution.[11] By the early nineteenth century when Dr Joseph Mason Cox, physician at Fishponds, a private madhouse near Bristol, condemned 'a blind, indiscriminate routine of practice' a substantial medical literature had laid down the guidelines for more selective treatment.[12] Publications by Cullen, Arnold, Ferriar, Haslam and other practitioners argued, on the basis of observation and experience, that professional judgement and a sensitive response to individual patients were required to assess appropriate therapy. Reinforcing this trend towards greater discrimination was a fresh perception of the insane patient.

Cultural changes made it easier by the late eighteenth century to view the lunatic as a patient: an individual to whom the doctor might relate, rather than an animal to whom he might administer a standard treatment. In its stress on the brotherhood of man evangelicalism helped break the intellectual fetters of the Great Chain of Being that earlier had strengthened the belief in the lunatic as an animal. Evangelical influence helped reintegrate the mad within humanity precisely because it emphasised the fundamental similarity of all human beings before God. To a certain extent early romantic sensibility harmonised with this in seeing the perceptions of the mad as authentic experience similar in its validity to that of the poet, and thus a means of extending mental horizons.[13] But perhaps the most potent influence was the associationist psychology of John Locke with its perception that the mad were within reach of the comfortable terrain of everyday thinking:

For they do not appear to me to have lost the faculty of reasoning, but having joined together some ideas very wrongly, they mistake them for truths, and they err as men do that argue right from wrong principles. For, by the violence of their imaginations, having taken their fancies for realities, they make right deductions from them.[14]

His views were embraced eagerly by mad-doctors, as for example by John Haslam, the apothecary at Bethlem, who defined insanity as 'an incorrect association of ideas'.[15] This fresh perception that the essential attribute of the mad was irrationality rather than animality was a pre-condition for a fundamental change in the treatment of insanity. Since madness now appeared to consist at least as much in mental as organic defect, psychological rather than physiological methods seemed appropriate. And central to psychological medicine was the concept of management.

The importance of management had been recognised as early as the 1750s and its theory was developed with increasing finesse and subtlety during the next half century. By 1792 William Pargeter was clear that 'the chief reliance in the care of insanity must be rather on management than medicine'.[16] But concepts of management differed. There was a limited consensus that it derived from the benevolent authority of the physician, apothecary or asylum superintendent who exercised judicious firmness towards his patients. Beyond this there was disagreement as to the best method of subduing or managing the mad. Dr Willis intimidated his patients – amongst them George III – through eye contact as well as more coercive methods. Haslam suggested in 1798 that he attained his 'ascendancy' over patients by means of decisive actions and a system of rewards and punishments. Thus:

> By gentleness of manner and kindness of treatment, I have never failed to obtain the confidence, and conciliate the esteem of insane persons, and have succeeded by these means in procuring from them respect and obedience.[17]

Here the notions of ascendancy and obedience appear to be incongruous with those of conciliation and mutual confidence. But this may be resolved if the moral dimension of management is examined more closely.

John Ferriar of the Manchester Infirmary and Asylum wrote with unusual penetration on this topic in the 1790s. He perceived that 'the management of hope and apprehension in the patient forms the most useful part of the discipline'. His experience had suggested to him that it was 'useful to remonstrate, for lunatics have frequently a high sense of honour, and are sooner brought to reflection by the appearance of indignity than by actual violence, against which they usually harden themselves'.[18] Although contemporaries were impressed by the mildness of this new kind of therapy Ferriar's statement indicated that this was partly an optical illusion. Although moral treatment was less overtly coercive than traditional methods of restraint – chains, manacles or whips – it nevertheless might involve deeper constraints within the mind rather than the body. Foucault's conclusion that 'a purely psychological medicine was made possible only when madness was alienated in guilt'[19] has a kernel of truth.

Psychological medicine was similar to physiological medicine in being in an intermediate state by the turn of the nineteenth century. Management was interpreted by some practitioners by reference to traditional ideas on the need to instil fear in the mad. Thus, Cox promoted his notorious swing as a means of gaining ascendancy over a patient since 'rather than repeat the ride in the whirligig, as he termed it, he submitted entirely to my wishes'. This was hardly surprising since such rides produced extreme vertigo and nausea. However, Cox justified this in terms of an older set of ideas concerning the insensitivity of the maniac:

Maniacs in general are not sensible to the action of the common oscillatory swing, though it affords an excellent mode of secure confinement, and of harmless punishment.[20]

But fear and surprise could also be justified in relation to the newer psychology of Locke since it might be argued that the association of wrong ideas needed to be jolted apart. Cullen, professor of physic at Edinburgh University, argued that fear was a useful tool in management because 'fear being a passion that diminishes excitement may . . . be opposed . . . to the angry and irascible excitement of the maniacs'.[21]

It was not maniacs but melancholics who were thought to be particularly appropriate subjects for such management. And melancholy was seen as a national disease, as in George Cheyne's *The English Malady* of 1734. This fashionable nervous disorder was associated with the sensitive susceptibilities and overcivilised lifestyles of the better-off in Georgian England.[22] And it was to the needs of the middle and upper classes that much of the expanded institutional provision in the treatment of the mad was directed. This was particularly obvious in the case of private madhouses, which, as part of the lucrative 'trade in lunacy', were directed at least as much to the profit principle as to the relief of the mad. The newly instituted public asylums emphasised their therapeutic objectives but focussed them on the relief of particular social groups. The Manchester Asylum spoke of the assistance that it hoped to give to 'Persons of middling Fortunes' and the York Asylum aimed to help 'persons of moderate circumstance'.[23] In the case of York and Liverpool this philanthropic aim was also extended to poorer patients and it was hoped that 'the increased payments made by the rich may serve to diminish, in some degree, the demands on the poor'.[24]

This contemporary evidence on the largely bourgeois clientele of the asylum is at variance with some modern interpretations – notably those by Foucault, Doerner and Scull. Foucault has suggested that during the seventeenth century the mad, along with the poor, were seen as a social problem because of their idleness. In this 'classical' period their confinement, as was that of other social deviants, was organised to act as both punishment and reform. That the institutionalisation of the mad was a social response to an economic problem is also stressed by Doerner. Removing the pauper insane from the community into institutions had practical utility in freeing others in their families from caring for them and thus allowing them to work. It also underlined the values of bourgeois society where rationality came to be identified with work and irrationality with idleness and poverty. For Scull too, the advent of the market economy was the principal cause of a weakening of the familial system of caring for the insane poor, and this resulted in the rise of the specialist institution – the asylum.[25] In these interpretations madness has lost its 'neutral' character as an illness and taken on a social resonance, and the asylum is seen as an agency of social control rather than of therapy.

These hypotheses are more obviously relevant to the larger pauper asylums of the mid- and late nineteenth century than to the small and fairly élitist institutional provision of the eighteenth century. Asylums in this earlier period catered for a tiny proportion of the population. At the end of the eighteenth century Bedlam housed about 250 inmates; St Luke's, approximately 300; Manchester, 100; York, 112; and Liverpool, about 60.[26] No accurate figures existed for those in private madhouses although an incomplete source of information, the Town and Country Registers, which enumerated only non-pauper patients, indicated that fewer than 500 patients were to be found in licensed private houses by 1800.[27]

These specialist institutions were a necessary, but not a sufficient, pre-condition for a therapeutic regime. Patchy evidence on treatment indicated that these were transitional institutions poised uncertainly between older custodial conventions and newer therapeutic ideals. Bethlem with its indiscriminate medication and mechanical restraint of inmates, exemplified the view of a lunatic as an animal. But even here an acceptance of change was discernible in 1770 with the exclusion of the crowds from their traditional entertainment of teasing the mad.[28] At St Luke's a more progressive view of madness as mental illness rather than spectacle had led to a welcome for the specialist visitor but not for the staring public. But even here insight into the possibilities of individual medication and of managing the patient coexisted with older ideas on the insensibility of the mad to cold and discomfort. Chained lunatics were to be seen lying on straw in unheated cells where unglazed windows exposed them to the extremities of the weather.[29] And at Leicester Thomas Arnold, physician to the asylum, accepted the view of associationist psychology that madness was a matter of disordered reason, but this did not stop physical restraint being applied to patients. This was an interesting, and not untypical, illustration of the way in which 'advances' in theory did not necessarily underwrite the development of more enlightened practice.[30] Underlying this fusion of varied, sometimes contradictory, systems within asylums was a curative optimism. The Liverpool Asylum was directed to the 'restoration of reason' for some if not all of its patients. The asylum at Manchester looked forward to the 'great prospect' of 'frequent relieving, if not perfecting the cure' of its inmates.[31]

At Manchester the patients were expected 'to live ... as one family, rendering one another mutual help and assistance'. They were to be resocialised under a highly developed system of management: the physician, Dr Ferriar, wrote that the discipline was to be mild but exact.[32] In his regime, selective medication on an individualised basis was useful in the acute forms of disorder but discipline was considered important during convalescence:

For in the cure of a disease of this nature, the patient must 'minister to himself:' medicine may restore him more early and more completely to the command of his intellectual operations: discipline must direct him in their exercise.[33]

Although Ferriar's emphasis on moral treatment foreshadowed better-known developments in the nineteenth century it is difficult to decide to what extent his writing reflected the actual practices of the Manchester Asylum. Evidence on the use of chains, straitjackets and straps suggests that some mechanical restraint continued to be used. Isolated reports in the local press on the keepers' brutality to patients indicated that there were some lapses from the 'Rules' of 1773. These had laid down that the patients were to be treated 'with all tenderness and indulgences compatible with the steady and effectual government of them'.[34] Thus, the relationship between theory and practice might be tenuous and ideals betrayed by reality. Nowhere did this gap between objectives and their fulfilment become more obvious than at the York Asylum.

An idealistic case was made for the York Asylum during the five years of local discussion that preceded its opening in 1777. Since the existing four English asylums could not accept all applicants there was a need for additional accommodation:

The birth of the asylum

Something should be done for the relief of those unhappy sufferers who are the objects of terror and compassion to all around them and whose cases lay a just claim to the benevolence of their fellow creatures.

Strongly impressed with a desire of alleviating the miseries of that unhappy part of the community, some humane persons have formed a noble resolution of affording an asylum.

In soliciting subscriptions the promoters played on the humanitarian sympathies of their readers: the lunatics were 'miserable and afflicted' or 'unhappy sufferers' and their 'deplorable situation' cried out for redress. One of the worst features of their predicament was financial:

Many persons of moderate circumstances, who, labouring under the terrible misfortune of an unsound mind, have no place to retire to but a private mad-house, where their cure stands a great chance of being protracted for the benefit of a mercenary keeper.

In contrast, the York Asylum, modelled on the 'excellent establishments' at Newcastle and Manchester, would be under men of 'principles and honour' who would ensure that 'the most humane and disinterested treatment was provided' for patients.[35]

The York Asylum was intended to be a medical institution, although a planned purchase of land for the asylum next to the County Infirmary did not prove practicable.[36] Its promoters had used as one of the justifications for erecting a fifth English asylum the unmet needs of prospective patients for medical treatment.

By this unavoidable exclusion or delay in the admission of objects many useful members have been lost to society, either by the disorder gaining strength beyond the reach of medicine, or by the patients falling into the hands of persons utterly unskilled in the treatment of their disease.[37]

At the York Asylum a regular physician was to give attendance and a house apothecary assisted by matron, head keeper and six servants was to care for the patients. Dr Hunter, promoter and sole physician, saw the basis of his expertise in the treatment of the insane as located in secret formulations of green and grey powders that he used as aperients and emetics. He saw psychiatry as an 'obscure branch of medicine':[38] unlike others in comparable positions – notably Battie, Haslam, Arnold and Ferriar – he produced no specialist writing. The admissions book for the asylum revealed little intellectual penetration on the classification of patients' symptoms. Most were described as 'flighty', a few as 'melancholic' and a very small minority as 'flighty and wild' or 'furious'.[39] An absence of case-notes may also suggest that he had little interest in either a systematic observation of patients or a scientific record of their treatment.

These internal features of the asylum were not discernible to the public, who were given occasional case histories and generalised descriptions of asylum practice that suggested that all was conducted on the most progressive lines. For example, at the Charity Sermon in 1783, on the occasion of an annual appeal for money at St Michael Le Belfrey, York, details were given of the remarkable recovery of one patient. Having entered the York Asylum in 1778 in a state of deep melancholy, he had endured a period of over five years in which 'everything was indifferent to him'. But during this period of insensibility he was treated with tenderness and his medicines consisted not of harsh evacuants but of tonics and a generous dietary, so that eventually he recovered and was restored to his family.[40] This kind of selective publicity enabled Dr Hunter to claim:

In this asylum the patients are treated with all the tenderness and indulgence that is compatible with a steady and effectual government; and the servants are enjoined never to use unnecessary severity.[41]

Thus the York Asylum appeared to offer its patients a progressive regime that included a judicious combination of medicine and management. Yet despite this favourable image there was unease in some quarters about the reality that existed behind the impressive Georgian facade of the York Asylum and the extent to which it was fulfilling its original, humane objectives.[42] For the local Quaker community evidence that institutional practice had betrayed the ideals of the asylum's founders was given by the circumstances surrounding a Quaker patient's death there in 1790, after a short stay during which access by members of the Society of Friends had been refused. Disquiet at this led to the foundation of a second York asylum, the Retreat, in 1796.

The laymen who initiated this small Quaker asylum were intelligent pragmatists. In deciding on the appropriate treatment for their patients they unconsciously followed the method of empiricism and observation developed by medical specialists. Having previously adopted humanitarian and evangelical ideals they were naturally predisposed in favour of milder treatments. And as members of the Society of Friends, brought up under a strict Quaker discipline, these lay therapists found ideas of management both congenial and familiar. Receptive to the more significant developments that had occurred earlier in the treatment of the mad, those at the Retreat were fortunately placed to synthesise them into a distinctive form of enlightened therapy. This 'moral treatment' was to make the name of the Retreat world famous.

2

The Retreat: a distinctive concept

'A place in which the unhappy might obtain a refuge – a quiet haven in which the shattered bark might find a means of reparation or of safety'.[1] This perceptive description of the Retreat after half a century's existence emphasised its function as a sanctuary or shelter for the afflicted and hinted at its singularity in seeking to realize to the full the concept of an asylum. Those who had begun this venture in 1792 had done so, not from a specialist knowledge of the insane or a desire to benefit financially from their plight, but from compassion for their afflicted brothers in humanity. The distinctive therapy of this Quaker institution followed from its reliance on the religious and moral principles that informed the lives of sane members of the Society of Friends; its robust rejection of contemporary prejudices regarding the treatment of the insane; and its pragmatic formulation of therapy as a series of responses to the everyday needs of its patients. However, the eventual success of the York Retreat, and the international fame of its moral treatment, were by no means assured in its early years nor were the methods it adopted immediately self-evident.

FOUNDING THE RETREAT

From a historical perspective the creation of the Retreat in the 1790s had an apparent inevitability. The 'new social spirit' that activated the Society of Friends to relieve suffering and help the oppressed had already led to practical attempts to end slavery and was shortly to lead to Quaker involvement in the relief of the London poor and to attempts to ameliorate the conditions of prisoners.[2] Yet the proposal by a York Quaker, William Tuke, to provide more enlightened care for another category of sufferers – those with mental illness – was far from being accorded immediate approval. Some queried the need for a Quaker institution since they considered that Friends had not 'experienced the least disadvantage or difference of treatment from the rest of the patients' on account of their religious persuasion. Others were uncertain as to its function: a York asylum would be too big for local needs and too small for national ones. There were strong objections from areas distant from York because of the expense that would be incurred in sending patients there; some would therefore have preferred the asylum to be set up more centrally in London. Concern was expressed over its financial viability and it was suggested that hiring premises would be more prudent than building a custom-made asylum.[3] The financial commitment involved worried William Tuke's own family. His wife, Esther, at first dismissed the scheme with the dry remark, 'Thee has had many wonderful children of thy brain dear William, but this one is surely like to be an idiot.'[4]

Fellow Quakers recognised that William Tuke possessed 'an uncommon degree of firmness of mind'[5] and this stubbornness of purpose helped him to persevere in the face of such criticism in order to achieve what he thought was right. His conscience had been stirred by the fate of Hannah Mills, the Leeds widow who had died in the York Asylum. Admitted on 15 March 1790 suffering from 'Melancholy' she died only six weeks later on 29 April. What was a matter of acute concern to local Quakers was the fact that the overseers from York Monthly Meeting had been refused permission to visit her in the asylum. She had therefore been bereft of any religious consolation during her last days, and no one knew whether the treatment she had received had contributed to her death. Anxieties about conditions in the asylum were being voiced locally, and suspicions about 'abuses of power' within a 'clandestine' institution were current.[6] Discussion in William Tuke's household on the asylum, and the conditions under which Hannah Mills died, prompted the question of whether more humane facilities could be provided. Ann Tuke asked, 'Father, why cannot we have an establishment for such persons in our own Society?'[7]

An apposite conjunction of individual personality and event meant that this casual remark acquired historical resonance. Tuke's own philosophy that 'I never could find that there's more required than there's ability to perform'[8] sustained him through early difficulties in launching and administering the Retreat. From his earlier experience in helping to promote Friends' schools at Ackworth and

York in 1779 and 1785, he had obtained skills in fund-raising and institutional organisation. His appointment as clerk to the national Yearly Meeting of the Society of Friends in 1783 had presumably given him a useful grasp of Quaker organisation and of prominent individuals in different localities whose support for the Retreat would contribute to its success. And his years running the Tuke grocery and tea firm since 1752 should have imbued him with sufficient business sense to balance philanthropic zeal against financial prudence. Tuke's practical idealism contributed to the successful inauguration of the Retreat and was also imprinted on the character of the new institution.

The launching of the Retreat was a prolonged affair involving intellectual debate to convert the sceptical, an adherence to formal and long-drawn-out administrative procedures in gaining support within the Quaker community, repeated fund-raising initiatives and practical problems in building the institution and recruiting staff. So six years elapsed between the death of Hannah Mills in April 1790 and the reception of the asylum's first patients in June 1796.

The proposal for the Retreat was first put in formal terms at the end of the Yorkshire Quarterly Meeting of the Society of Friends held in York during March 1792, although it is likely that William Tuke had previously discussed his ideas publicly at local Preparative and Monthly Meetings.[9] The Quarterly Meeting asked for an outline scheme to be presented at their next assembly in June of that year, when a blueprint was given:

> That, in case proper encouragement be given, ground be purchased, and a building be erected, sufficient to accommodate thirty patients, in an airy situation, and at as short a distance from York as may be, so as to have the privilege of retirement; and that there be a few acres for keeping cows, and for garden ground for the family; which will afford scope for the patients to take exercise, when that may be prudent and suitable.[10]

The scheme met with a generally, but not uniformly, favourable response. Further discussion and money-raising took place at these regional Quarterly Meetings in September 1792, April 1793 and June 1793 as well as at a special meeting called to coincide with a General Meeting at Ackworth School in July 1793. By this time £1,156 had been subscribed or donated, and so a committee was formed to buy a suitable plot of land. Before the close of 1793 eleven acres had been bought for £1,357.

An intensification of effort was discernible in 1794: the pressing need for funds led to redoubled efforts to publicise the nascent institution, to persuade Friends of its utility, and to urge on them the necessity of subscriptions. To the 1,000 copies of the proposals circulated in 1792, and 1,500 in 1793, a further 1,500 were printed so that they could be circulated 'within the compass of every Quarterly and Monthly Meeting in the nation'. A builder had prepared plans in the spring of 1794, and the cost for the central building and east wing was estimated at £1,883. As an act of faith a start was made on the building even though the funds to pay for it were then insufficient. By January 1795 the money had run out although the building was only half-finished. In spite of this, it was decided to build a west, as well as an east, wing to the asylum and to borrow whatever funds were required. Some additional money was given before the institution opened in June 1796, but notwithstanding this, £1,245 had had to be borrowed at interest in order to complete it.[11]

One reason for the slow influx of funds was doubt within the Quaker community as to whether it was a local institution intended primarily for the insane in Yorkshire or a truly national institution. The first circular in 1792 had given the unfortunate impression that Yorkshire patients would be admitted at preferential rates. Although this was later denied, it reinforced a feeling in some distant Quaker communities that the Retreat was too far away to be useful.[12] The discussions that had launched the Retreat, and those that settled its organisation, were always held within the county, a practice that further contributed to the detachment of Friends in other areas. In the lists of those who gave money to the Retreat, Yorkshire always outnumbered any other locality in both numbers and the amount subscribed. Although it was perhaps to be expected that in the first list of subscriptions all but a handful were from Yorkshire, it was still the case over half a century later that the county subscribed far more than any other area. By 1851, for example, Yorkshire had provided one-fifth of the donations, half the annuities, and nearly one-third of the subscriptions.[13] A circular of April 1793 admitted that Yorkshire Friends originally 'did not consider the institution as likely to accommodate the Society in the whole nation',[14] but although the implication was that this had been a misunderstanding, no direct indication was given that there had been a decisive change of mind on this point. The expense that travel to York occasioned Quakers in the south of England proved to be a continual irritant as was shown by an abortive plan to found a Southern Retreat in 1839.[15]

The most fundamental problem in these early days, however, was the unknown nature of the enterprise to which Yorkshire Quakers had committed themselves. A London Quaker, John Bevans, agreed to build the Retreat but admitted that previously the design of an asylum 'was a subject that never occupied my thoughts'. The uncertainties of design and of local costs meant that he refused even to provide estimates for the plans. Indeed, the earliest plans were provided by William Tuke and his son Henry, a point that has not been appreciated hitherto. Tuke visited St Luke's Hospital in London, and the structure of the building and conditions of its patients helped crystallise in his mind the distinctive elements that he wished the Retreat to embody. In the late autumn of 1793 he expounded his views to Bevans who was himself by this time better informed on his subject, having done some homework by reading John Howard on prisons and hospitals, and by visiting St Luke's.[16] Bevans accepted many of Tuke's ideas but omitted a third floor in favour of a lower, longer building that provided lengthier galleries where the patients could get exercise. He also substituted a central staircase for the two on each side of the building that Tuke had included, because Bevans felt that this facilitated supervision of patients. Finally, he substituted ordinary squared ceilings for the arched cells of Tuke's design because this increased the amount of air for patients. Tuke replied in some detail to Bevans, arguing for his original views in some cases, but deferring to the 'superior judgement' of Bevans.[17]

In the design of the Retreat financial stringency circumscribed ideals. William Tuke admitted that his original ideas were 'more than the finances will be likely to warrant us to construct at first'. Bevans rebuked Tuke on more than one occasion because he considered him overconcerned with 'how slender it might be built so as to stand'. He reminded him of the problems caused by poor construction at Ackworth, built by the London Foundling Hospital and recently taken over by Quakers as a boarding school. Eventually, it was decided that though the Retreat's galleries would

The Retreat: a distinctive concept

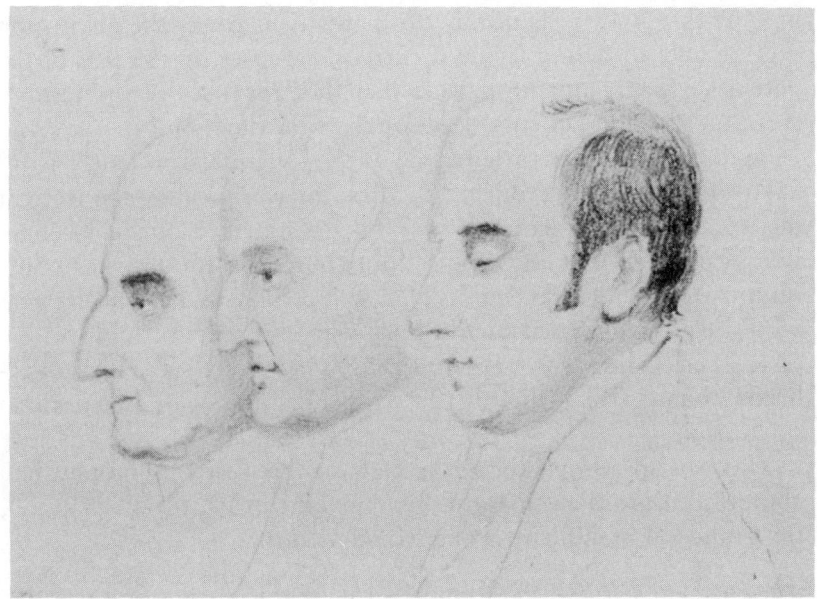

Plate 1. Pencil sketch of three generations of Tukes: William, Henry and Samuel (1826)

be reduced in width, the thickness of the walls would not be altered.[18]

Tuke's anxieties over the cost of the building were the result of a hesitant flow of funds. Whereas an appeal for funds for Ackworth School had raised £10,000 between 1778 and 1780,[19] repeated requests beginning in 1792 had raised only £5,346 for the Retreat by 1801. This may have been because of the comparative novelty of an asylum compared to a school, and also because fewer Friends saw this second institution as having direct relevance to their own families or acquaintances. As the institution began to prove its worth funds flowed in more briskly: £6,709 was contributed during the next decade from 1802 to 1811, and a further £9,704 by 1821. This increased scale was also due to the appointment of agents in 1817 who had the responsibility of stimulating local donations. Most of this money was devoted to capital expenditure on buildings that included an extension of 1803, the purchase of the Appendage in 1810, and the erection of the Lodge in 1816–17. But one-fifth of the subscriptions had to be used to balance the current accounts. The committee had expressed the hope in 1797 that 'when the number of patients increase, the institution will be able to defray its own current expenses by the pay of the patients'. It was not until 1802 that the 'expenses of the family' were met by the patients' fees for the first time. But in 1805 and 1806 deficits were recorded again as they were continuously from 1810 to 1821.[20] Thus, during the first quarter century the Retreat ran at a loss on its patients' account for nineteen out of twenty-five years. Without the £4,285 contributed by the Quaker community to balance the books it is doubtful whether the Retreat would have weathered the difficult wartime years of high prices, or the period between 1811 and 1822 when there were dual overheads arising from running the Appendage as well as the main asylum.

Those who administered the Retreat felt that this money had conferred more than financial benefits on the institution. Samuel, the grandson of William Tuke, concluded that

the general interest which this mode of support naturally occasions, and the constant stimulus which it must prove to those concerned in the management, to deserve the good opinion of the Society, cannot fail to have a salutary tendency.[21]

For the donors too, there might be more than the sense that a charitable duty had been done. One quarter of the money contributed before 1821 had been invested as a form of life annuity on which 5 per cent interest was paid.[22] And for those giving substantial sums – as in comparable subscription hospitals – there were important privileges in the right to nominate patients at non-economic rates:

A contribution of one hundred pounds, from any Quarterly or other Meeting in its collective capacity, or a donation of twenty-five pounds from any Friend, or a subscription of fifty pounds for an annuity, shall entitle such meeting, donor, or annuitant, respectively, to the privilege of nominating one poor patient at a time, on the lowest terms of admission.[23]

And Quaker subscribers of two pounds or more became eligible to attend the meetings for the government of the Retreat.

The government of the Retreat was modelled on the organisation of the Society of Friends. A General Meeting was to be held annually in June and was in certain respects similar to the Yearly

Meeting of the Society in that the meeting had the power to make and alter rules. In addition, the General Meeting for the Retreat had the power to appoint the treasurer, the directors, and the Committee of Management for the institution. The directors met every three months, usually during or after the Yorkshire Quarterly Meetings. They were chosen from subscribers to the Retreat and numbered forty, of whom eight retired each year. Like the Quarterly Meetings of the Society of Friends, which acted as the channel of communication between the local Monthly Meetings and the national Yearly Meeting, the Quarterly Meetings of the Retreat's directors possessed few executive functions. They approved the accounts of the committee, read minutes of their proceedings and, on occasion, advised them. Of greater significance was their power to appoint two male visitors and three female visitors who were charged with the responsibility of regularly inspecting the institution, and of recording their observations in a book to be inspected by the committee and the directors. The main executive responsibilities were shouldered by the seven subscribers chosen by the General Meeting as members of the monthly Committee of Management of the Retreat. They fixed the terms for the admission of patients, compiled the accounts, appointed officers and ensured that they administered the institution according to its rules.[24]

By January 1796 the buildings were sufficiently near to completion for appointments to be considered for 'the various departments in the family'.[25] Where were suitable officers to be found? Tuke's first-hand contacts with existing asylums seem to have been confined to York and to St Luke's and his fundamental reservations about each were such as to preclude approaches to any staff there. An obvious alternative was to look to the Quaker community itself, not least because it was assumed that the Retreat's ethos would be imbued with the religious and moral precepts of Friends. For the key appointment of superintendent Tuke turned to his brother-in-law, Timothy Maud, a Bradford Quaker who had retired recently from his life-work as apothecary and surgeon.[26] But his tenure was short lived: Maud was sixty-seven years old, in failing health, and died only one month after the Retreat had received its first patient. Then followed a difficult interregnum in which Tuke failed to persuade John Hipsley, formerly in charge of Ackworth School, to take over.[27] It was nearly a year before

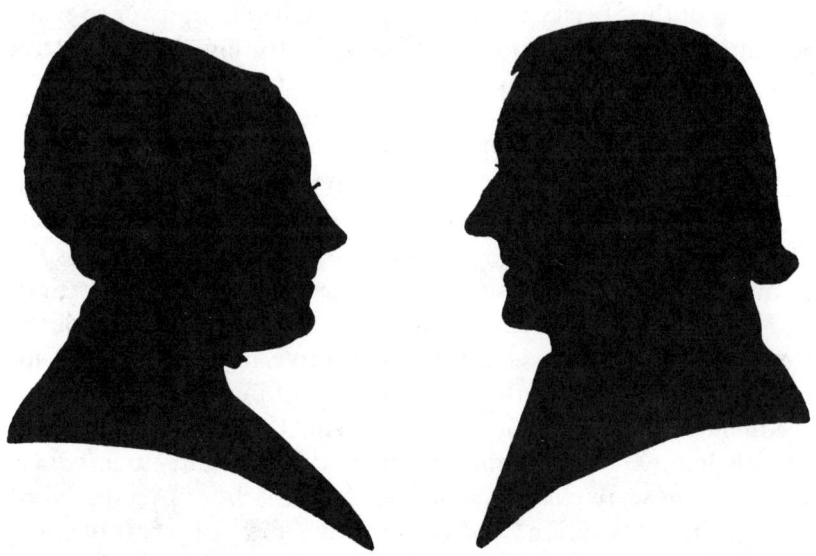

Plate 2. Silhouettes of George and Catherine Jepson

Tuke, who had shouldered the burden of office, was able to hand over to a successor — George Jepson.

Jepson was to become the foremost practitioner of moral treatment in early nineteenth-century England but at this early date he did not seem an obvious choice for the office of Retreat superintendent. Like many other medical practitioners he had had no formal training in his profession although his skill and experience were attested to by the confidence of local people in consulting him. In a lengthy letter of February 1797 that discussed Jepson's suitability for appointment, Tuke acknowledged that 'his knowledge of medicine would be of great use to the institution' and also that he was 'a steady religious friend'. A reference to Jepson's possession of 'talents superior to the station of keeper' suggests that Jepson had first been suggested for a subordinate position.[28] A replacement was needed as keeper of male patients for Joshua Cordingley, who had been dismissed for careless supervision of a suicidal patient during the previous month.[29] The importance of appointing the right man to assume overall executive control of the Retreat led Tuke to favour the cautious step of allowing Jepson to assist him at the Retreat for a trial period. This would give Jepson 'the opportunity of judging better of the proposal' and the Committee of Management that 'of forming a better judgement [of Jepson] than by hearsay'. The probationary period went well and on 26 June 1797 the committee approved his appointment as superintendent. His energy and steadfastness of purpose no doubt were soon tested since he must frequently have had to act both as superintendent and as keeper of male patients. This was because of the difficulty of finding suitable men for this exacting role: by 1800 there had already been six such appointments.[30]

Problems in staffing the male side of the home were equalled by those in the female division. At first there were two superior appointments: Jane King as housekeeper and Ann Relton as overseer of female patients were chosen in May 1796. By August the latter had been replaced as principal nurse by Catherine Allen, who also took over the former's duties in April 1797, thus effectively assuming the duties of the matron of the establishment.[31] Jane King had proved inadequate to the demands of her post, being of 'little use' in any emergency and with 'spirits often unequal to her situation'. Those at the Retreat welcomed her request to leave and were perhaps not surprised to see her return later as a patient on four separate occasions.[32] Catherine Allen had had previous experience with the mentally ill as a nurse at Cleeve Hill, a Quaker private house near Bristol, run by Edward Long Fox as a precursor to his more famous Brislington House. Dr Fox thought highly of her, and local Friends found her very good-natured and agreeable, although her dress was thought to be too smart for a member of the Society of Friends.[33] Catherine Allen's warmth of personality, compassion and dedication won the gratitude and admiration of her patients and their families. With the fortunate appointments of Jepson and Allen the domestic organisation of the Retreat was assured of humanity and efficiency until their retirements in 1823.

The choice of doctors was also opportune in relation to their skills and their perception of a professional role at the new institution. In June 1796 a respected York medical man, Dr Thomas Fowler, was requested to act as the non-resident physician to the Retreat. Fowler had worked for many years as a chemist in the city, before qualifying as a doctor at Edinburgh at the age of forty-two, and then holding an appointment as physician to Stafford

Infirmary. His scientific approach to his work was evident in the careful compilation of case-notes on his patients, and his experimental approach to the use of drugs was apparent in his two books on the effects of tobacco and the use of arsenic. Indeed, he became well known for 'Fowler's Solution', an alkaline solution of arsenic whose use in the cure of agues, fevers and headaches he had discussed in his second book. Fowler's professional ability and humane dedication to the Retreat's patients were much appreciated in the five years before his death in 1801.[34] At this time four applicants came forward for the post but William Tuke also encouraged his nephew, William Maud (at that time a surgeon and apothecary in Bradford), to apply. The Committee of the Retreat chose Dr Cappe, who like Fowler, was not a Quaker. He had had some practical experience in attending patients at the York Asylum,[35] and his library of medical books also suggested a strongly developed professional interest in mental illness.[36] This also proved to be a short-lived appointment since Cappe died the following year.

Dr W. Belcombe (another non-Quaker), who had assisted the institution during Cappe's illness, was chosen to succeed him and continued as visiting physician until 1822. Initially there had been some doubts as to his suitability to act even as a temporary stand-in, apparently because he had the reputation for using his own judgement and going against accepted medical practices when he thought this was necessary. However, Lindley Murray, the American grammarian whose intellect was universally respected among the York Quakers, argued eloquently in his favour:

> I believe Dr Belcombe to be a man of genius, research, and sound judgement, and a person who would do much more than is barely necessary to fulfil the duties of this office . . . a man of real judgement, and a comprehensive strong mind. Such a man is, I think, peculiarly proper for the office in question, where enlarged views and a solid judgement may be of very great importance.[37]

In the uncertain terrain of mental illness, where there was profound disagreement over its nature and its treatment, an ability to entertain new ideas and develop fresh practices was particularly valuable. And it was essential for a medical man to be flexible in his role at the Retreat since a pattern of *lay* therapy was being created there.

A DISTINCTIVE LAY THERAPY

> I am following up thy advice to me . . . In fact I do not remember ever being so well in health mentally and bodily as at this time. I find the greatest advantage to result from silent meditation and the perusal of the Holy Scriptures, and can experimentally say, there is no Physician like the one in Gilead, he is both able and willing to apply a sovereign remedy for all our maladies, and knows the precise character thereof better than any human eye can penetrate.[38]

This extract from a letter by an ex-patient of the Retreat to the second lay superintendent, Thomas Allis, mirrored the characteristic philosophy of this Quaker institution. Faith in 'the Physician in Gilead', whose healing powers were transmitted most directly through religious activities, sustained both patients and staff. Reliance on beliefs that enriched the lives of ordinary members of the Society of Friends flowed logically from the circumstances that had led to the foundation of this York institution. Lacking expertise in the care of the insane and having cause to distrust the methods employed in existing asylums it was natural to have recourse to familiar remedies. It was hoped that the religious framework that had supported Friends when sane would prove even more efficacious in meeting the greater needs of those who had in some degree lost their sanity.

The first minute to approve the establishment of 'A Friends Institute for Mentally Afflicted', that of the Yorkshire Quarterly Meeting of June 1792, emphasized its dominant Quaker character. On the subject of insane Friends it resolved that

> persons of this description . . . are often from the peculiar treatment which they require, necessarily committed, wholly, to the government of people of other societies: by which means the state of their own minds, and the feelings of their near connexions are rendered more dissatisfied and uncomfortable . . . It appears therefore very desirable that an Institution should be formed, wholly under the government of Friends . . . This would . . . alleviate the anxiety of the relatives, render the minds of the patients more easy in their lucid intervals and consequently tend to facilitate and promote their recovery.[39]

At this time the asylum was referred to as 'a retired habitation' – hinting both at a sense of apartness from secular pressures and at its non-institutional character. In the following year, William Tuke's thoughtful daughter-in-law, Mary Maria, supplied its enduring name of 'Retreat',[40] thus encapsulating the distinctively religious character of this withdrawal.

Faith rather than specialist knowledge sustained the laymen who planned and administered the Retreat. This kind of religious philosophy was exemplified by Samuel Tuke's private prayer:

> What a blessing it is to possess a sound mind!
> Lord make me sufficiently thankful for this . . .
> Let me prove my gratitude by earnest endeavours
> to alleviate the sufferings of those who labour
> under the most awful of thy permitted visitations.[41]

At a time when most doctors learnt about the treatment of the mentally ill through their professional practice rather than specialist training, the untutored ministrations of laymen at the Retreat were unremarkable. But their pragmatic therapy was distinctive precisely because it was imbued with the values of the Society of Friends. Before we turn to the principles that informed treatment it is helpful to review briefly the way in which Quakers perceived the nature of mental illness, and the manner in which recovery could take place, in order to understand what role the Retreat was seen to perform.

Convinced of the God-given nature of the universe and of the experiences that occurred within it, Friends sought to come to terms with sombre events such as the onset of insanity. Correspondence by friends and relatives of Retreat patients indicated submissiveness when this happened and patience in enduring it. Hannah Blose wrote to William Tuke that 'the account of dear James' mind being in a more tranquil state is a cause of thankfulness and [I] hope to acquiesce with what Providence sees meet in future in this Dispensation'.[42] Although it was appropriate to hope for recovery it was acknowledged that this would occur as a result of divine, rather than human will. A Friend wrote to George Jepson that 'the issue must be left to that Gracious Being who will (I believe) in his own time proclaim "it is enough" '.[43] Thus, those who worked at the Retreat were seen as instruments of God's will, as in this letter acknowledging the recovery of a patient:

It appears her faculties are (through permission of kind providence without which all human aid would fail) restored, a-mercy. I hope her relatives and friends together with herself will remember with grateful hearts, and I sincerely wish she may continue to enjoy the blessing of her faculties thus restored. I also desire to notice the good management and kind attention she [has] met with at the Retreat which I think is due to those who have the oversight and care of the patients placed there, and who have been so effectually instrumental in the recovery of many.[44]

To be an effective instrument of God's will in the care of the insane therefore required more than scientific medicine. It is significant in this context that Samuel Tuke referred to 'the divine art of healing' in discussing the character of the moral treatment that had been pioneered at the Retreat.[45] After many years associated with the institution his considered view was that it was essential for a moral manager of an asylum to have an elevated character:

A ready sympathy with man, and a habit of conscientious control of the selfish feelings and the passions, ought ever to be sought as carefully as medical skill . . . he should be one who knows experimentally the religion of the heart; who can condescend to the weak and the ignorant, and who, in the best sense of the phrase, can become all things to all men.[46]

And the man who above all others at the Retreat was acknowledged to have known 'experimentally the religion of the heart' was George Jepson, the first lay superintendent. Caring for the insane was seen as a practical expression of religion: it partook in specialist form of the general Quaker view that a life is one's testimony. It was logical therefore for those staffing the Retreat to have sought a Quaker like Jepson, 'a wise good man, who would religiously exercise his faculties and affections for the welfare of his charges'.[47]

Although the focus given by the religious spectacles worn by the Retreat's therapists gave clear pragmatic definition as to immediate methods and aims it provided more strictly circumscribed intellectual vision on less immediate, but equally important, issues. 'I have happily little occasion for theory',[48] observed Samuel Tuke, accurately expressing the practical, rather than abstract, preoccupations of the Retreat. Speculation and debate about the nature of insanity appear to have been conspicuous by their absence among those who managed the Retreat: such brief observations as were made occurred between much more substantive passages describing treatment and were used only to explain why such methods were employed. But some tentative inferences may be drawn from these scattered comments about the Quaker perception of mental illness.

In the early years of the Retreat its therapists kept an open mind on the nature of insanity. In 1813 Samuel Tuke spoke of 'the present imperfect state of our knowledge' on insanity and a consequent inability 'to ascertain its true seat in the complicated labyrinths of our frame', and thus to decide whether such 'disease originates in the mind' or, alternatively, whether 'in all cases of apparent mental derangement, some bodily disease, though unseen and unknown, really exists'.[49] However, by the mid-nineteenth century Drs Thurnam and Kitching, the first and second medical superintendents, were giving greater weight to the physical origins of insanity, and this reflected an increasing emphasis in contemporary psychiatric debate on the somatic nature of mental disorder. But this discourse also retained what Michael Clark has aptly referred to as a 'quality of *sustained metaphysical ambiguity*'.[50] Kitching's discussion of the interaction of mind, soul and body revealed this ambiguity very clearly in a discussion on the death of the insane:

The insane die of, or with, diseases involving the material organ through which mind and soul manifest themselves, and the resultant insanity covers all the faculties with its dark and confusing pall. This dark pall remains to the end, and is only removed when the spirit emerges from the trammels and infirmities of the flesh into the light of eternity.[51]

As a pious Friend Kitching's apparent materialism was heavily qualified by his view that the soul had remained essentially inviolate and could still be a means to receive God's grace.

The impact of this 'inner light' upon the soul had been central to the beliefs of the Society of Friends since its founder, George Fox, had experienced his 'spiritual birth' in the seventeenth century.[52] His *Journal* had recorded his mission 'to turn people to that inward light, spirit, and grace, by which all might know their salvation and their way to God'.[53] Those who managed the Retreat were concerned not to ignore any indications that this inner light still continued to shine in their patients, and soon became aware that not all of them were 'deprived of right religious sentiments'.[54] Access to religious books, conversation on spiritual topics and attendance at religious readings were therefore made an important part of most patients' lives, and convalescent patients might be allowed to attend a Quaker Meeting in York.[55] This perception of the 'divine spark' within the mad was exceptional in an era when those who administered public asylums and private madhouses were 'progressive' if they saw the insane as partaking not in animal but in human creation.

Convinced of the full humanity of their patients Jepson and his colleagues developed the implications of this principle so that it formed the basis for an all-embracing code of practice that later became known as moral treatment. Central to this was the belief that

> the patient on all occasions should be spoken to and treated as much in the manner of a rational being as the state of his mind will possibly allow. By this means the spark of reason will be cherished.[56]

They believed that the patient could be influenced through his understanding, and further, that a large proportion of those cared for were sensible of the distinction between reasonable and unreasonable conduct towards them.[57] Locke's associationist psychology, with its view of the restricted nature of the disorder in minds of the insane, reinforced their own evangelical feelings that the insane were the brothers of the sane and led them to delimit the boundaries of mental illness in their patients. 'Their intellectual, active, and moral powers, are usually rather perverted than obliterated; and it happens, not infrequently that one faculty only is affected.'[58] It seems likely that these beliefs on occasion acted as self-fulfilling prophecies: the high expectations of the therapist stimulated some patients to live up to them. William Tuke's affectionate description in December 1796 of the initial progress of the Retreat's third and seventh patients suggests the encouragement that was given them to adopt normal patterns of living:

> He is now so well as to sit with the other patients without the [strait] jacket and with common clothes . . . Mary Evans has also today manifested an inclination for a particular set of tea cakes. I am not certain whether we understand her meaning but we have sent such as I suppose she wanted.[59]

The singularity of this approach to the insane can be gauged by some reactions of visitors to the Retreat in the early nineteenth century. Many of these left comments in the visitors' books suggesting that what they had seen at York contrasted most favourably with other asylums with which they were familiar in the United Kingdom, Europe and North America. The mildness of its regime, its minimal use of restraint, together with the cleanliness and good order of the establishment, were subjects of frequent comment.[60] The Retreat thus exemplified the unusual belief that the comfort of patients outweighed the convenience of keepers. This testimony suggests that at the Retreat reality reflected rhetoric and that practice did not fall too far short of its ideals. It is not suggested here that such humane ideals were confined only to the Retreat, but it is argued that the institution was actually seen by contemporaries to have implemented these ideals successfully. A further, fundamental, element in this interpretation of the special features of the Retreat is that its objectives and practices stemmed from, and were manifested in, a pervasive religious morality. It was this religiosity that gave distinctiveness to the Retreat – and also surprised its visitors. John Griscom, an American Quaker, recorded his impressions of his visit of 1819:

> We first entered the room of the convalescent men. The peculiarity of their condition was very striking. A company of grave-looking Friends, dressed in the costume of the Society, and presenting the image of sober and rational reflection, formed so remarkable a contrast, with the noise and vehemence of a French lunatic hospital, as to make it difficult for the imagination, to realise the fact of their mental alienation.[61]

Yet the Retreat's methods were not unique: they formed part of a wider impulse towards psychiatric reform in Europe. However, it is important to appreciate that there is no evidence that the Retreat's therapists were aware of these similar initiatives when they began their work in York. Prominent reformers included Chiarugi in Italy and Pinel and Daquin in France. Joseph Daquin directed the Chambéry institution and published *Philosophie de la Folie* in 1791. His humanity towards the insane had obvious parallels with that of those who administered the Retreat, as did his belief that one should 'rid one's self of all the prejudices one has about the various types of insanity and apply moral treatment in all cases'.[62] Vincenzo Chiarugi's three-volume work, *On Insanity*, came out (in 1793–4) later than Daquin's publication, but it needs to be read in conjunction with an earlier work of 1789, the *Regulations* for the Hospital Bonifacio in Florence, which Chiarugi had directed since its opening in 1788. Daquin had been touched by the state of the mad. Chiarugi asserted boldly that 'it is a supreme moral duty and medical obligation to respect the insane individual as a person'.[63] In order to do this he thought that it was essential to gain the patient's confidence and trust, provide a kind, comfortable regime and use restraint only on a minimal basis. His symbolic breaking of the chains of the mad occurred in 1788, some time before Pinel's better-known drama at the Bicêtre in 1793.[64]

Philippe Pinel's work at two Parisian institutions – the Bicêtre (from 1793) and the Salpêtrière (from 1795) – had some similarities with that of Chiarugi. However, Chiarugi's published work showed a greater academic emphasis and reliance on earlier writers such as Cullen in formulating his threefold clinical classification. In referring to Chiarugi, Pinel adopted his usual dismissive tone in referring to other practitioners and stated inaccurately that 'it was Chiarugi's lot to follow the beaten track'.[65] It was unfortunate for Chiarugi's work and for his reputation that he had no successors to follow him and build on his work as did both Pinel and the Tukes.

Pinel[66] took issue with the 'blind routines' of traditional medical methods of treating the insane, preferring a much more discriminating use of medication and greater emphasis on the moral side of treatment. He preferred to equate moral not with psychological states but more narrowly with emotional ones and saw knowledge of his patients' emotions as the key to diagnosis and cure. Believing that patients should be treated with 'kind and compassionate firmness' he advocated a regular and comfortable regime, with good food, plenty of exercise, minimal restraint and with some work provided as therapy. As a qualified doctor, he adopted a scientific approach to his work with the insane, stressing the need for controlled experimentation in the choice of medicines, for careful observation of patients and for the compilation of systematic case-records. His emphasis on precise distinctions in diagnosis and treatment was linked to his aim 'to discriminate accurately between the different species of the disease'[67] and was to result in his fivefold classification of mental diseases. This work of Pinel was better known than that of either of his contemporaries, Chiarugi or Daquin, and is often linked with that of the Tukes at the Retreat in providing a major influence on the development of moral treatment.

What was the relationship between the work of Pinel and that of the Tukes? There were some obvious similarities in that both used an apparently mild regime for patients, minimal restraint, selective medication and exercise and work as therapy.[68] But there were important differences too. Pinel believed that religious activities should be restricted because they promoted dangerous ecstasy[69] whereas these activities were seen as a central element in therapy at the Retreat. At York a much broader definition was given to moral states that were seen as synonymous with psychological, rather than Pinel's narrower definition of them as emotional, ones. The role of the Retreat's lay therapists contrasted with that of Pinel: the former were intimately involved in the day-to-day details of their few patients' lives; the Parisian doctor, working in a much larger institution, was more of an aloof investigator. This was linked to a fundamental difference of attitude and methodology. Pinel adopted a systematic approach to study the symptomatic states of his patients and construct a scientific nosology of mental diseases. The Retreat's lay therapists were more pragmatic in working out their treatments and more selective in recording their cases.

Pinel did not mention the work of the Retreat in his *Traité Medico-Philosophique sur la Manie* of 1801. This book was included in the 1803 bequest by Dr Cappe to the Retreat although there is no direct evidence that anyone there consulted it until 1812, when Samuel Tuke read it.[70] Dr D. H. Tuke later suggested that the Retreat's therapists had heard of Pinel's work by 1806 and that Pinel had learned of the York establishment five years after he had begun his own work, through Delarive's account of the Retreat in 1798. It seems likely therefore that similar yet distinctive methods for the moral treatment of the insane were worked out independently in Paris and York.

3

Moral treatment

It lies outside the town, surrounded by its beautiful gardens. Its internal arrangements are everywhere characterised by the most admirable order and refinement. The whole system of treatment pursued, is one of invariable mildness and benevolence, founded on the principle of kindness, as the only rational mode of influencing the insane.

This description of the Retreat by a visitor in 1844[1] is interesting precisely because of its stereotyped emphasis on what had come to be seen as outstanding ingredients in the Retreat's renowned system of moral treatment – kindness and good order within an attractive environment. It is the function of this chapter, and of Chapter 4, to see to what extent this image accurately reflected reality. I also intend to explore ambiguities hinted at even within this conventional description: the tension that may have existed between 'order' in the establishment, and the 'benevolence' by which those who were disturbed in mind were induced to conform to it. Chapter 3 discusses the therapeutic environment of the Retreat, the comfortable domestic regime in which the patients lived and the occupational therapy that gave them variety. Chapter 4 assesses the extent to which this apparently humane system, with its infrequent recourse to restraint and its attempt to re-create a sense of family, may nevertheless have contained inherently repressive elements.

Moral treatment as it was understood by its practitioners in the eighteenth and early nineteenth centuries meant that psychological methods were employed to help in what was seen as a mental disorder. Intrinsically they did not necessarily possess either a humane or an ethical character,[2] although historically such treatment might have these attributes in particular institutions. As we shall see, the Retreat's therapy embodied both of these qualities. However, the interpretation that was given to each ingredient within moral treatment, and also their mutual interaction at different times, was to result in a rather more complex and many-sided therapy at the Retreat than has usually been conveyed by its conventional description as one of mildness and kindness.

In adopting moral treatment the Retreat's therapists were influenced, as were many other practitioners of the day, by earlier philosophical psychologists, and particularly by Locke. As we have seen, he argued that madness was a form of disordered reasoning, in which random associations of ideas led to false judgements and thus to erroneous actions. Important in the formation of these associations were the education and environment of the individual: defects in either might cement by custom the arbitrariness of associations that were being created in the mind.[3] The Retreat's therapists accepted that a 'proper regulation of the mind is essentially connected with the prevention of the disease'.[4] In this they may also have been influenced by the discipline of the Society of Friends, which aimed to inculcate in the young a habitual Christian self-denial, moderation and uprightness of character.[5] Where such habits had not been satisfactorily achieved, or had later been lost, the Retreat might provide a surrogate home and family in which to resocialize the patient.

Elements in a therapeutic programme designed to fulfil this and related objectives were derived from a commonsense application of accepted elements in eighteenth-century moral management, but this was then transformed by the specific context of this Quaker asylum into a distinctive regimen. Pleasant pastimes devised for the Retreat's patients served as diversions from painful thoughts or obsessive chains of ideas and as such were fairly commonplace ingredients in late eighteenth-century therapy.[6] A distraction for the mentally afflicted[7] might also be provided by agreeable surroundings within Georgian asylums or private madhouses though such ideals were neither so elevated nor so fully realised in practice as they were at this York establishment. There the patients' comfort was felt to be 'of the highest importance' and considerable effort was made to achieve it.[8] Yet the Retreat tried not just to provide a comfortable and varied life for its patients but to create domesticity within an institution. The catalyst that blended these rather disparate elements into a successful – and unique – form of moral therapy was the common values of patients and therapists.

These shared attitudes and assumptions probably gave a crucial dimension to the moral treatment developed by Quakers. I would suggest that the Retreat's lay therapists drew on a Protestant dissenting tradition of religious healing that was non-institutional and had lasting popular appeal. George Fox had been extraordinarily effective as a spiritual healer: 'I was sent for to many sick people', his *Journal* records.[9] The people he treated were usually suffering from a physical complaint, but in a minority of instances the affliction was mental. The happy outcome of Fox's interventions was seen as both cure and miracle, since Fox was careful to recognise the assistance of divine power.[10] It was natural for appeals for help during sickness to be addressed to another member of the Society of Friends since Quakers' overwhelming experience of the indwelling light gave them a close and mutually supportive fellowship that was directed by a charismatic spiritual leadership of great power. As Fox acknowledged, such leaders could 'shake all the country in their profession for ten miles round'.[11] One effective exercise of this religious leadership was spiritual healing, probably by a combination of the laying on of hands and of psychological suggestion. Evidence for a continuation of this tradition of spiritual healing amongst eighteenth-century Quakers is much more fragmentary than for the Methodists.[12] However, I would suggest that it is possible that George Jepson was such a healer.

Before he became the first superintendent of the Retreat Jepson had been held in considerable esteem by the countryfolk around Rawdon. They travelled to see him because of their belief in his healing powers.[13] Samuel Tuke hinted at the spiritual healing that Jepson practised at the Retreat when he praised the fact that Jepson was one accustomed to 'religiously exercise his faculties'.[14] A further clue to Jepson's powers was given in a letter to the Jepsons shortly before their retirement. This expressed the hope that you 'may continue to lean upon, and be supported by that divine power, which has qualified you to discharge the duties of your important station'.[15] Jepson's successors may also have attempted, though with less success, to continue this tradition. Thomas Allis believed, as we have seen, in the 'Physician in Gilead' and John Kitching referred to 'our Heavenly Father who alone is the great Physician'.[16]

The hypothesis that spiritual healing may have been an important element in the Retreat's moral treatment is not by its nature one that can be proved as an incontrovertible fact. The supportive evidence is necessarily fragmentary and elusive since in a positivistic age, where medical views were increasingly influential, such unorthodox practices were referred to obliquely. And because of this obliqueness and brevity it is also amenable to a more restricted interpretation: statements on 'the divine art of healing' may have been conventional expressions of piety rather than hints of a hidden, inner reality. One reason why such a restrictive view may be insufficient is that if the Retreat's moral therapy did indeed contain a hidden kernel that was spiritual healing, it helps to explain why the treatment was so successful at York and much less so in other institutions that attempted to copy it. Missing the central core of subjective experience and of shared beliefs, other asylums imitated only the objective and external characteristics of the Retreat's moral treatment.

We now turn to these apparently more accessible elements: a therapeutic environment, occupational therapy and a social milieu at the Retreat. But before we examine the detailed application of these important aspects in moral treatment we need to pause to consider the nature of the available evidence and to become aware of its limitations. Its most obvious characteristic was its one-sided nature. The annual *Reports* of the institution contained much useful material but it was selected to give a favourable impression of the progress that was being made, not least because reports were often used in conjunction with fund-raising efforts. This element of self-justification was also present in Samuel Tuke's influential *Description of the Retreat* as well as in much contemporary writing about the Retreat: it tended to argue the case for milder methods in the treatment of the insane and thus to gloss over any deficiencies in such an approach. It might be thought that an examination of a hitherto unexploited source, the medical records, and especially the case histories of patients, would give a more accurate view of the merits of moral treatment. However, it must not be forgotten that these again reflected the doctors' viewpoint and were tantalisingly brief on key issues such as the patients' own opinions or the efficacy of treatment. In pursuit of what is undoubtedly problematic, and may ultimately prove to be elusive, we now attempt to make an evaluation of certain elements in the Retreat's moral treatment.

A THERAPEUTIC ENVIRONMENT

The Georgian domestic style of the Retreat's buildings suggested an everyday accessibility that contrasted with the formal classical style and overpowering size of preceding asylums with their unspoken message that order would be imposed on those within. In its unostentatious style and appearance the Retreat differed markedly from the neighbouring York Asylum with its imposing facade and substantial complex of institutional buildings. The Quaker establishment was sited some distance from the built-up area within York city walls, and its elevated, rural position was enhanced by the gardens created around it. Occupying eleven acres of grounds, which were soon well planted with trees and flowering shrubs, the asylum fulfilled the ideal of its promoters as a 'retired habitation'.

Those who built the Retreat were perceptive in seeing that architectural style made an effective ideological statement.[17] They aimed to have 'studiously avoided that gloomy appearance, which frequently accompanies places appropriated for those who are afflicted with disorders of the mind'.[18] John Bevans, the builder-cum-architect, appreciated that in an asylum the medium was an important part of the message. He commented at an early stage that 'if the outside appears heavy and prison-like it has a considerable effect upon the imagination'.[19] Believing that the insane retained their essential humanity and were aware of their surroundings it became important to emphasise that an everyday normality was inherent in the patients' environment. Not only should any suggestion of a penal environment be avoided, but a positive effort was needed to create civilised surroundings for the mentally ill.

To appreciate how radical a departure this was from existing practice we need only look at St Luke's Hospital. Those planning the Retreat visited St Luke's on more than one occasion, taking from its design and practical arrangements what they felt was useful, but rejecting what they saw as inhumane. Created in 1751 as a more progressive alternative to Bedlam, St Luke's still exemplified many traditional assumptions about the animality of the mad. Its absence of heating, lack of warm water, and partially glazed windows indicated that the insane were thought to be immune to cold, and its straw bedding and minimal provision of clothing suggested that they had no need of comfortable surroundings. Whereas the use of chains for acute cases was justified on the alleged grounds that they provided more movement for the insane than did a strait-jacket,[20] their continued deployment seems also to have symbolised a brutish conception of the mad. William Tuke was distressed by the sight of these acute cases chained in straw,[21] and it seems probable that this deepened his resolution to provide more congenial and humane arrangements for Quaker patients. John Bevans visited this London asylum several times and enquiring 'minutely' into its arrangements, was given 'an opportunity to inform myself of everything I wished'.[22] What he had learnt helped him to formulate certain elements in his design, notably those concerned with the classification and security of patients, and seems also to have acted as a spur in devising less coercive, and more comfortable, alternatives for many aspects of the asylum.

In attempting to create a homelike setting for Quaker patients it might be thought that the domesticity of the Retreat owed something to the private madhouses that had proliferated since the seventeenth century. But these private houses were not purpose-built as was this York establishment.[23] Any domesticity they possessed seems likely to have been an incidental by-product of their buildings rather than a deliberate element in a therapeutic scheme. Thus, it is important to appreciate that one aspect of the Retreat's originality lay in this planned paradox – an institution that aimed to be a surrogate home.

Designed to give 'comfort combined with economy',[24] the Retreat's buildings and furnishings were planned along simple lines. Built in common brick and Welsh slate the Retreat was broadly rectangular in plan: the central portion had greater depth, and two wings extended at the rear on the south-east and south-west. The front elevation had windows arranged symmetrically round a front door graced with a small pediment, which was the sole concession to ornament. To 'prevent the Patients Ground from being overlooked by strangers' four airing grounds were placed at the rear of the buildings where patients could also benefit from available sunshine and command fine views over Walmgate Stray and the countryside beyond.[25] Inside the building, patients' rooms were arranged round long galleries, which were designed to give them exercise; strong barred gates at each end stopped them from wandering away from the eye of their keeper. Each gallery had a communal day-room that also doubled as a dining-room. In the central portion of the building were the superintendent's quarters from whence he had ready access via the central staircase to all parts of the building. And at either end of the main block were domestic rooms (including a bake-house, brew-house and laundry) and farm buildings.[26] Taken as a whole the design functioned reasonably efficiently in these early days when the Retreat 'family' was small.

The rooms were simply furnished with wooden furniture, much of it constructed specially for the Retreat. Visitors were impressed by the cleanliness, neatness and comfort of domestic arrangements. Great efforts were made to sustain this domestic illusion and to disguise overt signs of the security precautions of an asylum. The windows were not the unglazed barred openings of the traditional institution, but had the appearance of ordinary windows, although in fact the wooden sashes cased iron bars within their structure. The glass panes were only eight by six and a half inches square, a size chosen because it was thought to be too small to allow a patient to escape through, and was also cheap to replace at the cost of sixpence per broken pane.[27] This practical humanity also led to the bolts on bedroom doors being cased in leather, and later replaced by mortice locks, since the sound of them crashing shut at night might upset patients.[28] This sensibility on behalf of the insane was noted by an architect, William Stark, after a visit in 1810. He felt that 'a great deal of delicacy appears in the attentions paid to the smaller feelings of the patients' in making these arrangements and that as a result there was 'an air of comfort and contentment'.[29]

Stark's panopticon plan for the Glasgow Asylum of 1814, and James Bevans's dual panopticon design for the West Riding Asylum of 1818, led to some re-evaluation of the criteria for asylum design. Samuel Tuke, who had advised in the planning of the latter, was critical of the Retreat's design, considering that its extended wings were too far from the centre and comparing it unfavourably with the more compact, cruciform shape of the panopticon. He also felt that the Retreat's windows were too high in patients' rooms, that galleries were chilly, airing courts too small and surrounding walls too high.[30] In short, by 1814 the domestic plan of the Retreat was already seen as falling short of the ideal therapeutic environment for patients. And as time went on such criticisms of the cramped, old-fashioned layout became more insistent. An appeal for funds to build new wings in 1852 castigated the old for embodying 'in a solid form too many of the old ideas which experience has subsequently exploded'.[31] Although it proved feasible to build new rear wings for male and female patients, the original north front of the building remained, no longer seen as attractively domestic but 'behind the age'.[32] Certain features within it, notably the seven-foot-wide galleries, had been retrograde because of their narrowness even when they were constructed. Their unappealing darkness was lightened gradually by inserting larger end windows and creating additional wide and well-lit spaces through removing some patients' rooms on each side of them. And during the second half of the nineteenth century, large plate-glass windows replaced smaller sash windows in the principal, communal rooms giving better views and 'additional cheerfulness'.

A change in style occurred not only in the structure but also in the interior during Kitching's vigorous superintendency. In 1855 he defiantly reported that he wished the rooms to be furnished more aesthetically, even if Quakers did not ornament their homes, and justified it on the therapeutic grounds that this would arrest the attention of patients.[33] In ensuing years the dull blue-grey paint in the corridors gave way to more cheerful colours and elegant wallpaper and pictures adorned the upper surfaces. This process was gradually extended to other accommodation; new coloured carpeting replaced matting, and more plants, photographs and lithographs added variety.[34] Meanwhile, gas lighting had lightened the scene after 1843, electric lighting first appeared in the 1880s and a central heating system had been extended to all galleries by the 1860s. Attempts to improve the water supply[35] and modernise sanitary amenities were virtually continuous from the 1860s to 1890s. By 1874, when Kitching retired, his pampered patients lived in a cosy cluttered cocoon of material abundance.

By the late nineteenth century piecemeal alterations had transformed the therapeutic environment of patients. They no longer inhabited a rather austere, yet recognisably Quaker, domestic establishment but resided in a much larger institutional complex. Each set of buildings had a more clearly specified purpose that was defined largely by medical criteria. At the same time earlier Quaker inhibitions about the degree of comfort or the range of amusements permitted to Quaker patients had been relaxed in favour of

Moral treatment

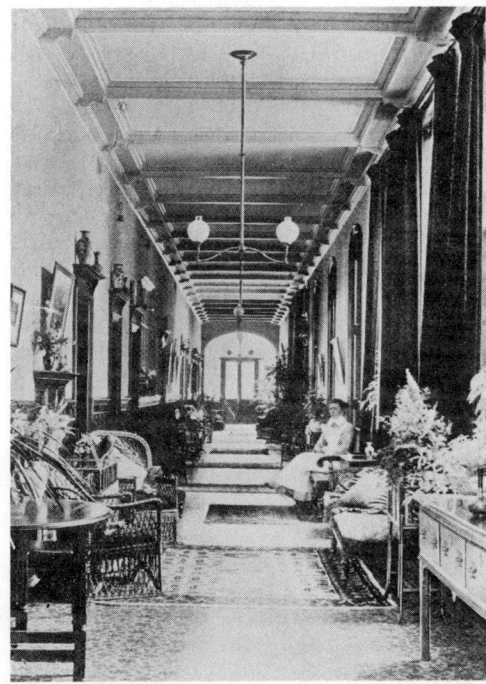

Plate 3.
The Sixth Gallery in 1900

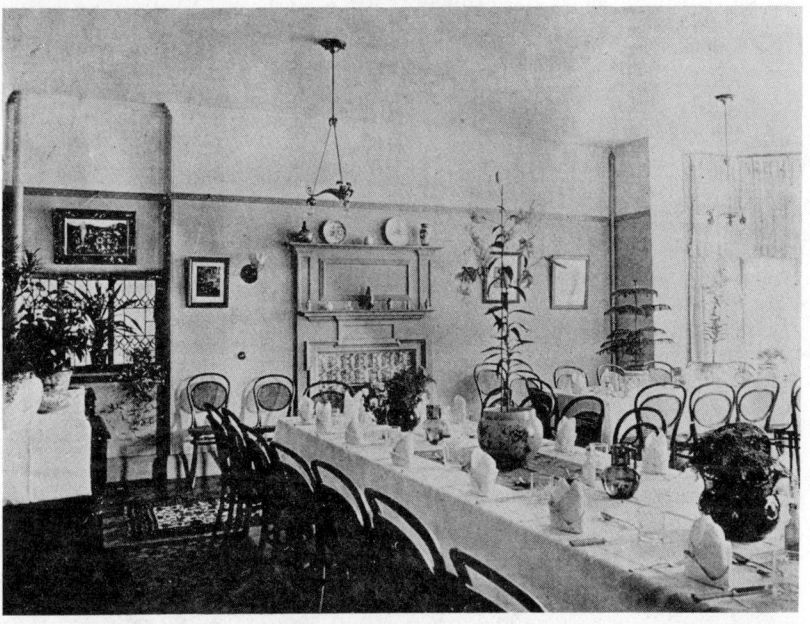

Plate 4. New dining-room for ladies, 1899

a more materialistic, even hedonistic, regimen. In part this was a result of an increasing proportion of high-fee-paying patients who were not Quakers and who might reasonably expect luxurious standards of living. It was also due to higher material standards in Victorian society that were reflected in more elevated expectations of the surroundings appropriate for insane patients. It may be conjectured that to some extent this growing stress on material comfort may also have stemmed from a less optimistic climate of medical opinion. With a declining recovery rate there may have been some compensation in emphasising the increased well-being of the large numbers of chronic cases left within the asylum. A further element in this 'well-being' consisted of a planned programme of patients' amusements and employments.

OCCUPATIONAL THERAPY

In describing the particular benefits of this undertaking it seems proper to mention that of occasionally using the patients to such employment, as may be suitable and proper for them, in order to order to relieve the languor of idleness, and prevent the indulgence of gloomy sensations [36]

The employment of patients was informed by the theory of distraction and was seen as being particularly appropriate for melancholics who needed to be diverted from 'favourite but unhappy musings'. Occupational therapy was also seen as being valuable in other cases, particularly convalescent ones, where it would encourage the growth of mental abilities and especially the power of concentration. And since the Retreat's lay therapists were convinced that patients should as far as possible be treated as if rational,[37] it followed logically that the patients should be induced to occupy themselves with the kind of pursuit they might well have taken up at home. Under Jepson's judicious guidance there was no elaborate programme of employment or amusement, but a straightforward attempt to involve patients in domestic activities and outdoor exercise. This policy was also continued under his successor, Thomas Allis.[38]

Some of the female patients helped in such tasks as polishing furniture in their gallery, assisting in the kitchen, churning butter or mangling clothes, and a few of the men pumped water, chopped wood or cleaned shoes. Many women seem to have enjoyed participating in sewing circles, made up of staff, visiting Friends from

Moral treatment

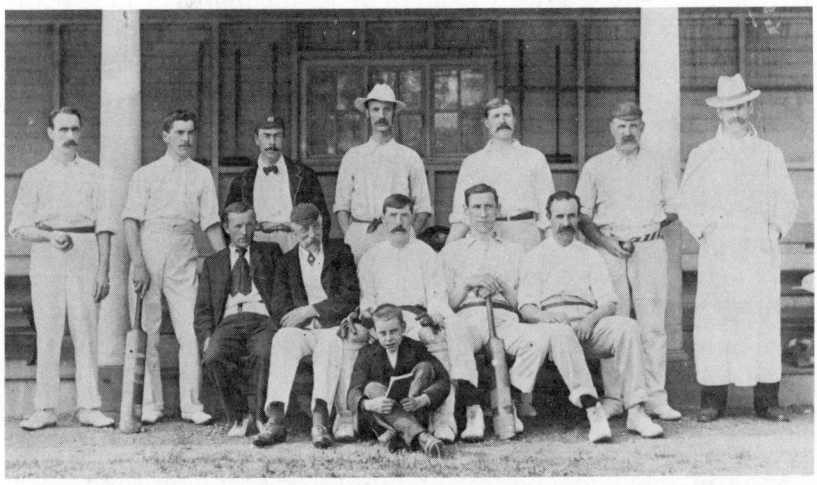

Plate 7. Cricket team, 1901

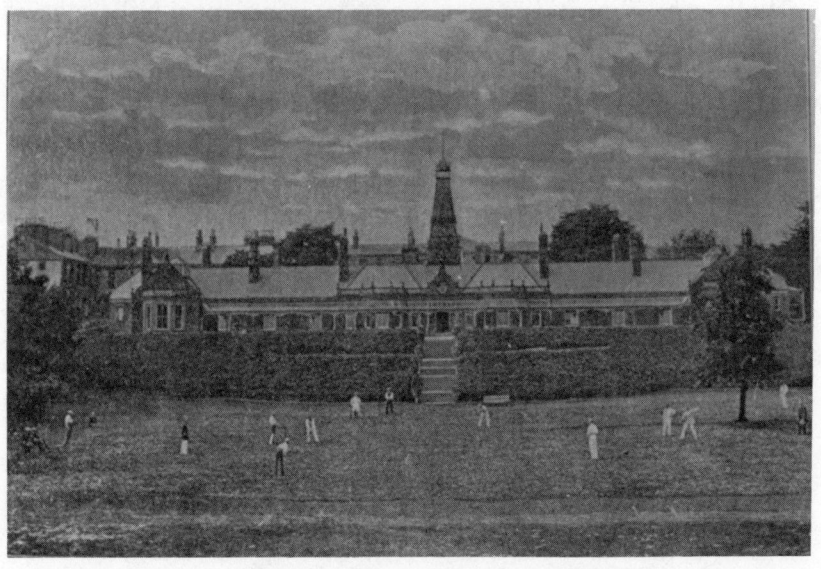

Plate 8. The Lodge (rebuilt in 1875) with cricket match

to any kind of employment or recreation.[52] Even the somewhat specious statistics of patients' employment in the annual reports of the institution disclosed, despite their optimism, that two or three out of every ten patients had not been employed in any way. The remainder were described as 'more or less' employed. In part the therapists explained this away by speaking of the high proportion of aged or infirm cases who could not be expected to be occupied. Such defensive explanations were thought to be necessary in the competitive world of asylum publicity where comparative employment statistics were scrutinised carefully by other professionals. So the buoyant tone of the reports needs to be corrected by details of individual case histories. These suggest that another sizeable minority were incapable of the kind of activities recommended to them. Imbeciles or cases of dementia might devise their own amusements: placing stones one on top of another; playing with dolls, bricks, marbles or counters; whistling on comb and paper.[53] The matron's daily report books that have survived for the period at the turn of the twentieth century also qualified the optimism of public reports by indicating that for women the main occupations were still either domestic work or reading.[54]

Despite these limitations the Retreat's therapists continued to include employment as a means of treatment, apparently considering that it was the process of being employed, rather than the quality of the activity or end-product, that was important. This gives some credence to the view that the work ethic of bourgeois society was being imported into the asylum. (This type of interpretation is discussed further in the following chapter.) The evidence is also amenable to the alternative assessment that such occupational therapy was a worthy attempt to encourage activities in which individual patients showed interest. On the one hand this might involve tolerating patients making baby clothes because of pregnancy delusions or, like Penelope, knitting garters that were immediately unravelled.[55] On the other hand it might lead a female patient to write poetry of quality fit for publication.[56] This sonnet, called 'Mignonette', was published in *Good Words* in 1864:

> There is no rose, among the garden flowers
> A Queen in her own right, or lily fair
> The bride of Kings, that breathes upon the air,
> Such fragrance as the fragrance of these bowers.
> The sun has passed this way and laid the hours
> Of light and warmth, with all a lover's care
> Upon my garden's breast and everywhere
> Arise sweet answers. This, that overpowers
> O'er rose or lily and does least forget

> The sun that loved it, seeking to renew
> Its vows of perfume, as in deep regret
> That it by day held up no gold to view,
> Crimson or purple, is my Mignonette,
> Whose beauty is its *sweetness,* not its hue.

Unlike the patient's view of her mignonette, this analysis of occupational therapy at the Retreat concludes tentatively with the suggestion that its attractive appearance of purposive recreation may have outweighed its intrinsic value in patients' treatment. There were remarkably few comments in the case-books that indicated, as they did for one patient in 1815, that recreation was facilitating recovery: '[she] has diligently employed herself in knitting curious pincushions by which employment her recovery appears to have been materially promoted.'[57] And as early nineteenth-century optimism on the possibility of curing insanity by mild methods receded, an increased stress was placed on the recreational as well as the therapeutic role of diverse occupations and amusements. These

> have not only been of good service in relieving some of the dullness of hospital life, but they have occupied an important position in that modern treatment of the insane which utilises every means likely to attract and strengthen the mental powers of the patients and divert their thoughts from morbid self-introversion.

Here Dr Kitching's confident tone in the Retreat's *Report* for 1875 concealed an element of 'whistling in the dark' in the pursuit of 'every means' of therapeutic diversion for long-stay patients. Its bombastic language and pseudo-scientific style were also found elsewhere in publicity on patients' pastimes. Ironically, it would appear that as confidence in the curative potential of occupational therapy wavered, its perceived value in promotional literature increased. Thus, what had earlier been thought of as simple country rambles were described as 'the study of botany' and visits to the public library were depicted as 'literary employment'.[58] This was a far cry from the simplicity of the Retreat's early domestic regimen.

A DOMESTIC MILIEU

The earliest statements setting forward proposals for the Retreat spoke of those who would live there as 'the family' and its rules referred to the superintendent as the 'master of the family'. Although many Georgian institutions used this terminology it is clear that at the Retreat rhetoric and reality were closely related in its early years. At that time it was 'simply intended as a kind home'.[59] And the marriage in 1806 of its first superintendent, George Jepson, to its matron, Catherine Allen, seemed to set a seal on the close personal relationships that had been achieved there.

Correspondence between Jepson and relatives of patients gave the impression of the Retreat as a microcosm of the Society of Friends with its close ties of friendship and familial relationships. Families frequently paid tribute to the 'kind', 'judicious' or 'affectionate' treatment their members had received. For example, a father wrote in 1803 about his daughter who had then been in the Retreat two and a half years:

[I] am sorry d[aughte]r Mary's faculties continue so weak but it is a great favour she is so healthy and comfortable, so pleasantly attached to those she is with [and] whom I have no doubt of their kind care and attention when needful.[60]

At about the same time an ex-patient wrote to George Jepson with similar sentiments:

I often think of you, and should be glad to hear from thee at some convenient opportunity . . . [and] conclude with kind love and due respect to thee and Catherine Allen and all my acquaintance at the Retreat. P.S. Please to give my love to William Tuke.[61]

Although this sense of affectionate intimacy at the Retreat was conveyed most vividly and frequently in letters from the earliest years, when small numbers of patients must have facilitated this sense of family, it was not confined to it. A letter to George Jepson from another old patient in 1819 stated, 'I hope my dear H. Ponsonby is very well. I often think on you and her for your . . . very kind behaviour towards me.'[62] Hannah Ponsonby acted as Catherine Allen's assistant from 1816, before becoming matron in 1823, when she worked alongside Jepson's successor, Thomas Allis. And during this later partnership patients and their families continued to some degree to feel this sense of togetherness as was suggested in 1833 by a man whose wife had been in the Retreat for a short time:

York, and patients, which mended bed linen and clothes while conversation brightened the passing hours.[39] Indeed, it was much easier to employ female patients in their customary pursuits of sewing, knitting, crochet and fancy work than it was to involve male patients. Some of the latter read or wrote letters and a few condescended to do some gardening or help on the farm during haymaking. But a later attempt in the 1830s to extend casual gardening into regular 'spade husbandry' was not wholly successful.[40] Unlike the county or borough asylums, where manual work was practised with mainly pauper patients, the Retreat's patients came predominantly from a trading, artisan or professional background,[41] which made them see such work as unappealing if not degrading.

The Retreat's rural situation was a natural stimulus to country walks and many patients went out with their attendants to walk on Walmgate Stray and to neighbouring villages such as Heslington or Fulford. For more enervated cases an occasional drive in a chaise was employed, and this change of scene seems to have been successful in raising some patients' spirits.[42] For most inmates, however, the beauty of the extensive grounds around the Retreat provided sufficient variety. Carefully laid out with walks, wooded glades, gardens and orchards the original eleven acres of land had been extended to twenty-seven by 1839: this formed a tranquil setting in which patients could hope to regain their serenity. Encompassing the highest land near York the Retreat gave unrivalled views over the surrounding countryside as well as over the town to the Minster. Thus, patients could live in a sheltered environment yet see over the low surrounding walls to the wider world beyond.

This controlled openness was an early distinguishing feature. In part a product of its history (since it had been set up in reaction to the closed institution of the York Asylum), it was also a positive element in its therapy. Visitors to the Retreat were welcomed, so long as prior notice was given and the visitor was accompanied by the superintendent. 'Indiscriminate admission', it was felt, might adversely affect patients' progress.[43] Friends from York took tea at the Retreat on Sundays, young female Friends participated in Thursday sewing circles, and during Quarterly Meetings in York long tables were provided to entertain numerous visitors to dinner and tea. This principle of accessibility to the Retreat was empha-

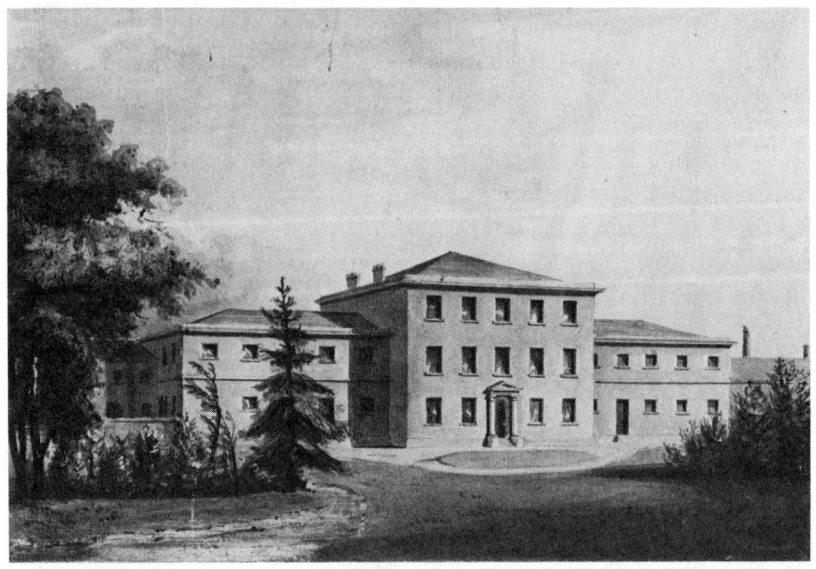

Plate 5. Perspective view of north front of the Retreat

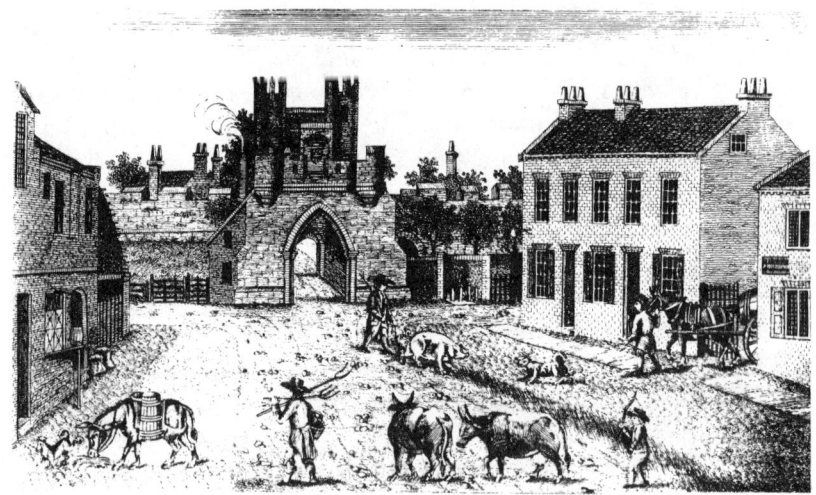

Plate 6. The Appendage (shown on right)

sised by its gates and front door standing open to the world.[44] Convalescent patients were encouraged to find their way back into a wider social world: they were invited to visit the homes of local Quakers, to take tea at the York Quaker schools, and to attend First Day Meetings. Their readiness to resume a normal life was sometimes tested by staying for a week or two as a boarder with a local Quaker family.[45] And in 1811 a 'half-way house', the Appendage, was opened for convalescent patients. It stood down the hill from the Retreat, just outside the town gates of Walmgate Bar, and was intended to give patients a greater opportunity to participate in normal patterns of life. However, this experiment was unsuccessful and ended in 1822, partly because of the expense and partly because convalescent patients were reluctant to leave familiar surroundings.[46] That these surroundings were sufficiently attractive and varied for patients to wish to stay was, in some sense, a tribute to the success of moral treatment at the Retreat.

A desire to overcome the monotony of asylum life through the provision of increasingly varied and ambitious forms of employment and recreation led in the mid-nineteenth century to a departure from the simplicity of earlier pastimes. This increasingly sophisticated pattern of living paralleled the changes that we have seen were taking place in the physical environment. In the early days reading matter was confined to the Bible. Later, newspapers and magazines, poetry, even plays and novels were perused. Music played an increasingly important role: individual patients played the piano, violin, harmonium or accordion and in the 1850s musical soireés and concerts were begun. Earlier references to chess were later supplemented by those describing enjoyable games of billiards, whist, draughts, bagatelle, backgammon and skittles. Rides for a few patients in a chaise were extended by the purchase of a coach in 1856 and additional carriages in the 1870s and 1880s. A concern to employ male patients more successfully than had been achieved hitherto led in the forties and fifties to the opening of printing rooms where patients printed magazines and also to the establishment of a joiner's shop where the more enterprising might make picture frames for the Retreat or carve chessmen or ships for their own delight.[47] Anxiety in mid-century that most of the occupations were 'mindless'[48] led to more patients being encouraged to take up more intellectual tasks: individual case-notes recorded a few learning, reading or translating French, Latin and Hebrew, and pursuing studies in chemistry or mathematics.[49]

For the majority, lighter entertainment was provided on an increasing scale. By 1875 the Retreat's *Report* recorded 'Concerts, Dances, Exhibitions of Dissolving Views, Lectures, Readings and Recitations, and Conjuring and Ventriloquist Entertainments'. With such a varied programme having been instituted by Dr Kitching it was perhaps difficult for his successors, Drs Baker and Pierce, to make their professional mark in developing moral treatment. However, they discerned a gap in the provision of physical recreation and so in the last decades of the nineteenth century improved facilities for cricket, tennis, football, hockey, golf, croquet and bowls were developed. By the twentieth century the Retreat was fielding elevens in competitive games of cricket and hockey, and these were made up not only of patients but also of staff. Involving doctors and nursing staff with patients in more ambitious schemes was also found in other spheres. Thus, the Retreat boasted a choral society, a minstrel troupe, a dramatic society, and the Lodge Shakespearians.

A more enterprising recreational programme within the Retreat was matched by more adventurous excursions and diversions outside its gates. Selected patients were permitted to visit exhibitions and flower shows, use libraries or even go to the theatre in York. Beginning with the experiment of a few patients visiting the Great Exhibition in London in 1851, occasional visits were made to places of interest farther afield than York. For example, a steamboat excursion on the River Ouse in 1871 and a drive to Castle Howard in 1894 were enjoyed by many of the patients. Thomas Allis's experiment of sending a very few patients for a short convalescent period in Scarborough boarding-houses was also gradually extended to cover longer periods and more patients, until in 1887 a convalescent home was established in Scarborough.[50]

A melancholic patient, after recovering his spirits in the Retreat, commented to his doctor on his discharge that

> whilst with us he had no time to think of himself and his feelings, and he feared that without the continuous change of employment that he had been having, he would be in danger of relapse.[51]

Not every patient proved as easy to divert from his depression. The case-books revealed a number of patients who could not settle

It is really pleasant to hear with what satisfaction and pleasure she talks of you all and the time she spent among you . . . if there is one subject more than another she likes to converse about it is that.[63]

Thus the belief that 'social affections' continued to exist in the mentally ill,[64] a conviction that was strongly held by those administering the Retreat, seemed to have been confirmed by the amicable relationships created here.

What were the key features of domestic life that appealed so much to patients and their families and that so impressed visitors? The most obvious characteristic was the unexpected *normality* of life there: the appearance of a comfortable, clean, well-ordered establishment evoked the sense of home more vividly than that of an institution. Also evident was a tranquil atmosphere engendered first by the attractively rural surroundings and confirmed by a calm, confident demeanour amongst its officers. Within this environment patients were encouraged, as far as their illness allowed, to participate fully in a domestic pattern of life: to dress in ordinary clothes, eat well-cooked and varied meals and to employ themselves in everyday tasks and amusements. And within this seeming normality each patient in the early years was seen as an individual who retained his or her identity rather than being viewed as an anonymous component administered by an impersonal bureaucracy. An important implication of this was that mechanical restraint was used sparingly and operated in conjunction with 'a code of honour'. Whether this physical mildness also involved a hidden mental subjugation is discussed in the following chapter.

The social relationships that existed between staff and patients and the potential that these had for therapy are an elusive topic. It appears that a valuable element in the early years of Jepson and Allis was the positive and affectionate response that was given to the patients' predilections. One who considered himself to be 'Duke John' was occasionally carried round the garden shoulder high, wearing a hat decorated with tinsel and peacock feathers, which he considered the Almighty had given him.[65] Other patients were allowed to devote themselves to pet white mice, or canaries, and to have formal funerals for the animals that processed in state from the committee room.[66] Some melancholics were given special privileges to encourage them to overcome their introspection and the problems this caused. A female depressive was drawn into the domestic bustle of the superintendent's house, which 'she very much enjoys and expresses much gratitude for'.[67] A male patient who was so miserable he refused to eat at mealtimes was allowed to go in the kitchen whenever he wanted and sample what took his fancy, until finally his repugnance to food was quite overcome.[68] Such individual preferences were acknowledged by staff, who continued to regard their non-convalescent patients as children to be indulged in their harmless singularities within the Retreat family. The extent to which this 'patriarchal' attitude towards patients might also constrain or demean patients is discussed in the next chapter. However, the habit of viewing the patients much as if they were children was an enduring one at the Retreat.

One reason for continuity in certain attitudes is to be found in stability of staffing. For a century four generations of the Tuke family were intimately associated with the institution. William, his son Henry and grandson Samuel gave many years of service as members of the Committee of Management and as directors. In addition, William acted as treasurer from 1792 to 1820 and Samuel from then until 1852. And William's great grandson, Daniel Hack Tuke, was secretary from 1847 to 1850, then assistant medical officer from 1854 to 1858, and finally a valued adviser until his death in 1895. Links with the earliest days of the asylum were also forged by its officers. When George and Catherine Jepson retired from their posts as superintendent and matron in 1823, Catherine was succeeded by Hannah Ponsonby, who had been like an adopted daughter to her and who also had been her assistant. Hannah continued as matron until 1841 when she retired at the same time as the second superintendent, Thomas Allis. Allis had had an apprentice for a time called John Kitching, who felt that Allis 'had been as a father to me'.[69] Kitching returned to the Retreat and served as its fifth superintendent from 1849 to 1874, and his son became assistant medical officer in 1871. Kitching's successor was Robert Baker, the nephew of Jonathan Burtt, who had been a director since 1852 and treasurer since 1866. Among visiting and consulting medical officers there was a comparable pattern. Dr Belcombe, physician from 1802 to 1826, was succeeded by his son, who held the same office until 1854. And the visiting surgeon,

Caleb Williams, was associated with the Retreat for nearly half a century from 1824 to 1871.

Cumulatively these familial links and overlapping periods of service must have been a force for continuity rather than change. Indeed, an element of stagnation was also the product of such a small accession of 'new blood'. Until the end of the nineteenth century the institution continued along essentially traditional lines that had been progressive when it had pioneered them at the turn of the nineteenth century but that became tired conventions as the years wore on.[70] Admittedly, there were some modifications in later years but these were perhaps less obvious in moral therapy than in patterns of living.

The sense of domestic intimacy was easier to maintain when numbers of patients and officers were small than in later years. At the end of its first year, December 1796, it had fifteen patients and by 1799 it had the thirty patients it had been designed to hold. By 1823, when Jepson retired, there were sixty-eight, numbers increased to over a hundred during the 1830s but then fell back, so that on Allis's retirement in 1841 there were eighty-seven patients. By this time, the larger numbers had inevitably led to some changes of atmosphere. One patient commented sadly that 'to one that has always been used to a small family, this is just like being in a show'.[71] Parallel with this increase in patient numbers came additional members of staff. In the early years there had been little sense of hierarchy among the officers, or of the separate worlds of staff and inmates. In a real sense the Retreat's patients *were* the family of the childless George and Catherine Jepson, and their accommodation was used by patients and staff alike. With the advent of the family man, Thomas Allis, the superintendent's domestic accommodation became more distinct. Growing numbers within the Retreat family inevitably led to a larger building with more specialist accommodation, which also weakened to some extent the original feeling of domestic intimacy. The growth in the establishment reinforced this: in 1797 there were seven officers or servants resident at the Retreat, in 1813 there were sixteen, by 1828 this had grown to twenty-six, and by 1840 to thirty-five. Associated with this growth was a more defined hierarchy: by 1840 both the superintendent and the matron had acquired assistants and so had some of the attendants.[72]

In addition to these trends there had been present from its inception some divisions within the Retreat's family. William Tuke, corresponding with John Bevans on the original design, had made clear that

> this is intended for persons in profession with us of all ranks with respect to property and that those whose circumstance will afford it, may be charged more than they cost the Institution in order to reduce the terms for the poor. It seems reasonable that such patients be in some respects differently accommodated.[73]

Samuel Tuke's *Description* revealed the extent of these differences in that affluent patients of a superior class had more comfortably furnished chambers on the top floor with 'delightful' views afforded by unusually large windows. They used the officers' dining-room as a day-room and also dined with them.[74] In 1816 the Lodge was built as a self-contained unit of more luxurious character to attract male patients who could pay high fees. Isolated by a long corridor from the main buildings it faced south over pleasure gardens,[75] and its patients were separated both geographically and socially from patients of a different class. With the advent of increasing numbers of high-fee-paying, non-Quaker patients in the mid- and late nineteenth century this process of differentiation accelerated. In adopting such a hierarchical system the Retreat merely reflected inequalities in nineteenth-century society. And in later implementing the hospital villa system, which in separating patients also weakened a sense of family, it is arguable that some compensating advantages were given patients in making available more specialised treatment.

The continuation of a patient's treatment in 1860 was justified on the grounds that she

> may fitly be compared to a hot-house plant as regards both body and mind, requiring for the conservation of the health of the one, and the tranquillity of the other the protecting and judicious care which an establishment such as this can and does supply.[76]

In seeing the asylum as a refuge John Kitching was echoing the sentiments of the Retreat's founders although in emphasising that a patient was 'a hot-house plant' he was unwittingly indicating one change that had taken place from earlier Quaker simplicity. There was a marked contrast between the homelike buildings and natural gardens of the original establishment and the late nineteenth-century asylum (replete with Turkish baths, a saloon for sophisticated evening entertainments and billard room) and surrounded by pleasure grounds (which featured amongst other amenities tennis-courts, a croquet lawn, a bowling-alley and a miniature golf-course). It seems possible that this increased emphasis on material components in moral treatment was compensation for a decline of psychological elements within it – the loss of 'family' within an expanding institution.

Yet changing emphases within moral treatment did not fundamentally change its objectives. Although the Retreat's lay therapists would not perhaps have expressed it in these terms they would probably have endorsed the conclusions of Pierce in the annual *Report* of 1908:

Patients tend in course of time to adapt themselves to their surroundings. If the rooms be dull and featureless, the patients will certainly sink into a deeper state of mental enfeeblement than they should do; if there are few interests their conduct will deteriorate.

He prefaced this statement with the remark that 'it is now accepted as a truism', and the fact that that was indeed the case was in part a testament to the Retreat in its early pioneering years. Tranquil surroundings, pleasant occupations, friendly relationships and a gradual return to normal patterns of social living apparently contributed to high recovery rates. And by this criterion, and that of the uniformly admiring comments of visitors, the success of moral treatment seemed to have been established to such an extent that it was widely imitated by other institutions in the early nineteenth century.[77] But what was difficult to transplant were the intangible human relationships that informed the early development of a milder therapy at York. Ultimately, the Retreat was itself to find difficulties in perpetuating this elusive, but crucial, ingredient in moral treatment.

A subtle transformation of the Retreat's ethos was discernible during the middle years of the nineteenth century. Early lay therapy had been informed by personal insight into individuals' problems and by a commonsense practicality in alleviating them. This was shown in Thomas Allis's suggestion to a patient worried by the iron casings in the windows that these served to protect him from burglars.[78] That this comfortable reassurance was accepted may suggest the friendliness and mutual confidence that arose from daily contact in the Retreat 'family'. This kind of relationship became more difficult, if not impossible, as numbers grew. When Jepson took office he had 15 patients to look after but Allis had 70, Kitching 110, Baker 135 and Pierce 151. The increased impersonality that resulted from a growth in numbers was resented by one patient. She argued in 1878 that it was desirable to replace distant medical officers with an old-style lay superintendent and wife because they

> would feel a genuine pleasure in trying to do good to the poor creatures under their care and not treat them as though the main object was to preserve an appearance of order.[79]

Here the implication was that patients were no longer subjects to be treated but objects to be managed. And it is to a discussion of moral management that we now turn.

4

Moral management

Traditionally the Retreat's therapy has been seen as the embodiment of sweetness and light. That apostle of non-restraint, John Conolly, described it in 1856 as 'the first in Europe in which every enlightened principle of treatment was carried into effect'.[1] The verdict of Victorian psychiatrists and reformers has been continued in a Whiggish tradition of historiography such that a modern, standard history of mental institutions can conclude that the Retreat's achievement was that it 'removed the final justification for neglect, brutality and crude medical methods. It proved that kindness was more effective than rigorous confinement'.[2] More recently an iconoclastic interpretation by Michael Foucault has challenged these well-worn assumptions: he has argued that a more repressive regime was concealed by its 'mythical values' and that 'madness was controlled, not cured'.[3]

This chapter will consider these contrasting views in relation to the Retreat's moral management by looking at three crucial areas: patients as children within the Retreat family; educating the insane; and the use of rewards and punishments. It ends with a brief assessment of the changing character of moral therapy at the Retreat.

PATIENTS AS CHILDREN

Images of the family and of the role of children within it are often contradictory or confused. At one extreme the family unit may be depicted as warm and loving: its supportive atmosphere nurturing its members and helping them to come to terms with their problems. At the opposite extreme the family may be seen as a more negative, even destructive, force: its claustrophobic inner life inhibiting independent growth and its authoritarian parental control constraining the individuality of children. In the case of the Retreat 'family' these difficulties are intensified by problems of interpreting opaque and ambiguous historical evidence. Nevertheless, the idea that York patients were children must be discussed since it was a metaphor whose significance struck both a contemporary and a modern commentator as penetrating to the inner reality of the asylum.

Two years after the institution had opened its doors, a Genevan visitor, Dr Delarive, provided a detailed analysis of the Retreat's practices:

> They do not consider them as absolutely deprived of reason; or, in other words, as inaccessible to the motives of fear, hope, feeling and honour. It appears, that they consider them rather as children, who have too much strength, and who make a dangerous use of it. Their punishments and rewards must be immediate, since that which is distant has no effect upon them. A new system of education must be adopted to give a fresh course to their ideas. Subject them at first; encourage them afterwards, employ them, and render their employment agreeable by attractive means.[4]

His views have recently been given emphasis, even notoriety, by Foucault, who concluded that 'madness is childhood' and that 'everything at the Retreat is organized so that the insane are transformed into minors'. He argued that the legal status of the lunatic as minor was translated from its juridical function of protecting the insane individual to a practical situation that made him vulnerable to domination and sovereignty by others.[5] Patients at the Retreat were thus allegedly subjected to the authority of a patriarchal, bourgeois family. Foucault's ideological standpoint imposed a clear-cut interpretation. Whether this cuts through the Gordian knot of historical complexities by ignoring much that would give an alternative reading of the situation must now be considered.

Other references to patients as children help to clarify in what sense this analogy may have been made. On two occasions (in 1813 and 1846), Samuel Tuke referred to the 'parental' role of the Jepsons: first in reference to the 'judicious attention' paid to patients' comfort and then more generally in relation to their influence over their charges. He saw this as a two-way relationship and felt that patients in turn had 'an almost filial attachment' to the Jepsons.[6] Fifty years later on the occasion of the Retreat's centenary, the daughter of Thomas Allis (George Jepson's successor), who had grown up at the Retreat in the 1820s and 1830s, remembered that it was then thought that patients had a claim 'to all the loving truthfulness and sincerity which we should show to our children'.[7] These public references suggest a tender solicitude for patients' welfare rather than the domineering parental role suggested by Foucault. Other, more private testimony gave some support to this kind of interpretation. One visitor, in 1811, recorded his belief that 'at the Retreat they [the patients] were nursed like children'.[8] And further references in mid-nineteenth-century medical case-books substantiated the impression that patients were seen as dependents who needed to be looked after like young children. 'His food has to be put into his mouth. He has to be dressed and undressed and served like a child' was the description of a patient in a state of deep melancholy. And of a comparable case it was said that she 'is in great distress of mind, fretful and crying like a child – is capable of being soothed by a firm, kind manner'.[9]

There were, however, clear limits set to this analogy by both patients and therapists. Patients objected to some visitors because they were 'very apt to converse with them in a childish, or, which is worse, in a domineering manner' and 'seemed to imagine they were children'.[10] Although some patients might feel demeaned by such behavior and reduced in stature because of it, others might themselves adopt non-adult patterns of behaviour. A maniac was described by her doctor as one who does 'many harmless, silly pranks, sets the nurse at defiance and conducts herself like a wayward child'. Such neutral tones might give way to moral disapproval in other comments as in, 'He remains childishly playful and incapable of self-control.' In a few cases a significant interpretation of childish behaviour was put forward: 'To describe the state of J. H. W. since his admission is to describe that of a spoiled child; or of an undisciplined mind, in which the passions have never been brought under control.'[11] Childishness in this sense – that of inappropriately infantile patterns of behaviour – was thus deprecated and a more authoritarian tone coloured the comparison of the insane with that of children. So how was such inappropriate behaviour to be modified?

A useful guide to the way this question could be answered was given in Samuel Tuke's *Description* and is worth quoting at length:

There is much analogy between the judicious treatment of children, and that of insane persons. Locke has observed, that 'the great secret of education, lies in finding the way to keep the child's spirit easy, active, and free; and yet, at the same time, to restrain him from many things he has a mind to, and to draw him to things which are uneasy to him'. It is highly desirable that the attendants on lunatics should possess this influence over their minds; but it will never be obtained by austerity and rigour.[12]

In seeing patients as in some sense schoolchildren this passage drew attention to a central function of the Retreat in educating or re-educating those who had been sent there. We have already seen the influence of Locke's associationist psychology on York therapists' belief in disordered reasoning as an explanation of insanity. Education, in its broadest sense, would help to re-create correct patterns of thinking and thus establish appropriate standards of behaviour. This would accord with the strong emphasis on self-disciplined living within the Society of Friends that was usually established by an education conceived in terms of both religious truth and correct principles of behaviour.

It is therefore hardly surprising to find strong parallels between the therapeutic objectives of the Retreat in seeking to resocialise its patients and that of Quaker education. There was little difference between its rationale of mild therapy and the objectives that previously had been laid down in 1778 for a Yorkshire boarding school:

By gentleness, kind and affectionate treatment, holding out encouragement and approbation to the deserving, exerting the influence of the fear of shame . . . to bring forward into the Society and its service a number . . . acquainted . . . with the discipline of wisdom.[13]

At both Ackworth and the Retreat gentle treatment was preferred but where positive inducements failed there was a hint of more peremptory methods. These alternatives were brought out clearly in an influential book on Quaker discipline where the young were to be brought to good habits 'by persuasion and warning, by rewards and punishments, by alluring to good and deterring from evil, by precept and instruction'.[14] At the Retreat it is clear that at least some patients were cast in this same role of pupil: 'Her conduct is more that of an ill-brought up child than anything else to which it can be compared.'[15] It may also be surmised that the moral manager of an asylum saw himself as the teacher and disciplinarian of such patients. D. H. Tuke, who was an assistant medical officer at the Retreat in the 1850s, collaborated with another

Moral management

notable psychiatrist, J. C. Bucknill, to publish in 1858 a standard work on psychological medicine. This defined the abilities desirable in those who practised moral therapy:

A faculty of seeing that which is passing in the minds of men is the first requisite of moral power and discipline, whether in asylums, schools, parishes or elsewhere. Add to this a firm will, the faculty of self-control, a sympathising distress at moral pain, a strong desire to remove it, and that fascinating biologising power is elicited, which enables men to domineer for good purposes over the minds of others.[16]

A comparison of D. H. Tuke's views with those of his father, in the *Description of the Retreat* (previously quoted), reveals a highly significant shift from influencing the minds of patients to domineering over them. This difference in the therapist's motivation gives a further clue to the changes that had apparently occurred in the Retreat family between the second and sixth decade of the nineteenth century. In the previous chapter it was suggested that by mid-century the close-knit, non-hierarchical family, with its friendly daily contact between staff and patients, had been weakened. It is interesting that at the same time as these behavioural changes were occurring parallel changes were taking place in the semantic description of treatment, in which there was a growing preference for the term 'moral management' rather than 'moral treatment'. The former hints at a more systematic organisation of patients and a more pervasive authority over them than does the latter. Such changing nomenclature may reveal to a sensitive ear an underlying shift both in the distribution of power and in the nature of social relationships. And this somewhat tentative supposition receives further corroboration from the changing style of medical case-notes. John Kitching's observations on patients, in the quarter of a century that marked his superintendency from 1849 to 1874, were obviously much more concerned with controlling and disciplining patients, as well as with moralistic censure of their behaviour, than were those of his predecessors. How did Kitching, and other therapists, attempt to alter undesirable behavioural patterns in their patients?

EDUCATING THE INSANE

Proper regulation of the mind is essentially connected with the prevention of the disease. It must be acknowledged in several instances, its foundation appears to have been laid in an injudicious indulgence in early life; by which the ill trained mind has been brought into contact with the oppositions and difficulties of the world without the habits of endurance or self-government.[17]

This discussion of one cause of insanity is highly significant in relating it to morality and to a preceding lack of moral discipline in the insane individual. It points towards the duality inherent in the Retreat's moral treatment of insanity: its practice was informed by ethical beliefs as to what were right or wrong standards of behaviour. These principles of morality were derived from those current at that time within the Society of Friends.

'To bear witness by practice, as well as by profession' of the fruits of their faith was a constant objective of Quakers.[18] Upright behaviour was essential both from an individual's point of view and also lest moral lapses reflect badly on the Society of Friends. So it is perhaps predictable that one should find friends and relatives making censorious ethical judgements on prospective Quaker patients. A fifteen-year-old boy, suffering from mania, was thought to have 'an unsubdued self-inflicted perverse disposition, originating in over-indulgence', and an imbecilic girl was accused of 'pride and highmindedness'.[19] Relatives anticipated that these kinds of ill-regulated or passionate habits would be corrected at York. 'I sincerely wish he may be favoured with a steady, calm, eveness of mind', wrote a father. A sister concluded that her brother's improvement at the Retreat 'may in part be occasioned by the more regular mode of living and greater subjection which we expect he has experienced, since placed under your care'.[20] And two important educational means to these ends were work and religion.

Employment was considered of the 'utmost importance' in moral therapy, a conclusion that was justified, as we have seen, by varied rationales. Prominent amongst these was the moral value given to work: 'to relieve the languor of idleness, and to prevent the indulgence of gloomy sensations'. For the curable, and especially the convalescent, employment was thought to be an important bridge on the road back to recovery and the resumption of life outside the asylum. Thus, work should be 'adapted to their previous habits, inclinations and capacities'.[21] This would not only revive the technical skills of earlier employment but also strengthen the moral faculties. Outside the asylum, Quakers regarded work as more than a means of livelihood. 'Whatsoever thy hand findeth to do, do it with all thy might' was felt to be an important religious injunction. An evangelical Quaker interpreted this in characteristically extreme terms:

> To give ourselves, without reserve, to the occupation provided in the order of Providence . . . is . . . a good *moral* habit of incalculable importance . . . If we fail . . . how is it possible that we should render to the judge of all the earth a *good* account of our stewardship?[22]

And amongst some relatives of patients there was a feeling that physical work, even for the mentally ill, would provide a 'merciful coercive discipline' that would undo the 'manifold bad consequences' of idleness.[23] Work was therefore seen as involving moral discipline, which included an element of self-control and the shouldering of responsibility. Thus, amongst more intelligent convalescents, one patient took charge of all the plants in the house, another assisted in dispensing drugs and also made picture frames for the house and a third assisted Dr Thurnam in the compilation of his statistics.[24]

Foucault has suggested that asylum employment possessed

> a constraining power superior to all forms of physical coercion, in that the regularity of the hours, the requirements of attention, the obligation to produce a result detach the sufferer from a liberty of mind . . . and engage him in a system of responsibilities.[25]

While we may accept that work did involve concentration and responsibility, the conclusion that this necessarily had a harmful effect may be more questionable. In deciding whether employment was coercive it would be relevant to consider patients' own feelings, their stage in convalescence and the suitability of occupation for the individual. There is evidence that some patients were reluctant to engage in activities. One patient protested to the Committee of Management:

> T. Allis wishes to know why I do not employ myself. I am not able to do so or at least to my advantage otherwise I would gladly [do so]. Remaining tranquil gives me an opportunity to fit myself for business hereafter.
>
> Meditation and retirement are a source of great enjoyment and peace to a happy and contented disposition. And not dangerous, irksome, or frivolous as some suppose.[26]

Because this patient was diagnosed as a religious melancholic it might well have been considered beneficial to divert his thoughts from his self-concerns. However, there was a change of thinking at the Retreat on the suitability of employment for every case: the enthusiasm of the early years gave way to an appreciation that greater selectivity was necessary.[27] In spite of this a moral presumption continued that some employment was desirable for all save acute cases and hence patients in other categories might incur censure for their 'idleness'.[28] In part, censorious remarks may reflect disappointment since care was taken to encourage patients to seek recreation or employment that accommodated their individual preferences.

While Foucault's view that work was 'imposed as a moral rule' may be accepted as one valid interpretation of the Retreat's employment policies, his more fundamental critique of the subject must be rejected. Foucault ignores his own warning 'Let us not forget we are in a Quaker world' in failing to recognise that for Quakers it was part of normal life to accept a moral injunction to work. For Quaker patients the path to recovery and the resumption of the habits of the outside world might therefore include work. Thus in this context alien values were not imposed on patients since they shared the same assumptions as their therapists. Another reservation about Foucault's analysis concerns the way in which he condemns the Retreat for forcing *adult* responsibilities on patients in the work situation but criticises it elsewhere for demeaning them to the status of *children*. It becomes difficult to see what model of social therapy the institution could have adopted that would not have attracted such indiscriminate censure. Foucault's opinion that religion occupied an important pedagogic role is one from which no one would dissent but his view that religion was also 'a constant principle of coercion' is more problematical and needs further discussion.[29]

Quakers believed that the soul could rise above disease and therefore felt that patients' religious feeling was the key that might unlock the door of insanity. Every encouragement was therefore given to patients to participate in religious activity, and their demeanour at such events was carefully evaluated. Many patients attending the New Meeting House were considered to be 'deeply imbued with religious feeling', and patients who attended a religious Reading were said to have 'behaved with great propriety, many of them evincing a serious deportment, listening attentively'.[30] The self-restraint that religious meetings involved had been commended from the early years of the Retreat:

> Several attend who are disposed to various irregular actions, and the restraint which such impose upon themselves, forms an important part of that moral discipline which, even in a curative point of view can hardly be too highly estimated.[31]

Formal religious exercises were only part of a more pervasive moral milieu. Doerner's view that its rural situation symbolised the Retreat's acceptance of a moral social order in accord with nature is perceptive.[32] But it was nature as part of a divinely ordered universe that most appealed to Quakers, rather than, as Doerner also suggests, the countryside in opposition to the industrial capitalism of the city. It was in this former sense that the York establishment could be seen as a romantic institution. Close contact with nature through walks or physical outdoor exercise conferred the kind of tranquillity on patients that the Lake poets themselves extolled in their deistical view of nature and its benign influence on humanity. One patient's brother revealed the kind of thinking that linked employment to the moral order and to the 'healing' process:

> As he [the patient] himself used to say farming and agricultural occupations were the natural employment of man, so do such pursuits best recommend themselves to the mind . . . to a weak or diseased mind what can possibly be more likely to soothe, to strengthen and under proper discipline to restore, in measure, that capability for usefulness which assuredly exists wherever there is bodily strength. The flower garden for some, the plough, the spade, the hoe for others, seedtime and harvest, summer and winter, have their various allotted labours and happy are those who . . . find moderate employment here in the least vain of all the idle vanities of this life and are therewith content.[33]

Here it was evident that apparently discrete elements in the lives of patients were integrated into a cohesive, underlying synthesis. But was this a 'healing' process or one of 'coercion'? What kind of weight should be given to recurring words like 'discipline' and 'restraint'? We now turn to a fuller discussion of these and related issues in an analysis of the system of rewards and punishments at the Retreat.

REWARDS AND PUNISHMENTS

Classification

As we have seen, Dr Delarive had suggested as early as 1798 that the patients were seen as children in that 'their punishments and rewards must be immediate, since that which is distant has no effect upon them'. He described the system of promotion used after a patient had exhausted his fit of mania in the ground-floor cells:

> If he behaves well, he is preferred to a chamber on the first floor: this is a kind of honourable promotion, which excites his emulation. These rooms, larger and more agreeable than the cells and provided with more furniture, display throughout the picture of neatness.[34]

The description is interesting in linking the stages of recovery both with material comfort and with the patient's attitudes: this progression became a standard feature of the psychiatric hospital. Erving Goffman, in his sociological analysis of the asylum, describes how it later operated:

> In this system the attendant is likely to be the key staff person, informing the patient of the punishments and rewards that are to regulate his life and arranging for medical authorisation for such privileges and punishments. Quiet, obedient behaviour leads to the patient's promotion in the ward system; obstreperous, untidy behaviour to demotion.[35]

Andrew Scull in his historical study of the asylum's development attributes to the Retreat the 'invention of these techniques'.[36] Did the Retreat originate them and did it operate them in the manner that has been outlined?

By the 1790s the techniques of managing patients through a system of rewards and punishments had already been established elsewhere. At Manchester Asylum, Dr Ferriar was accustomed to remonstrate with a violent patient and appeal to his sense of honour before secluding him 'till he shows tokens of repentance'. John Haslam, apothecary at Bethlem, operated a comparable system of psychological deprivation:

> Where the patient is in a condition to be sensible of restraint he may be punished for improper behaviour by confining him to his room, by degrading him, and not allowing him to associate with the convalescents, and by witholding certain indulgences he had been accustomed to enjoy

Moral management

... they are rendered much more tractable by wounding their pride than by severity of discipline.

Ferriar would have agreed with this conclusion since he referred to the 'high sense of honour' of patients and believed that 'the management of hope and apprehension in the patients forms the most useful part of discipline'. He provided accommodation for convalescents because this 'would act powerfully in creating a habit of self-restraint, the first salutary habit in the mind of a lunatic'.[37] Thus, classified accommodation was one instrument within a system of rewards and punishments that was outlined in publications of 1795 and 1798. In organising a system of classification the Retreat was operating within a spectrum of existing ideas on the moral management of patients, although within this general context it may well have developed distinctive practices.

Classification became more elaborate as the size of the Retreat grew and as knowledge of patients' disorders and of managing them increased.[38] At first the separation was along the lines of what seemed the most obvious points of difference – sexual and social – rather than medical. Men were accommodated on the east, to the left of the central administrative block, and women to the west. Propertied members of the Society of Friends, who paid higher fees, were housed, as we have seen, in superior accommodation separate from the general class of patients. It was only among this ordinary category that demarcations began to be made according to their behavioural state.

On both sides of the house the more 'difficult' patients were housed farthest from the central block, presumably so that their behaviour would not disrupt the communal social life of the establishment. These patients were thought of as consisting of two distinct groups: first, disorderly or noisy patients, and secondly, fatuous or imbecilic patients. Each group had its own accommodation, and nearby were seclusion rooms for the confinement of more violent patients. Much later, in 1888, it was decided to utilise the villa system of separate accommodation to provide for more specialised accommodation of acute cases and the West Villa was built for them.

Male patients were divided into three categories by the mid-nineteenth century, each with day-rooms, airing courts, and with exercise galleries for two of the classes. Apart from the two cate-

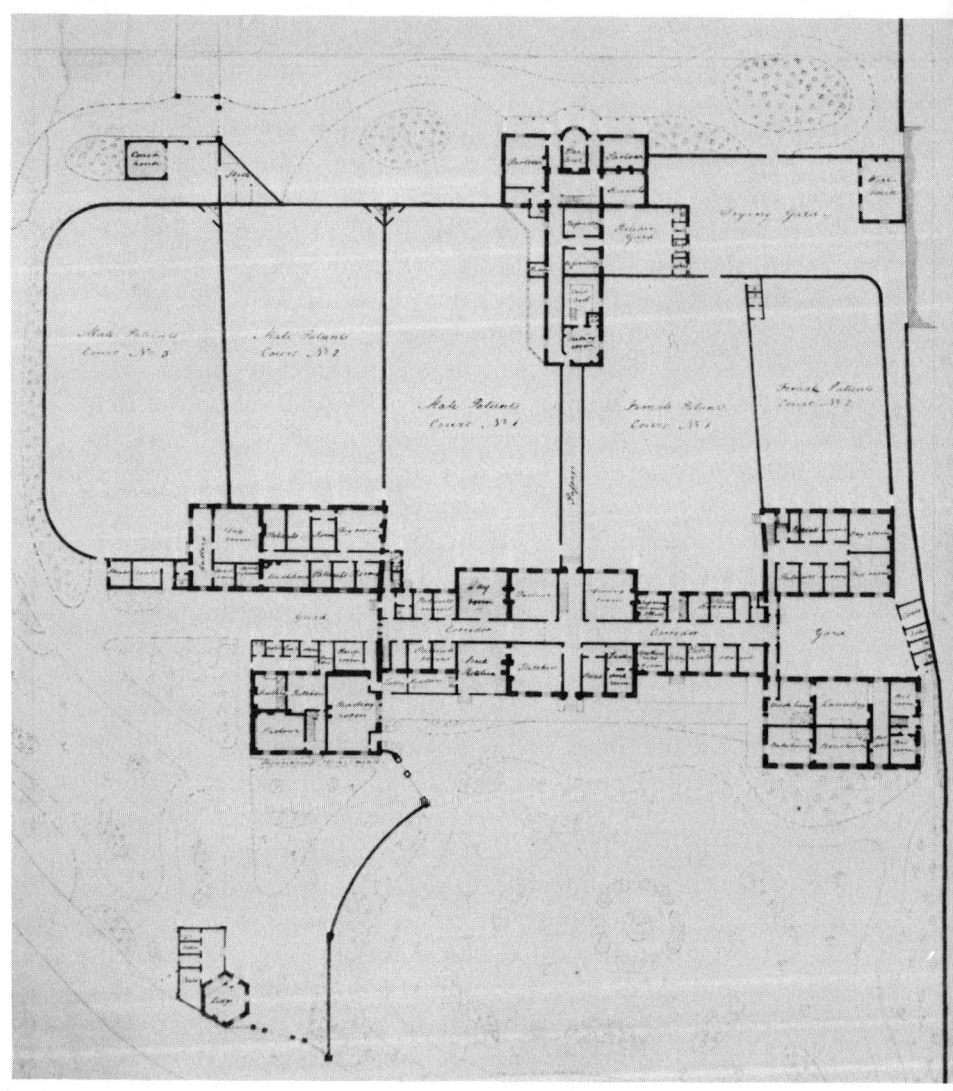

Plate 9. Plan of the Retreat in 1827

gories already described the first class was seen as 'capable of much rational enjoyment' and therefore as convalescent. Among women there were more categories: the fourth one included the two subgroups[39] just described; then there were a further three classes. Earlier, when there had been two rather than three classes, Tuke had described how allocation was dependent in part of patient preference: 'if a patient finds the society in one room unpleasant she is removed to the other.' Dr Thurnam admitted in 1840 that the threefold classification of women was 'less precise' than that operating on the male side of the house.[40] Convalescent women were fortunate in having had separate accommodation provided for them on the first floor of the new domestic wing in 1827, and the front garden was converted into 'pleasure grounds' for them. As we have seen the Appendage had been opened in 1811 for convalescents of both sexes so that they would have easy access to the town. Convalescent patients were so reluctant to move down the hill into this strange accommodation that it became filled with chronic cases, and the experiment was abandoned in 1822. A more successful innovation for convalescents was the short stay by the sea in Scarborough lodging-houses begun in the 1830s, and later extended in 1887 and 1903 with the leasing first of Gainsborough House within the town, and then the more secluded Throxenby Hall outside Scarborough.

The flexibility of the Retreat's system of classification was a product both of inherent problems in categorising patients on the basis of behavioural symptoms, and of a deliberate desire for an arrangement that would allow an easy transition from one class to the next. Samuel Tuke therefore recommended a provision of adjacent day-rooms and galleries so that patients could keep their own bedchamber but transfer to different daytime accommodation.[41] Although this fluidity may originally have been motivated by a simple therapeutic desire to match the type of accommodation and care to the stage reached on the way to recovery, its potentiality as a tool in moral management soon became apparent. The outline of such a scheme was implicit in Tuke's *Description* of 1813 where it is discussed only in relation to the segregation of violent patients:

Those who are violent, require to be separated from the more tranquil, and to be prevented, by some means, from offensive conduct towards their fellow sufferers. Hence the patients are arranged into classes, as much as may be, according to the degree in which they approach to rational or orderly conduct.

They quickly perceive, or if not, they are informed on the first occasion, that this treatment depends, in great measure, upon their conduct.[42]

An organised extension of this principle – exploiting to the full the potentiality of classification into a system of regular demotions and promotions linked to patient behaviour – appears to have been

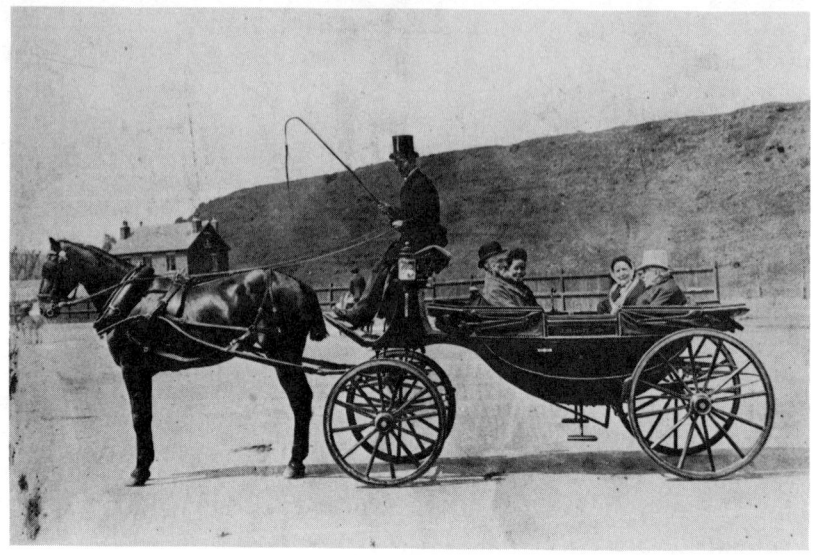

Plate 10. Patients taking the air at Scarborough

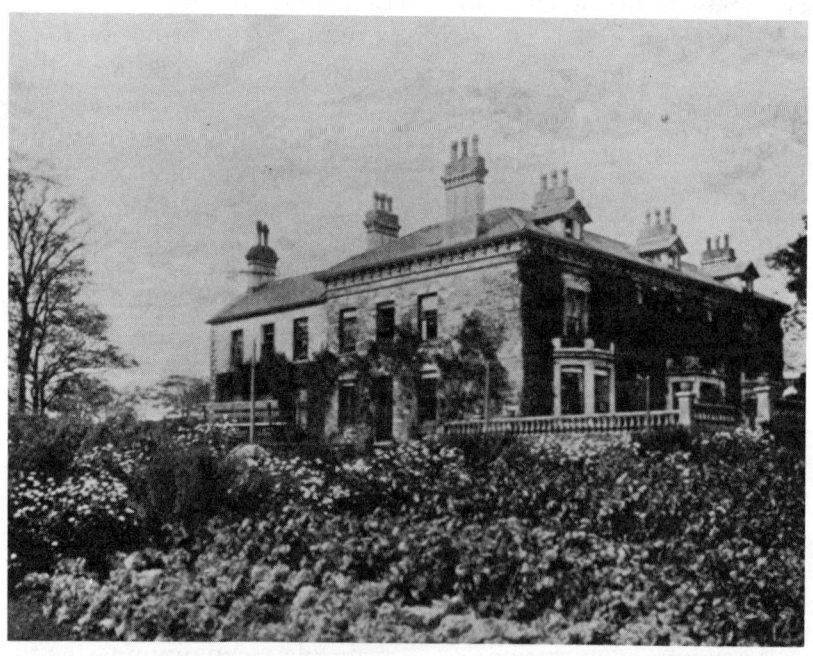

Plate 11. Throxenby Hall, 1904

Moral management

due to Dr Kitching's arrival. Take, for example, a patient suffering from dementia whose case-notes for 1855 were not untypical in their explicit use of mobility to influence behaviour:

1 June. Very dirty in her habits, and has been placed in the Low Gallery today – temporarily . . .

11 June. Remains in the Low Gallery, destructive to her clothing and dirty in her habits.

1 July. Not appearing to derive benefit from being in the Low Gallery, she has been placed for some days past in an upper one – and she has made considerably more attempt at self control. She is much more engaged in sewing, and is more cleanly in her habits. She says she is determined to get home, and that this appears to be the only way of doing so.[43]

Sometimes it was found to be unnecessary to actually move a patient because showing her alternative accommodation was a sufficient threat, as for case 963, a melancholic. 'The discipline of sending her to see the other gallery in the evening is probably beginning to have a good effect.'[44] In other instances, promotion within the wards was combined with other inducements, as in this example of a patient suffering from remittent mania in 1855:

1 January. Promised a mug of porter for his supper if he would work today: he has agreed to do so.

14 January. Has not been materially influenced by reward in the way of porter etc. – Is very dirty and destructive.

11 June. Has been promoted to the Higher Gallery for a day or two, and conducts himself well.[45]

Such promises were an important element in the Retreat's treatment. That trust between patients and therapists was essential had been implicit in the institution's social philosophy from its earliest days but was formally set out in 1847 in the 'Information and Suggestions for the Friends of Patients'. This stated that 'false representations in the management of the insane are on all grounds objectionable'. It insisted that prospective patients should know that they were being taken to the Retreat and that relatives should not try to involve its officers in any deceptions that had been used to get patients to come to York. The document stressed that it was of 'the first importance that patients should enter the establishment free from any moral distrust of those to whose care they are about to be entrusted'. Nearly half a century later Dr Bedford Pierce pleaded again for truthfulness by relatives when a patient was brought to the Retreat and explicitly stated that treatment was impeded if a patient lost trust in those who looked after him.[46]

It was hoped that trust could be built up from the first seconds of a patient's arrival. It was Jepson's genius to have begun the tradition that impressed on newcomers that they were not lunatics who had lost all claim to kindness and respect but human beings who would be assisted to live in a community. He insisted that all means of restraint should be removed from a patient on arrival, he should be spoken to as if he were a rational being and should be assimilated into the social patterns of living by taking a light meal shortly after arrival. The practice of gaining trust through kind treatment on arrival continued, as we can see from this description of a patient's arrival in 1870: 'On the evening of her coming she had a warm bath and some tea and tea cake and was put to bed.'[47]

Internal restraint

It was a cardinal belief that patients were aware of their treatment and also that they could be involved in their own therapy. One example of this will be cited at length, because it was unusually explicit about a form of therapy that was so pervasive that it rarely achieved much comment or analysis from the pragmatists at the Retreat. In 1839 Dr Thurnam, the new resident medical officer, took a patient (diagnosed as a maniac) into his confidence and explained to him the lines on which his treatment was proceeding:

John Thurnam thinks it desirable, in reply to W. R.'s numerous notes, to endeavour to explain a little of the views, as he understands them, of the medical officers and the Superintendent in the present mode of conducting W. R.'s case.

They consider that W. R. labours under a degree of restless activity of mind, which, whilst it does not incapacitate him from correct reasoning, yet imparts so much of enthusiasm to his will and of exuberance to his feelings as to frequently demand that restraint and moral discipline, which W. R. has happily the power of commanding from his friends at the Retreat, whose moral duty it is to impose this in the kindest, most considerate manner possible. J. T. hopes that W. R. will perceive the propriety of his co-operating so far in this plan of treatment as to exert all the self-control of which he is capable; which will be the only effective way of hastening the period of his restoration to his usual intercourse with his fellow patients and his exemption from every species of restraint beyond that essential to the good order of the establishment.[48]

Here moral management was depicted to the patient as a two-way process that involved both the imposition of a 'moral discipline' by therapists and also the development of a 'self-control' by the patient. Eventually, it was assumed that internal restraint would replace external restraint.

One way that this therapeutic pendulum worked was through a code of honour that was either imposed on, or adopted by, patients:

The principle of honour is often very strong in the minds of lunatics: I have often known patients who were under a voluntary engagement of good behaviour, hold a successful contest for a considerable length of time with the strong wayward propensities of their disorder, and even conceal all aberrations of mind. The attempt is highly beneficial to the patient and ought to be sedulously encouraged by the attendant.[49]

Evidence on how this system operated came most clearly from reports on patients who broke the code and attempted to escape. The first example comes from 1861:

24 June.   The last time he was trusted out in the grounds he broke bounds, went to a public house for some ale, on which account he was confined to the inner court, but promised liberty as soon as he would undertake not to leave the premises. A few days ago he gave vent to violent feeling, so much so as to attack the Medical Superintendent, for which he was put into seclusion the rest of the day.

8 August.   Having about a month ago given an implied undertaking that he would not abuse his liberty he was allowed to resume it, and has been more comfortable and quieter since.[50]

Here the code of honour was linked to rewards and punishments but an element of judgement was used to evaluate the patient's disposition. An example from case-notes dating from 1880 suggests that this discretion was replaced later by a legalistic parole system:

30 November.   Yesterday Miss R. attempted to escape, but was secured before she had got into the open air. Refusing to sign 'parole', she has been removed from the Centre to the 4th Gallery.

30 December.   Having signed 'parole' Miss R. was yesterday brought back to the Centre.[51]

Attaining the right balance between freedom and constraint was a pivotal point in moral management. 'Too much liberty . . . is an obvious evil. On the other hand, if caution is carried to timidity and seclusion to excess, the minds of patients will deteriorate', as Kitching acknowledged.[52] Building on, and extending, healthy affections and faculties was seen as central to patients' recovery. Important in this respect, from the earliest days, was a social therapy that involved a sensitive appraisal of patients' readiness to participate in, or withdraw from, communal living. A particularly interesting case in this context was that of Samuel W., a long-stay patient suffering from remittent mania, who was in the Retreat from 1803 until his death in 1824[53] (see the Appendix). The nature of his illness meant that several intervals of apparent sanity each year were divided by periods of violently antisocial behaviour when he tore blankets, broke windows or attacked his attendant. He was physically restrained by a strait-jacket during his most aggressive phases and his behaviour was carefully monitored. 'This afternoon he appeared less violent and at his own request with promises of good behaviour had the waistcoat taken off.' He did not always manage to fulfil his promises, but the staff invariably accepted his word, thus emphasising the mutual trust on which moral treatment was based. As Samuel W. became by slow degrees calmer and more rational Jepson allowed him into company: 'he was a little calmer, smoked his pipe in the upper dining room in the evening very quietly. Yesterday and today was at liberty and quiet.' After another period of normal social living in which he was able to attend Meetings in York, go shopping, or partake in local Friends' hospitality his illness would recur. Often Jepson would detect early warning signs of an impending paroxysm: a flurry of letter-writing, malicious comments, volubility at Meeting or a singsong tone of voice. Sometimes an attack, like the one during a stay at Henry Tuke's home, took everyone by surprise when suddenly he 'seemed to have lost the government of himself in a great degree'.

Contemporary visitors to the Retreat marvelled at this self-government by patients within a social community. Yet more recently it has been suggested by Foucault that this system of individual responsibility was fundamentally repressive. Ignoring the more rhetorical flourishes and metaphorical obscurities of some of his writing on the Retreat let us concentrate on his more fundamental criticism. He suggests that such an imposition of moral responsibility created anxiety and guilt in the mad. The formal social occasions in which patients participated imposed on them alien social personalities; it forced them to act as strangers to themselves because of the roles that observers expected them to adopt.[54] Unfortunately, neither Foucault nor anyone else can have a definitive answer as to whether such accusations are valid or invalid, because relevant evidence on patients' states of mind does not exist in sufficient detail. The most appropriate response to Foucault would probably be to ask how a madman could re-enter the world of everyday living without at some stage participating in ordinary social events? If it is accepted that at some stage the mad, or some of them, might wish to leave the 'freedom of unreason' for the world of reason (and even Foucault speaks of 'cure'), then a second question follows from the first. Were patients introduced into communal activities prematurely when their state of mind was unprepared for it? If this were the case then patients might well suffer anxiety about their capacity for self-control in a social situation, and perhaps guilt later on, if their behaviour was seen as inadequate.

The impression gained from reading the early case-books of the Retreat is that therapists were sensitive to this issue and attempted to the best of their abilities to suit the situation to the patient. Take for example the notes on one of the first female patients, who suffered from mania with melancholy and whose fluctuating condition necessitated frequent changes in her therapeutic situation:

18 October 1803. She has been for ab[ou]t a w[ee]k growing more calm. Has now got on her usual clothing and been walk[ing] in the garden where she behaved very well tho' not yet quite herself.

21 November 1803. Has been in the parlour since the above date (and conducted pretty well, but never quite herself being too talkative) till the 19th when she became very high and irrational, was confined to her room, this morning is more calm.[55]

Here the patient assumed a social personality when fit to do so, withdrew to a more secluded situation when in a manic phase and gradually participated in communal living again as she recovered, at first in the comparative freedom of the gardens and then with other patients indoors. Clearly, mistakes were made in evaluating a patient's condition as this later entry for the same patient implicitly acknowledged:

> 18 March 1805. Has been getting better a few weeks and is now pretty even in her spirits. N. B. More than usual care has been taken during her present recovery in respect to bringing her forward into company with great caution which has been attended with a good effect.

Not every therapist, doctor or attendant possessed Jepson's sensibility and therapeutic skill in assessing patients. Later, a more oppressive system of moral management was to be imposed that involved greater insensitivity to patients. Symptomatic of this change was the fact that from the 1850s patients' case-notes referred much more frequently to 'discipline' and 'control'. For example, it is startling to read the initial observation on a patient admitted in 1851, suffering from monomania: 'On the following day [i.e. after admission] she strove for the mastery but was made to yield, and since that time has been tractable.'[56] Remarks on other patients revealed that a change in priorities appeared to have taken place: to a much greater extent the patient was now slotted into a fixed environment rather than a social context being created for the individual. Everyday routine was rigidified into the 'rules of the house', which patients were expected to obey. In 1855 a non-conforming male patient 'underwent a little discipline in the form of a shower bath for refusing to conform to the rules of the house in regard to hours etc. It has had a decidedly beneficial effect'.[57] Even imbecilic patients were not immune as a later entry for 1874 revealed: 'Has continued very much the same – the dread of shower baths has kept him in better order, and he continues in better order and spirits'.[58] It is revealing that although there were two references to the order that reflected the interest of the institution there was only one reference to the state of the patient's own feelings.

Other references reinforced this impression that patients increasingly were regarded rather less like children (to be treated indulgently) and rather more like untrained animals (to be domesticated), as in the eighteenth-century view of the lunatic. 'After the first day or two when she made some resistance to any restraint she has settled in comfortably and is becoming quiet and

Moral management

tractable' were the opening remarks about a patient suffering from delusions who entered the Retreat in 1872.[59] A comparable comment was made the following year about a case of dementia, when the patient had been at York a month:

> 27 February 1873. He continues untidy and uncouth in his manners and language. He is also very mischievous and will turn other patients violently out of any seat he wishes to occupy. But he is settling down gradually to conform to our rules.[60]

The desirable patient seems to have become a docile subordinate as in this reference from 1892: 'So far she has given very little trouble and seems quite anxious to obey all the rules of the institution.'[61]

Anxiety, but this time within a moral rather than social context, was also revealed by a melancholic patient. Before losing her nerve and failing to implement her plan of drowning herself in a pond in the grounds she left a suicide note:

> I . . . constantly feel that I am greatly out of place amongst all the unblemished moral characters in this house and fear that my having been here at all will bring much trouble on you. I therefore feel compelled to take this desperate and dreadful step.[62]

Such anxiety and guilt within a moral world appear at first to give concrete corroboration of Foucault's assertions. Yet the letter ended with sentiments that must make us pause before we accept such criticism. 'I do wish to thank you with as much sincerity as I am capable of for all your kindness towards me. Nothing could have exceeded it.' Some patients undoubtedly continued to feel that the Retreat was in some way a kindly, even protective, institution. One such patient evidently felt that any internalised constraints that the asylum involved were much less than he would face in the outside world: 'when returning home is mentioned to him, he evidently shrinks from it, from a sense of the amount of self-control required in mixing again in society.'[63]

What we have been considering is the process by which patients internalised the norms of an institution. Ultimately this was a unique experience dependent on the conjunction of individual patient (each having a distinctive personality and type of illness) and therapist (each possessing varied skills and sensibility). These encounters took place within an evolving institution with changing ethos, values and environment. The dynamic and fragmentary nature of such experiences exacerbates the already acute problem of generalising about such an intrinsically elusive topic as self-control. However, a further dimension must also be considered before an overall assessment of the degree of repression in such moral management is attempted. Fortunately, this additional perspective is slightly more accessible: the use of mechanical restraint or seclusion in the overt coercion of patients. Such restraint had a pervasive effect: its resonance was an essential element in 'the principle of fear' that linked external restraint to internal self-control.

External restraint

The principle of fear, which is rarely decreased by insanity, is considered as of great importance in the management of the patients. But it is not allowed to be excited, beyond that degree which naturally arises from the necessary regulations of the family. Neither chains nor corporal punishment are tolerated, on any pretext, in this establishment.[64]

Samuel Tuke then clarified the extent to which this 'principle of fear' could be used. He was clear that it should not be utilised to justify 'the barbarous practices' of traditional lunatic management, that over-reliance on it tended to delay recovery by contracting and debasing the understanding, and that it should therefore be used as a final resort when other methods had failed. For both the types of patients categorised by contemporary medicine – melancholics and maniacs – Tuke was clear that mild methods were most likely to promote recovery and should constitute their normal treatment. He explicitly rejected the idea that lunatics, like wild animals, should be subjugated through fear.[65]

This lengthy analysis in the *Description of the Retreat* of 1813 was not intended merely as an abstract discussion of the merits of the traditional 'terrific' management of the mad versus the 'mild' methods more recently developed. It was also depicted as a faithful representation of what occurred at the Retreat. Yet a comparison of this account of 1813 with the later one of 1828 in *A Sketch of the Retreat* revealed an important inconsistency. In the former Tuke stated that the accepted wisdom 'of its being necessary to commence an acquaintance with lunatics by an exhibition of strength, or an appliance of austerity is utterly erroneous'. The later account acknowledged that those at York at first assented to 'the general correctness of these views' and only the experience of Jepson later led him 'to abandon the system of terror' in favour of influencing patients through their understanding or affections.[66]

In what did this early 'system of terror' consist? I would argue that it is a misreading of what Tuke wrote to suggest, as did Michael Fears recently, that those who began the Retreat believed that 'in some cases of violent excitement, the cudgel and the whip were the most suitable instruments of coercion'.[67] Tuke wrote that the Retreat subscribed generally to contemporary ideas of terrorising the lunatic, of which these instruments were a part. But he then went on to say that these practices were modified by the 'good sense and feeling' of the Committee of Management. And neither in the internal records of the asylum nor in the comments of visitors was there any hint of this kind of brutality. What was present was the occasional use of overwhelming force in cases of violent mania, such that the patient would see the hopelessness of struggle against restraint, and thus harm himself less than if he were approached more tentatively. For example, 'in the evening he had become quite outrageous and was by three men jacketed by force'.[68] Such 'heroic' measures to restrain patients were used as little as possible. There was a determined effort to replace the chains of traditional practices with milder and more discriminating methods of restraining violent patients.

Mechanical restraint was the ultimate resort when other methods of moral management had failed. Regarded as essential in a few instances, its use in others was seen by Jepson as the result of the inadequate management practised by attendants over their patients.[69] In cases of violent excitement – when injury would occur to the patient himself, or to the attendant or other patients – a strait-jacket was used. Jepson stated, 'We do at times use the strait-waistcoat when it appears necessary to prevent the patient from doing mischief'.[70] Such jackets, made of ticking to the Retreat's own design, were later replaced for the less excited cases by leather straps, attached from the waist to the arms, which allowed patients to use their hands to some extent.[71] 'We do not think ourselves justified in trusting him at present with the use of his hands' because he tore clothes and struck another patient, so 'G[eorge] J[epson] has therefore ordered them to be confined to his sides with a belt and straps.'[72] A later alternative for violently excited patients was to restrain them in a chair. A manic-depressive 'made

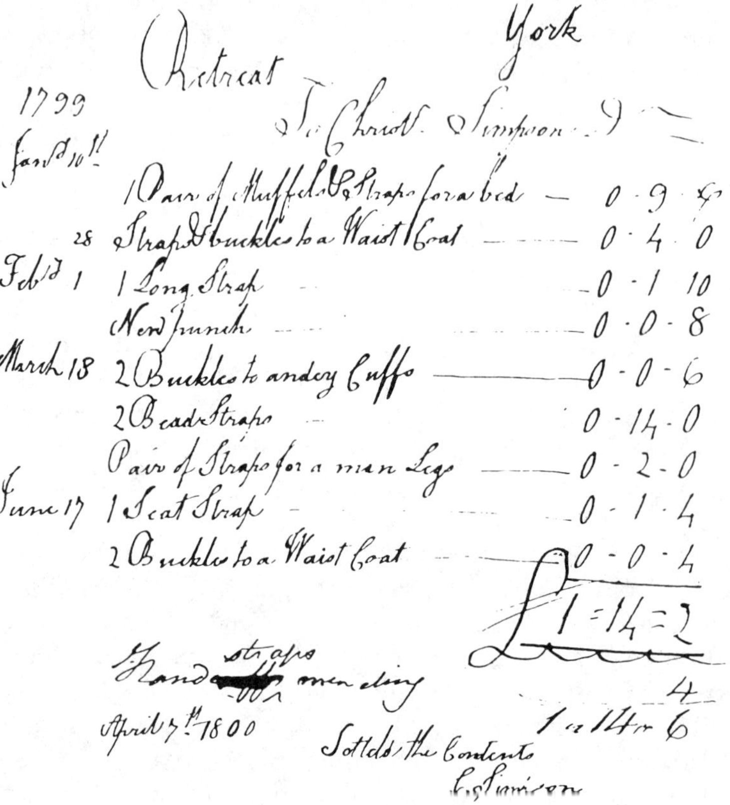
York
Retreat
1799 To Christ. Simpson Dr
Jan.y 10th 1 Pair of Muffels & Straps for a bed — 0 · 9 · 6
28 Straps & buckles to a Waist Coat — 0 · 4 · 0
Feb.y 1 1 Long Strap — 0 · 1 · 10
New punch — 0 · 0 · 8
March 18 2 Buckles to andery Cuffs — 0 · 0 · 6
2 Bead Straps — 0 · 14 · 0
Pair of Straps for a man Legs — 0 · 2 · 0
June 17 1 Seat Strap — 0 · 1 · 4
2 Buckles to a Waist Coat — 0 · 0 · 4
£1 = 14 = 2
Hand straps mending — 4
1 = 14 = 6
April 7th 1800 Settled the Contents
C. Simpson

Plate 12. Early bill showing purchase of means of mechanical restraint

an attempt to strangle herself, and has been kept in a chair and manacled'. Another patient, this time a maniac, 'has a strange disposition to be mischievous and is therefore obliged to be tied to her chair'.[73] These incidents dated from the 1820s (when Jepson had been succeeded by Allis) and are interesting in showing a continuing use of mechanical restraint for excited or violent patients.

The most violent patients were secured firmly in bed lest self-injury or the destruction of bedding and furniture resulted.[74] Special beds were constructed for the seclusion rooms as we can see from a bill for 1799: 'Making a strong bedstead, box^{t} [sic] round with one board in breadth at the top edge including all, £1-14$_{s}$-6$_{d}$'.[75] These beds were like chests in being a foot deep and were sometimes lined with straw or flock. The patient was 'restrained in bed by a kind of enchantment' because restraining straps attached to the bedstead were invisible to him as they were fastened to the back of his strait-waistcoat.[76] By 1815 the use of the jacket had been superseded as the regular Quaker Visitors noted. 'Four of them were under restraint in bed – only one had both the straps and jacket on – a new kind of buckle having been introduced which renders the waistcoat unnecessary.'[77] This spring buckle attracted much attention from other asylums in Britain and the United States, where it was imitated by more 'progressive' establishments.[78] For less violent patients, who needed some restraint at night in their own rooms, a complex linen and leather web of straps was employed that kept the patient in bed but allowed freedom of horizontal movement.[79] By mid-century this had been superseded by the simpler expedient of tying down the quilt tightly to the four corners of the bed.

How prevalent was mechanical restraint and did the frequency of its use vary over time? For the earliest years of the institution there is insufficient evidence to estimate its incidence. In 1813 no more than four out of sixty-four patients, or about 6 per cent, had been subjected either to mechanical restraint or to seclusion. Official Quaker Visitors found two, three or four patients restrained at any one time in the 1820s and 1830s, or between 3 and 7 percent of the inmates. This correlated well with the figure of 5 per cent, which Tuke estimated had been the case on Jepson's retirement in 1823. It is unlikely that any great degree of precision can be obtained since the definition of restraint was a fluid one. For example, a higher figure of 11 per cent was given for 1828 but this referred to 'any degree of personal restraint except those of the bounds allotted to them for exercise', and presumably may also have embraced not only cases of mechanical restraint but also of seclusion.[80]

Seclusion was itself an ambiguous term since it referred either to a formal period in a seclusion room or to a quiet time in a patient's own room. In either case it might be combined with mechanical restraint by straps or waistcoat but was not necessarily associated with it. Keeping a patient in a quiet, gloomy room minimised the disturbances to the senses from sight and sound[81] and hence, according to the sensationism of Locke's psychology, should subdue the excitement of patients. Informal seclusion for a short time in a patient's bedroom seems to have been used with discrimination but more frequently than formal seclusion in the refractory rooms. For example, no more than two patients were to be found in the latter at any one time between 1828 and 1834.[82]

The influence of the non-restraint movement was to decrease the official figures of seclusion employed at the Retreat as well as that of mechanical restraint. During the late 1830s and early 1840s Lincoln and Hanwell had apparently shown that asylums could be run without recourse to mechanical restraint.[83] Their success caused even the Retreat to review its minimal use of restraint:

> The Retreat, although its first principles of treatment at once abolished all cruel forms of restraint, and although it has undoubtedly been beneficially influenced by the experiment of entire non-restraint made at Hanwell and elsewhere, has not considered it wise to pledge itself to the non-restraint practice as a principle, conceiving that there may still be exceptional cases in which mild restraint is the best and kindest, as well as the most scientific mode of dealing with them.[84]

Those at York felt that the torment or degradation of the patient was not precluded by the abolition of such restraint, and that in some cases it might even be the kindest mode of treatment.[85] They preferred to determine pragmatically the individual needs of each case rather than abrogating their judgement under the force of absolute principle. Nevertheless, it was noticeable that the frequency with which mechanical restraint was used declined dramatically: from 1843 to 1852 there were only sixteen such cases (and these included cases of restraint after surgery), and thereafter it became even rarer.[86] It had become, as was stated in 1846, 'a serious deviation from the general practice of management at the Retreat'.[87]

The decline of mechanical restraint taken by itself does not necessarily mean that the custodial element in an asylum has been reduced since it may have been replaced by comparable practices. Chapter 6 will discuss the use of chemical restraint, which will add a further dimension to this analysis.[88] Here we are concerned with the use of seclusion in the second half of the nineteenth century. When systematic records of cases of seclusion began to be kept at the end of 1845 about 13 per cent of patients were involved. By 1850 this had been halved. The decline in the recorded incidence of seclusion was dramatic: from 787 cases during 1846, to 339 in 1850, 102 in 1855, only 16 in 1860 and negligible numbers thereafter.[89] The trend was clear even if these numbers were imprecise, having been obtained through aggregating weekly cases of patients secluded for different periods of time. Such figures tended to conceal as much as they revealed, as was shown when Dr Pierce explained to the Lunacy Commissioners in 1893 that the nine cases of seclusion recorded actually meant that seclusion had been resorted to for nine patients on fifty-four occasions totalling 335 hours in all.[90] Certainly the official medical journals and the annual *Reports* indicated that seclusion was resorted to only in cases of excitement during mania or epilepsy. Dr Kitching stated confidently that its use in other cases was very brief. Interestingly, he commented that the patients must understand its use, otherwise they would regard it as punitive.[91] Was seclusion so employed?

In some instances seclusion does seem to have been used as punishment. One of the very few cases minuted in the medical journal for 1865 was for 'extreme insubordination'. Earlier, Dr D. H. Tuke referred to the 'discipline of seclusion' having affected a behavioural change in a case where an excited patient used abusive language to his attendant. The patient himself stated defiantly that seclusion was no punishment to him (itself a revealing comment), and that 'My mind to me a kingdom is'.[92] A comparable instance of a patient who used bad language to her doctors indicated a sequence of repeated incidents and seclusion. 'Altho' complaining of the discipline she underwent yesterday – she is decidedly affected beneficially by it.'[93] It is evident that seclusion was part of a wider scheme of rewards and punishments: an essential ingredient in the system of classification and a useful technique in moral management:

1 January 1855. J. B. has been inclined to defy all authority – and refuse compliance with the ordinary routine of the house. He has consequently been placed in seclusion, which in conjunction with kind but decided expostulation from the Superintendent has been beneficial and has broken through the taciturnity which he had adopted.

5 March 1855. Has conducted himself agreeably and has been allowed to go to the large library and read there, a privilege he has not abused.[94]

Tuke considered that the 'principle of fear' had a 'salutary effect' when 'moderately and judiciously excited' in general society.[95] In this context what was the impact of external restraint upon the patients within the smaller society of the Retreat? There is evidence that some patients welcomed the use of seclusion as in this comment of 1850: 'Has many times lately desired to go into the seclusion room, where he walks about for several hours, and sometimes is unwilling to come out to his meals.'[96] In contrast, mechanical restraint was generally disliked and resisted by patients. This dislike was a useful element in the technique of moral management since it meant that the psychological impact of restraint, and its coercive effect on patients, was much greater than its actual deployment. Thus, psychological resonance was a crucial hidden dimension in the principle of fear. And the visual impact of mechanical restraint must have been such as to suggest to inmates that a punitive mechanism existed in the institution. In 1828 the case-books referred to a woman patient being manacled to her chair; in 1836 the official Quaker Visitors commented that an inmate was wearing iron handcuffs; and in 1835 a keeper described how his patient managed to escape in spite of a waist strap and ankle chains.[97] These disparate incidents are also quoted here because the language utilised appeared to be that of a penal institution.

The impact of the non-restraint movement was sufficiently great to make the Retreat much more circumspect in its language and practices by the 1840s and in later decades. The desire to be seen as a progressive institution meant that statistics were massaged to give a favourable impression, as in recording numbers of patients under restraint, rather than the actual incidence of its use over time. The Lunacy Commissioners who periodically visited the Retreat also criticised the asylum on more than one occasion for omitting to record instances of restraint.[98] An alternative strategem was to utilise practices that, although constraining a patient, did not formally qualify as restraint, as in the increased use by the Retreat of strong dresses and suits rather than camisoles or strait-waistcoats. And it is a reasonable supposition that cases of seclusion were usually recorded when they involved a formal removal to a seclusion or padded room, and thus that the much more widespread practice of confining patients to their own bedrooms for short periods was not always acknowledged publicly.

MORAL MANAGEMENT AND MORAL TREATMENT

The patients are considered capable of rational and honourable inducement; and though we allowed *fear* a considerable place in the production of that restraint, which the patient generally exerts on his entrance into a new situation; yet the *desire for esteem* is considered, at the Retreat, as operating, in general, still more powerfully.[99] [S. Tuke, *The Description of the Retreat*]

Since traditionally fear had been a more potent means of subduing the mad the Retreat's greater reliance on the desire for esteem appeared to contemporaries to constitute a mild form of therapy. For nineteenth-century reformers and twentieth-century administrative historians this establishment's minimal use of external restraint seemed automatically to confer a badge of enlightened practice. More recently an anti-institutional critique has questioned this progressive interpretation and drawn attention to repressive elements inherent in social relationships established in an asylum. Evidence that has been reviewed in this and the preceding chapter suggests that the Retreat was in this context Janus-faced: its treatment was both repressive and rehabilitative.

While acknowledging the danger of an overgeneralised and monolithic interpretation of the asylum that pays insufficient regard both to individual reactions and to changes in the character of the institution within our period, it seems useful to reach some conclusions on the ambivalent character of moral management at York. The balance between internal and external restraint to which Tuke alluded was a changing element in the Retreat's therapy in the period under consideration. In its first half-century its mode of external coercion was openly practised through mechanical restraint and its attempt to develop self-control in its patients was performed in a kindly manner utilising social patterns of behaviour familiar to its Quaker patients. Less obviously the ethos of these early years did include a disciplinary and moralistic element but this was not so much a systematic imposition of institutional rules as an expression of shared Quaker values. In mid-century the asylum experienced a subtle transformation as a result of a number of interrelated factors: its growing size, a change in therapists, increasing numbers of non-Quaker patients and most importantly, the need to replace the overt coercion of mechanical restraint with more pervasive but concealed techniques of social management. A more organised use was now made of methods that had been used previously in a less developed or centralised manner. Classification, seclusion and privileges became part of a cohesive moral management in which rewards and punishments were used systematically to influence patient behaviour.

In the 1870s one patient was sufficiently articulate to protest against what she saw as the control of patients to the superintendent, Dr Baker:

> I told him one day that I believed what he meant by 'better' was a nearer approach to that subdued and helpless condition below the power of complaint, which I saw in many of those around me.[100]

But not every patient was so aware of the psychological control that had replaced physical coercion. Twenty years earlier another patient had written home to contrast the Retreat's mild therapy unfavourably with that of other establishments where he had been treated:

> So far from disliking this place, the only fault I find with it is that the treatment is too mild. I have been accustomed to severity . . . It did me all the good in the world . . . [This] seems [like] a man dallying with disease instead of attacking it.[101]

These comments suggest the diverse nature of patients' responses to the Retreat's moral management. Therapists also saw patients in varied ways. The patient was seen as a minor although the balance between freedom and control in his treatment varied according to the stage of his illness. For the very sick there was indulgent nursing as for an infant; for those on the road to recovery there was a kindly but regulated framework suitable for a schoolchild; and for the convalescent there was imposition of a moral discipline such that the patient accepted responsibilities appropriate to one emerging from childhood into adult life. This systematic regulation of patients' lives had been implicit in the Retreat's moral treatment from the earliest years. Its underlying philosophy was revealed starkly in a private letter written by Samuel Tuke in 1814. He considered that it was essential to erect in any asylum 'as complete a system of espionage as possible' under the authority of an officer who was 'a sort of head spy'.[102] And not only was there this close supervision but each aspect of life at the Retreat had a function within an overall pattern. Delarive noted perceptively, shortly after the Retreat had opened, that the comfortable living arrangements there had a hidden psychological dimension: 'This neatness has attached to it ideas of order, decency, happiness, and respect both for oneself and for others.'[103] Informing these and other aspects of therapy were the attitudes of the Society of Friends. Inherent within them was a fundamental tension between the desirability of humanity towards the weak and the importance of encouraging moral self-discipline in the hope that the weak would become strong. Thus, the ambiguity at the heart of the Retreat's moral management stemmed from the restrictive contemporary code of Quaker conduct.

5

A Quaker institution

As the disorder is a mental one, and people of regular conduct, and even religiously disposed minds, are not exempt therefrom, their confinement amongst persons in all respects strangers, and their promiscuous exposure to such company as is mostly found in public institutions of this kind, must be peculiarly disgusting; and consequently augment the disorder.[1]

This desire on the part of the Retreat's founders to separate Friends suffering from mental illness from the social contamination of patients with different backgrounds and beliefs was part of a more general trend in which eighteenth-century Quakers had become isolated from a wider society.[2] Prominent among the causes of this social isolation were the disownment or expulsion by the Society of Friends of members who married outside its ranks and the 'seclusive influence'[3] of numerous prohibitions enshrined in a strict code of discipline that governed the moral education of the young and the everyday behaviour of the adult. 'Peculiar' forms of archaic dress and language retained by Quakers were both a witness to this social separatism and a contributor to it.[4] In a popular handbook J. J. Gurney explained the value of this separation:

Our plain language, manners, and dress, may be regarded as forming an external bulwark, by which Friends, considered as a religious community, are separated from the world, and, in some degree, defended from its influence.[5]

And in his view this plainness should be seen as the *'little fruits of great Christian principles'* and hence given great importance by Quakers.[6] The upright Friend would therefore see

The importance of an entire abstinence from those customs, prevalent in the world, which are necessarily impregnated with moral evil, for example from, profuse and extravagant entertainments – from unnecessary frequenting of taverns and public houses – from excess – in eating and drinking – from public diversions – from the reading of useless, frivolous, and pernicious, books – from gaming of every description, and from vain and injurious sports – from unnecessary display in . . . style of living . . . and, generally from all such occupations of time and mind as plainly tend to levity, vanity, and forgetfulness of our God and Saviour.[7]

Henry Tuke, the most theologically inclined member of the Tuke family, commented perceptively on Quaker discipline that it included the duty of 'private advice, for the reformation of those who walk disorderly'.[8] This responsibility might be exercised on behalf of the Society collectively lest its good name be impugned: traders who went bankrupt, or merchants who armed their ships in time of war, could be disowned because they had departed from the standards of honest dealing or betrayed the pacifist principle. An even more powerful reason for the exercise of Quaker discipline was the rehabilitation of the individual. Thomas Clarkson – the great slave abolitionist who was a sympathetic observer of Quakerism – argued against the view that it was 'a system of espionage, by which one member is made a spy' upon another. Instead, he suggested that it was a 'Christian duty' that was intended 'not to persecute but to reclaim'.[9] However, seriously delinquent members were disowned from the Society. This practice was justified by St Paul's words to the Thessalonians, 'We command ye brethren, in the name of our Lord Jesus Christ, that ye withdraw yourselves from every brother that walks disorderly.' Alternatively, the individual whose deviant behaviour was thought to be the result of illness might be termed insane and be sent to the Retreat.

Ambiguity characterised the way in which moral failure was related to insanity at the Retreat, since its therapists were ambivalent on the question as to how far each overlapped the other, as we can see, for example, in the following three cases. Dr Thurnam commented about a maniac, Quaker schoolmaster James M., that

his conversation was further distinguished by what would appear to have been *involuntarily* erroneous and exaggerated statements. These were evidently the result or manifestation of an excited imagination, and did not proceed from moral turpitude, as after narrating a story in this false or exaggerated manner, he would break off saying 'and yet it was not exactly so, but so and so' – and would then repeat it in terms more nearly, if not altogether coincident with truth.[10]

This passage reveals a paradox in that the patient was acquitted from a charge of 'moral turpitude' first by the 'involuntary' nature of his illness and then by his own 'voluntary' perception that he had not been entirely honest. Thurnam's successor, Dr Kitching, addressed himself to the same issue over the sexual behaviour of one of his patients, Eleanor K., a non-Quaker whose family had intimate connections with the Society of Friends:

Last evening she made a communication to the effect that she had for many years been in the practice of self-pollution. This has been intimated by her before, but was classed among her self-incriminating delusions. Some circumstances observed by the nurse, however, strongly confirm the suspicion of the truth of her statement. The above description, now applicable to a person who has been regarded by a large circle of friends as a woman of great refinement and superior moral attributes but who is now addicted to falsehood and masturbation, suggests the painful enquiry how far her present moral degradation may have subsisted and been successfully concealed for a long period, or how far it may be the pure result of insanity.[11]

Significantly, the patient appeared to have suffered 'moral degradation' whether she was considered sane or insane, so that the doctor had taken as an assumption, what might have appeared a problematic area for his 'painful enquiry' to solve. And despite an increasing emphasis on the organic nature of insanity as brain disease, and a growing reliance on chemotherapy to treat it, Retreat doctors seemed even more prone than alienists elsewhere[12] to indulge in moral judgements on patients. For example, in 1877 a Quaker patient, Elizabeth N., 'had some paroxysms of excitement but it seems rather from a moral baseness than . . . insanity'.[13] These extracts from case-books suggest that the behaviour of the insane was still often judged by the moral standards of the sane.

This was particularly evident in the censorious way in which the sexual behaviour of patients was regarded. In some respects this was merely a reflection of more general attitudes since nineteenth-century doctors saw 'self-abuse', 'self-pollution', 'vicious habits' or 'onanism' as a cause of mental illness. The methods used to combat it at the Retreat were also unexceptional:[14] moral exhortation, cold showers and sponging or, rarely, surgical intervention through circumcision or silver rings inserted through the penis.[15] Yet the repugnance with which masturbation was viewed at the Retreat seems to have been unusually strong as was shown by the inhibited references in early admissions registers that were written in Greek. Retreat patients might suffer anguished guilt when contemplating their deviant behaviour. William R., a Quaker, disclosed to his doctor there that 'The cause of my insanity is onanism . . . I have striven and prayed again and again to conquer it but in vain'.[16] Another Quaker patient had become melancholic because of his secret practices. 'For 14 years he had been in the habit of self-pollution, for which he is now exceedingly penitent, and remorse for this vice has preyed upon his spirits.'[17]

'If reason and conscience do not rule the body . . . there will soon be an end to health and respectability', counselled an influential book on Quaker discipline. 'Should the drunkard see before him a glass of ardent spirits, and be assured that the salvation of his soul depended on his abstaining from the draught, the liquor, nevertheless would, in all probability, be swallowed in a moment.'[18] Alcoholism was at first seen not as a form of mental illness at the Retreat but as a borderline area, rather a matter of moral failure than physical disease. The case-notes on a Quaker patient, Mary S., in 1817 indicated the kind of thinking behind admitting an alcoholic:

[She] has for several years, been in the habit of taking strong drink and to great excess, and so extravagantly attached was she to this injurious indulgence that all endeavours to restrain her proved ineffectual. As a last expedient therefore her husband and friends got her admitted to this institution. Though a doubtful case it was perhaps one of monomania of drunkenness.[19]

By the 1820s this kind of ambiguous case was admitted as a voluntary boarder, not as a patient, as happened with a female Friend, Phoebe B., in 1829. She had become addicted to both opium and gin, and her friends felt that she needed the moral discipline of the Retreat to break her of her habits. The directors of the Retreat, however, clearly did not see her as suitable for certification as an insane patient. A way through was found in Phoebe's signing a statement undertaking 'to submit to such restrictions as you may think most calculated to benefit me . . . and I also engage to remain in the Retreat as long as you may be inclined to keep me and it shall appear in your judgement right for me to stop'.[20] The directors became increasingly reluctant to take such cases and by 1835 were refusing to do so. However, an interesting letter in 1832 requesting the Retreat to take an alcoholic as a boarder indicated the kind of reputation as a moral reformatory that the asylum had gained by this time. A Huddersfield man wrote that his brother

> having accustomed himself to the use of spiritous liquors to such an extent, that there seems no hope of reclaiming him but by absolute restraint, his friends are very desirous that he may be got into the Retreat for a while, in the expectation that by regular habits and absence from temptation he may be restored.[21]

It is significant that the institution's own Committee of Management continued to believe that it should be 'used as a retreat' for 'ambiguous cases of insanity connected with extreme moral weakness or apparent depravity of conduct'.[22]

Given that Quakers had an unusual 'completeness of view respecting good and evil' it was predictable that the Retreat should be seen in part as a moral instrument to reclaim those members who had failed conspicuously to live up to the comprehensively high standards of the Society of Friends. The force of Quaker principle was felt by all patients at the Retreat, and a non-Quaker inmate, Joseph P., complained in 1882 that 'the Quakers are too strong in their own belief'.[23] Comments in patients' case histories reflected Quaker orthodoxy on the undesirability of wasting time either on one's appearance or on frivolous reading. A revealing comment made in 1809 about a female maniac hinted at the relationship between straying from the narrow path of moral probity and losing one's mind in insanity. Mary R. had been 'much addicted to novel and romance reading, and . . . appears to have cultivated her imagination too much and her judgement too little'.[24] Some seventy years later another Quaker patient, William E., was the subject of medical comment that implicitly linked moral failing to a lack of progress towards recovery since he 'reads a good many novels but does no useful work'.[25] A comparison of two cases in which Quaker patients displayed an unhealthy interest in their clothes tentatively suggests that aberration from Quaker discipline in this respect had shifted from being an indication that an individual was not himself but was suffering from mental disorder, to the view that this deviation constituted part of insanity itself. In 1807 the previously sober William S. suddenly began to evince 'gaiety in dress and behaviour',[26] but his illness was diagnosed as 'mania with melancholia'. In 1829 Caleb A. was seen as suffering from 'monomania of vanity'; he was 'fond of showy dress, and wears a most preposterous head of hair and a beard that would make a Turk jealous'.[27] Since diagnosis had a symptomatic basis it was all to easy to progress from moral censure of deviant behaviour to a belief that in extreme cases it constituted insanity. The clearest examples of this process occurred in those cases deemed to be morally insane.

Moral insanity was seen by alienists as an affective disorder that could coexist with unimpaired intellect. Dr Arnold discerned it in the late eighteenth century, but it was left to Pinel (with his *manie sans delire*), and Esquirol (with his *monomanie – instinctive*) to categorise the concept, and to James Cowles Prichard to develop it.[28] In this context it is interesting to note that Prichard was born into a Quaker family although he later renounced his membership.[29] In what was to become a much-quoted passage Prichard stated that moral insanity was

a form of mental derangement in which the intellectual faculties appear to have sustained little or no injury, while the disorder is manifested principally or alone, in the state of the feelings, temper or habits. In cases of this description the moral and active principles of the mind are strangely perverted and depraved; the power of self-government is lost or greatly impaired; and the individual is found to be incapable . . . of conducting himself with decency and propriety in the business of life.[30]

Prichard later acknowledged that it was 'often very difficult to pronounce, with certainty, as to the presence or absence of moral insanity',[31] but in the mid and late nineteenth century mad-doctors pronounced on the 'disease' with a surprising self-confidence. Among them were the Retreat's doctors, who took a particular interest in the subject – and none more so than John Kitching, the second medical superintendent.

In his book, *The Principles of Moral Insanity,* Kitching stated that the scepticism and vagueness in the public mind on this subject needed to be dispelled in order 'that all misconception should be removed as to what results from disease, and what from guilt'. As a believer in George Combe's work in phrenology he found no difficulty in believing that the intellectual and moral faculties could be unevenly developed, and that one could detect this in the bumps on the head. If the coronal part of the head was narrow and shallow one would conclude that the moral feelings would be weak. If moral faculties were undeveloped – either congenitally or through disease – then the individual was deprived of self-control and was 'morally an animal'. Thus, he argued that the morally insane who were involved in vice or crime must be distinguished from criminals who could control their actions.[32]

Although some of Kitching's contemporaries feared that this effectively put the mad-doctor in the role of God,[33] Kitching himself had no such self-doubts. In his contribution to the Retreat's *Report* of 1855 he saw his work as an advance in psychiatric medicine in which it was now possible to see certain types of behaviour as the product not of wickedness but of organic defect. He hoped that his Quaker readers might be able 'to recognise as mental disorder, what they may have been accustomed to consider, the evidence of perverse temper or irregularity of conduct'. Sending such individuals to the 'kind control' of the Retreat would be beneficial. In his *Report* two years earlier Kitching explained why this should be the case in that 'the orderly habits they are compelled to observe in the asylum' promoted recovery.

Twenty-two individuals with a confirmed diagnosis of 'moral insanity'[34] were treated at the Retreat. Of these, eighteen were Quakers or connected with the Society and four belonged to other religious affiliations. The cases spanned the entire nineteenth century, but fifteen of them were diagnosed in the period of 1838–55, when interest in this disease by Drs Thurnam, D. H. Tuke and Kitching was most pronounced. In addition, five earlier cases, admitted between 1806 and 1833, were rediagnosed as morally insane by John Thurnam, who wrote additional 'modern' interpretations of previous cases in the institution's registers and case-books. The last case at the Retreat to be labelled as 'moral insanity' on admission occurred in the 1880s. But by the early twentieth century moral insanity was seldom referred to in psychiatry, and alternative diagnostic descriptions such as moral imbecile, psychopathic personality or sociopathic personality were preferred.

Attention is confined here to the eighteen Quaker patients with moral insanity. Their case-notes were written in heavily moralistic terms. Diagnoses were facilitated by clear perceptions of how an upright member of the Society of Friends should behave and

Table 5.1. *Characteristics of Quaker moral insanity cases*

Specific criticism	Number of cases
Self-willed	8
Irritable	7
Idle	7
Unsuitable sexual behaviour[a]	4
Abusive	3
Deceitful	2
Violent	2
Dirty	2
Intemperate	2
Sullen	2

[a] Included are one case of masturbation, one of venereal disease, two of overfamiliarity with the opposite sex.
Source: BIHR J/1/1 and K/2 case-books.

therefore in which ways there had been a departure from the norm. Their main behavioural defects – as described in medical registers and case-books – are summarised in Table 5.1. In addition, singularity on the part of an individual in the form of eccentricity, a liking for practical jokes, a love of solitude or a propensity to wander about also attracted censure.

'Industrious, temperate, and regular in his conduct' were the standard terms of approbation used in the case-books to describe Quaker patients before the onset of mental illness in all its varieties. In contrast, four of the cases of moral insanity were described in general terms as having irregular habits. Irregularity stemmed from self-will and this was emphasised for nearly half of the group of these non-conforming individuals labelled as morally insane. They were 'obstinate', 'capricious', 'intractable', and 'wayward'. In two of the cases, their determination to pursue their own aberrant conduct, against the advice of Friends, had earlier led to disownment from the Society of Friends. Case 737 had made an unsuitable marriage with a servant girl outside the Society, and case 739 had been expelled for persistent drunkenness.[35] Case 675 also drank but not to the same point of delirium tremens. Instead, 'as he grew up he fell into idle habits, became somewhat intemperate, and addicted to low and improper female society . . . and is at present suffering from gonorrhoea'.[36] This young patient was kept at the Retreat for six months in spite of the fact that the doctors could find 'no signs of mental disorder'. They deferred his departure until a situation was found for him but admitted that they were prolonging his stay because it was 'highly important that restraint should be so long continued as to have a permanent effect in establishing other habits of mind, and in deterring from a recurrence of similar conduct'.[37] Here the Retreat was clearly being used as a moral agency rather than a hospital.

For other patients, too, moral discipline rather than medicine was the preferred treatment.[38] Case 716 was 'very self-willed and obstinate – indisposed to follow medical or other advice'. He was put on a plain diet and sponged vigorously with cold water every morning.[39] Case 651, whose case-notes are reproduced in the Appendix, suffered from a 'strange perversity of the moral feelings' and was placed under the 'watchful care of the nurse'.[40] This patient was in the Retreat on three separate occasions, totalling over eight years. On leaving, after her second spell, the superintendent overoptimistically congratulated himself on her recovery and attributed it to the 'orderly habits'[41] of the asylum, which had made her 'altogether better regulated in herself'.[42] But he warned her about her 'follies and imprudences' and suggested that if she persisted in such conduct she would suffer 'the entire loss of character as a virtuous woman'.[43]

Women were particularly prone to be consigned to the borderland of insanity in the Victorian period because of mildly deviant or independent behaviour.[44] The eight female Quaker cases of moral insanity provided further corroboration of this. Case 158 was consigned to the Retreat for nervous instability and for not being a paragon of domestic virtues. She was 'remarkably stingy and ill-natured . . . half-starved her children and hen-pecked her husband'.[45] Case 716 had an ill-regulated mind and manifested undefined eccentricities, and case 722 was flighty and passionate. Case 724 suffered from the same failing as the aforementioned case 651 and was overfamiliar with the opposite sex. She was abusive too, as were cases 748 and 776, who both also failed on the count of personal cleanliness.[46] It is noticeable that none of the male cases of moral insanity were defined by reference to such a strict behavioural code.

'Insanity is not something fixed and definite; it is relative to the requirements of society – the standard of sanity in the class the person belongs to.'[47] This open admission that madness could be a social construct was given in the *British Medical Journal* for 1885. It is interesting to set beside it Clarkson's earlier conclusion in his monumental portrait of Quakerism that 'Nothing is of more importance to an individual than a good character, during life'.[48] He discussed the way in which Quaker discipline was a restraint but one with a 'moral good' as its object because it aimed at 'the preservation of moral character'.[49] Kitching's encouragement to parents and teachers to send to the Retreat those with an 'unhealthy condition of the moral faculties'[50] drew on the same kind of justification. The Retreat was seen as a moral training-ground for those whose early educational discipline had been neglected, as was said to be the situation in cases 199, 675 and 676. This was hardly surprising for case 676 since he was deaf and dumb. Nor was it unexpected for case 675, who had a below-average intellect, or for the comparable cases of 651, 724 and 748.

By the late nineteenth century discussion on moral insanity in general psychiatric literature merged into a wider concern over the extent to which insanity was linked to heredity.[51] Doctors at the Retreat were particularly interested in this general question since it had been apparent from the early years of the institution that many of the Quaker patients were related to one another. Dr Thurnam discovered that of 415 Quaker patients admitted between 1796 and 1840, 142 had inherited a predisposition to insanity from their parents. If collateral blood relations were included the proportion rose from one-third to one-half of the Quaker patients.[52]

A hereditary predisposition to insanity appeared to answer the issue that surprised contemporaries, 'that seeing "Friends" as a body are so regular and temperate in their lives . . . there should be so large an amount of insanity'.[53] Friends themselves were preoccupied with the further question of whether their own marriage patterns had contributed to the incidence of insanity. Had 'generations of inbreeding'[54] – arising from the prohibition on marriage outside the Society – increased a hereditary predisposition to mental illness? Several families of patients sent to the Retreat shared this belief. For example, in the Bland family, three of whose younger children became patients, 'the older daughters always said the insanity in their family was owing to their parents being first cousins'.[55] Dr Kitching tended to agree that intermarriage had led to a 'degeneration of vital and cerebral power'. And he took the analysis a step further by suggesting that the rule on marriage had increased the proportion of Quakers who had remained single and related this to evidence that the incidence of mental illness among celibates in Victorian society was higher than among the married. At the Retreat at this time, four-fifths of the male and three-quarters of the female inmates were unmarried.[56] Contrasting viewpoints were put forward by his successors. Dr Baker concluded that the incidence of insanity was at a lower percentage of 8.8 compared to the 10.4 per cent in society generally.[57] And Dr Pierce suggested, with some justification, that the reason why nearly two and a half times more cases at the Retreat exhibited a history of insanity in the family compared to society as a whole was that the Retreat had much fuller case histories than was usual.[58] One explanation for this was that Quakers preferred to send their mentally ill relatives to the Retreat rather than to a range of institutions. This was because they believed that the moral and religious character of the hospital aided recovery.

The founders of the Retreat emphasised the necessity of a religious environment for the recovery of patients:

When returning reason indicates a restoration of the mental powers, it may greatly tend to advance and establish this desirable event, to be under the direction of persons who are . . . concerned . . . to cherish in them the strengthening and consolatory principles of religion and virtue, instead of dissipating these impressions, by such diversions as enfeeble the mind, and disqualify it for that solid reflection which leads to substantial peace and comfort.[59]

The Quaker character of the institution was presumably appreciated by the families who sent patients there although it was a fact taken so much for granted that it seldom attracted comment. One such observation was that of the father of a patient in 1845 that 'it is a source of much comfort to us that he is in the Society of Friends'[60] at the Retreat. Certainly the correspondence between families and those administering the Retreat was of an unusually friendly and intimate character giving ample evidence of shared assumptions and objectives in the care of mentally ill relatives. As we have seen the requests in these letters to give remembrances to other Friends in their mutual acquaintance strikingly indicated the way in which the Quaker community itself was like an extended family. In a very real sense the Retreat was a microcosm of this larger community in its reflection of religious values and aspirations.

At the Retreat religion was all-pervasive and not confined merely to particular times or functions. It was therefore essential to choose as staff those who did not so much practise their religion as live it. One 'who knows experimentally the religion of the heart' and who could therefore practice the 'divine art of healing' was how Samuel Tuke expressed this in discussing the qualities needed in an asylum director.[61] To facilitate this Friends were always chosen to fill the positions of superintendent and matron, and in the early years, particularly, there was a greater concern to appoint those of right character to these positions than those with medical skill or experience. As far as possible Friends were recruited to fill other posts and contact was made with nearby Meetings to see if suitable members could be persuaded to take up employment at the Retreat.[62] In spite of this policy it proved difficult to recruit Friends to more than a minority of the vacancies arising among attendants and servants.[63] That this situation worried the directors is suggested by their comment in 1827 that the number of Quaker attendants was greater than for some years past.[64] When recourse was had in appointments to those who were not Friends there was concern to recruit upright individuals. 'Excellence of character was the test',[65] as William Waller remembered from his interview in 1843. A Wesleyan, not a Quaker, he was an attendant until 1856 and his journal eloquently testified that he saw his work as a religious vocation. Verses – more notable for sentiment than poetry – that he wrote about his patients referred to the human sympathy that drew him to them and the divine love that redeemed their lives together:

> Heaven bless all who enter here
> Shine on their darkness dispell their fear
> Let light and mercy from above
> Proclaim the brotherhood of love[66]

It is clear that Waller was an intensely religious man and it is not suggested here that other attendants necessarily saw their work at the Retreat in the form of a religious vocation as he did. But that Retreat attendants were at least sympathetic to the moral and religious ethos of the institution is suggested by their unusually long average duration of service.

Those who administered the Retreat believed that among those suffering from mental illness were those who 'were not deprived of right religious sentiments'.[67] One case that justified such a belief was Sarah G., whose conversation 'shows that religious affections are not or do not *appear to be* uncultivated, and her ideas of what is called "consistency as a Friend" are decidedly high'.[68] Convalescent patients found that reading the Bible was a constant solace: many carried it around in their pockets and referred to it frequently. Informal conversations with visiting Friends were also valued. For example, a patient suffering from melancholy found talking to Samuel Tuke comforted him because Tuke reminded him that 'the grounds of mercy are independent of the sinner's conviction of them'.[69] In the earlier years of the Retreat three-quarters of the patients attended the scriptural readings held every Sunday afternoon. Later there were twice-weekly Meetings as well as daily Bible readings in the wards.[70] For a convalescent minority of about one in six of the patients there were also much-welcomed opportunities to attend York Meetings.[71] 'I was much struck with the force and beauty of his language', wrote John Bright about a Retreat patient who had addressed such a meeting.[72] Attendance was dependent on seemly behaviour and the privilege was withdrawn if the patient was not up to the demands of the occasion.[73] Although adults at the Meeting were impressed with the demeanour of these patients,[74] girls from the Mount School viewed them with a mixture of 'dismay and interest'. The girls were intrigued by one patient who invariably 'put on a turban made of a red pocket-handkerchief' and then took out a second handkerchief and proceeded to lay snuff across it.[75]

How unusual was the Retreat in emphasising religion in its patients' lives? An enquiry was conducted by Bethlem Hospital in 1817 on the 'expediency of appointing a chaplain', which elicited a number of replies from other asylums as to the provision of religious services. This revealed that many English mental institutions encouraged convalescent patients to attend divine service on Sundays, usually in the parish church but occasionally in a room or chapel within the establishment, and that some also issued Bibles to their patients. Most commented favourably on patients' reactions in terms of their conduct and the opportunity it offered

A Quaker institution

them to practise self-control. Interestingly, Dr Edward Long Fox stated that his Brislington House patients were 'tranquillized by the display of order and decorum'. The answers furnished by George Jepson and Dr W. Belcombe suggested that religion was more pervasive in the Retreat but that its effect on patients was perceived in similar terms to that of comparable establishments. Belcombe commented that its effects were 'favourable to convalescents', and George Jepson stressed its tendency 'to tranquillise their minds, promote orderly habits, and encourage virtuous principles'. Implicit in their testimony was the view that it facilitated recovery and reintegration of patients into a wider Quaker community.[76]

The Retreat was never an official concern of that wider community: the institution retained a formal independence from either control or judgement by the Quaker community. Nevertheless, the Retreat was dependent for its continued existence on substantial financial support from the Quaker community.[77] The annual *Report* for 1845 was not unusual in acknowledging that 'the institution cannot be supported upon its present plan without the continued aid of its friends, in the way of donations, annual subscriptions and legacies'. Deficits on the patients' accounts, with expenditure exceeding income from fees, were particularly common in the first quarter-century of the institution's existence. As we have seen, this was a result of the high price of provisions in the Napoleonic War period, and also to the dual set of overheads between 1811 and 1822 arising from the temporary experiment of running a half-way house, the Appendage, as well as the main institution. In later years substantial sums of money were also solicited from Friends for extensive building and modernisation programmes. These appeals for money were frequently associated in the annual *Reports* with a stress on the Quaker character of the Retreat. It is likely that this financial vulnerability would have acted in some degree to intensify its role as a buttress of moral values within the Society of Friends, since dissatisfaction with the character of the Retreat would have tended to cut off its financial life-support system. An interesting example of this happening was the stance of R. D. Alexander: 'I am not inclined to renew my sub[scription] at present to the Retreat not approving of so much money being spent on intoxicating liquor.'[78]

This kind of close scrutiny and involvement in the Retreat ebbed slowly during the second half of the nineteenth century. By 1889 the directors of the Retreat were sufficiently worried by lack of interest to consider adjourning the Yorkshire Quarterly Meeting to the Retreat, on the occasion of its Annual Meeting. They also decided to announce this in periodicals since 'it is important that Friends throughout the country should feel that the Retreat is one of the national institutions of the Society'.[79] Such a reminder would hardly have seemed necessary a half-century before. What had changed?

To a considerable extent the change lay in the Society of Friends, which in the third quarter of the nineteenth century had forged much closer links with other denominations. The sympathy between evangelicals in other churches, the optional nature of 'distinctive' speech and dress for Quakers after 1860 and the ending in 1859 of the prohibition on marriage with non-Quakers had all encouraged assimilation within a wider society.[80] By the 1880s half of the Friends who married chose non-Quaker partners. By this time too, a more liberal interpretation of Quaker discipline allowed members to attend the theatre, enjoy musical activities or read novels.[81] Taken together these factors reduced the attraction of Quarterly Meetings – formerly the focus of much social activity in a close network of families.[82] The 'small attendances'[83] that worried the Retreat's directors may also have stemmed from a perception among Friends that the field of mental illness had been professionalised: 'qualified' doctors had replaced lay therapists and medicine had been given primacy over moral treatment. The utility of well-motivated amateur interest and involvement at the Retreat may have seemed less obvious in the late nineteenth-century hospital than it had been in the early days of a 'retired habitation'.

The diminution of external interest in the Retreat as a Quaker institution was paralleled internally by an increasing proportion of patients who were non-Quakers (see Fig. 5.1). The decision in 1818 to admit affluent non-Quakers as a means of balancing the books had not been intended to 'invade the original design, of providing a place where Friends labouring under insanity, and particularly in a state of convalescence might associate with each other'.[84] The first non-Quaker patient entered in 1820 and in the next few decades when non-Quaker patients formed a small minority the ethos of the institution did not appear to have been altered significantly by their presence. But a portent for the future

A Quaker institution

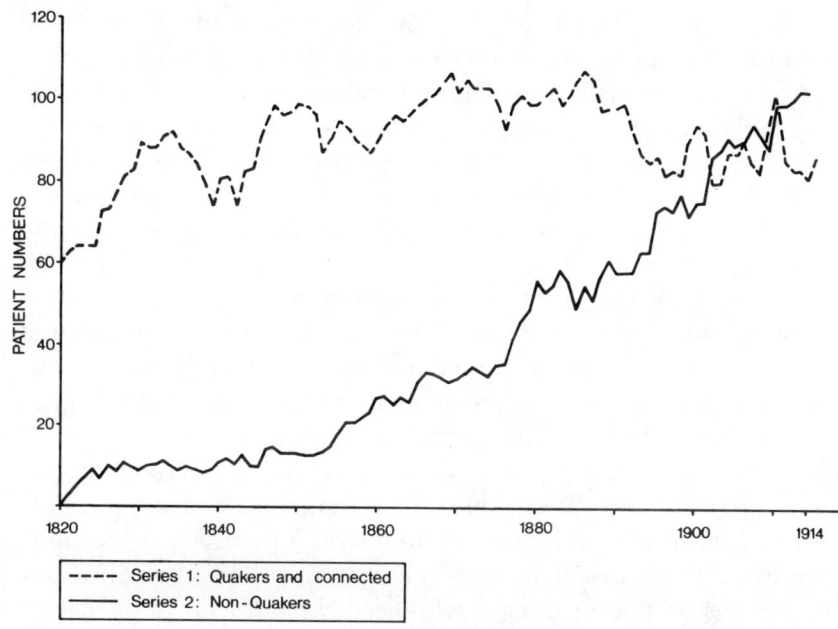

Figure 5.1. Quaker and non-Quaker populations within the Retreat, 1820–1914

was noticeable in that even during these early years the tone of the correspondence between the Retreat's officers and these patients' families was very different. Rather than the informal and friendly letters between equals, with shared assumptions and values, that were so marked a feature of the correspondence between Friends, this correspondence suggested an economic relationship based on the provision of satisfactory services. This growth in more detached relationships that can be associated directly with the increased number of non-Quaker patients was reinforced by other independent factors: the increase in institutional size and the transition from 'amateur' lay therapists to 'professional' medical personnel. The need to attract affluent patients from outside the Society of Friends may also have reinforced the pressures to provide luxurious features such as a billiard-room or Turkish bath and thus to speed the departure from a plain Quaker way of life. The influence of the growing number of non-Quaker patients was pervasive and difficult to isolate. However, it is clear that by 1902, the year when non-Quakers outnumbered Quaker patients for the first time (see Fig. 5.1), the ethos of the Retreat was much more like that of comparable institutions than it had been eighty years earlier when it was an institution run by Quakers for Quakers. And it is arguable that even by 1895 the Retreat was more of a Quaker institution in appearance than in reality since if the numbers of those patients 'connected' with the Society of Friends rather than 'in membership' are excluded, then non-Quakers already outnumbered Quakers.

It is remarkable that this transformation elicited neither comment in the published annual *Reports* of the Retreat nor minuted discussion by the administrative bodies that managed the asylum. But a related topic did surface in recurrent concern in the late nineteenth and early twentieth centuries over the increasing financial burden of subsidising poorer Quakers receiving treatment there. The growing cost of treatment – arising mainly from the improved staffing – led inexorably to the need to recruit more high-fee-paying patients if the principle was to be maintained of not turning away poorer Friends who needed treatment. In the event, it proved far easier to recruit these wealthy patients from non-Quaker families within the region than from the national network of Quakers. Paradoxically, it seems that it was in defence of the charitable impulse that had been central to its original principles that the Retreat lost an even more fundamental attribute – its overall Quaker character.

6

The ascendancy of medicine

The Retreat had been established as 'a retired Habitation' for those 'in a state of Lunacy' or 'Deranged in Mind', but a century later it was 'a Registered Hospital for the treatment of Mental Diseases'.[1] At its inception the Retreat was staffed by lay therapists, a half-century later it acquired its first medically qualified superintendent, and at the end of another half-century there was a well-defined hierarchy of medical superintendent, assistant medical officers and trained nurses. These changes involved a fundamental alteration not only in the Retreat's management but also in its rationale, ethos and patterns of treatment. This transformation produced changes that have been discussed previously – a transition from refuge to institution and a dilution of Quakerism – but its dominant feature was the medicalisation of the Retreat. The 'capture' of mental disorder by doctors, and the associated perception of derangement as disease, was not confined to the York establishment but rather was a general characteristic of the Victorian asylum.[2] However, the fame of the Retreat's lay therapy in the early nineteenth century, and its subsequent eclipse by other more innovative establishments in mid-century, gave a certain irony to this medical takeover.

FROM LAY THERAPIST TO MEDICAL PRACTITIONER

The success of the Retreat's lay therapy resided in the application of moral rather than medical treatment to the insane. It was George Jepson's genius to have discovered 'the almost infinite power of judicious kindness and sympathy on disordered minds' and to have applied this with 'real sympathy' and 'calm masculine [sic] reason'.[3] We have seen that it was the first superintendent's character, rather than his practical experience of healing, that constituted his main qualification for the post in 1796. 'What they sought, and what they found, was a wise good man, who would religiously exercise his faculties and affections for the welfare of his charges.'[4] Neither Jepson nor his successor, Thomas Allis, had any formal medical training. Allis in applying for the post in 1822 gave an honest account of his qualifications, which were personal rather than professional:

> Having no medical knowledge, whose nearest approximation to such knowledge is only a superficial acquaintance with chemistry as a science, possessing as he hopes just common rate abilities; with general knowledge, power of perception and habits of observation, attention and perseverance about on a par with the generality of persons occupying the middle rank in our society.[5]

Although the first superintendent had no formal medical qualifications, in practice he acted as the apothecary to the institution. Dr Fowler, the visiting physician, prescribed drugs for the patients that Jepson then made up.[6] In advertising for his replacement the Retreat wished to perpetuate this practice and in their advertisement stated:

> The person at present in that office acts as the Apothecary, and one qualified so to act, or at least to prepare the medicines under the direction of the Physician, would be preferred. The Superintendent also keeps the accounts of the institution, and has the general charge of the whole family.[7]

In his application Allis admitted lack of such experience but was optimistic to Samuel Tuke about his ability to soon master the simple essentials requisite:

> With respect to preparing the medicines I have had no experience of that kind yet from thy History of the Retreat I should gather that its *Materia Medica* was a very simple one, and should think that with attention knowledge of it, together with correctness and expertness in preparing the medicines might soon be attained.[8]

Since Tuke in the *Description of the Retreat* had written that the physician had 'perceived how much was to be done by moral, and how little by any known medical means', Allis was substantially correct in his thinking.[9]

The medical profession in the early nineteenth century was in a state of considerable fluidity in terms of status and qualification. The Retreat's practice of its apothecaries' learning on the job was unremarkable, as was the fact that its physicians also learned about mental illness by treating patients rather than from their prior medical training. Members of the Society of Friends who qualified as physicians in the late eighteenth and early nineteenth centuries were debarred from one method of qualifying since they could not in conscience take the religious tests that were part of the entry to Oxford and Cambridge. This was an advantage rather than a disadvantage since it forced them to study elsewhere (at first at Scottish universities or Leyden, and later at London) where medical training was more specialised and practical. And since such a procedure was expensive, those Friends who eventually qualified as physicians had often begun with humbler aspirations to train as surgeons. Such a man was the young Caleb Williams, appointed visiting surgeon to the Retreat in 1824. He was to hold the Chair of Materia Medica at the York Medical School where he trained distinguished pupils (including Sir Jonathan Hutchinson),[10] to give evidence on criminal insanity at notable trials[11] and eventually to qualify as a physician in 1855.[12] A similar – if more rapid – course was pursued by John Kitching. He served his surgical apprenticeship with Caleb Williams, before qualifying as a physician in London and returning in 1849 as Retreat medical superintendent – the successor to Dr Thurnam.[13]

It was John Thurnam's appointment as *resident* medical officer in 1838 that broke with the tradition of resident lay therapists and visiting doctors. At that time there were already two visiting medical men: Caleb Williams and Dr H. S. Belcombe. The latter had succeeded his father Dr W. Belcombe to the office of visiting physician in 1826. Dr H. S. Belcombe was, like Williams, a busy professional man. He was a physician at the York County Hospital, lectured on clinical medicine at the York Medical School, and was consulting physician to the Institute for Diseases of the Eye that had opened in York in 1831.[14] With a steady increase in the numbers of patients to around ninety by 1838, the Committee of Management found that the three or more medical visits each week were no longer adequate to meet the institution's needs. In an era when other asylums were appointing doctors as superintendents, and when insanity was increasingly viewed as an organic disease,[15] the role of the medical man was now seen as being much more central to an institution such as the Retreat. By 1838, according to one member of the Retreat's Committee of Management, it had

> after long deliberation determined that the interests of the institution required additional care being extended towards the patients and their attendants and that the records of the institution demanded more careful attention for the purposes of science and humanity than was then paid to them. For several years the Committee had been endeavouring to obtain what they considered important through the means which they possessed, but, being still dissatisfied with the results, they concluded to have a medical officer resident in the establishment.[16]

This private letter hinted at the dissatisfaction that was felt at the failure of the second superintendent, Thomas Allis, to 'grow with the job' and to develop new responsibilities to match the managers' enlarged concept of his duties. Allis had been a hosier and dairyman in the West Country and had applied for the post of superintendent in 1822 because of his financial difficulties during the severe rural depression of that time.[17] He confessed to having no 'natural predelection' for the work but felt that it would be possible 'to become as interested in the welfare of the institution and of the unhappy objects of his care as to become really fond of the employ'. Allis was fortunate both in having George Jepson advise and instruct him for several weeks on his duties,[18] and in working side by side with a very experienced matron – Hannah Ponsonby, who had been assistant to Catherine Jepson for several years.[19] In his role of master of the Retreat family Allis was efficient and kindly, though lacking Jepson's extraordinary skill in responding to the mentally ill. During his superintendency the Retreat grew in size from seventy patients in 1823 to ninety by 1841. Allis was responsible for the management of the household and the keeping of the accounts as well as the moral treatment of patients and their general welfare. On the medical side of their treatment he had Caleb Williams's assistance in surgery, Dr Belcombe's in prescribing medicines and that of Williams's pupil, John Kitching in dispensing drugs. Nevertheless, he was put under considerable strain by the growing extent of his responsibilities. It was this 'constant care and anxiety' that first made him take up natural history to 'relieve the mind'.[20] In this context it is not surprising that Allis failed to meet the Committee of Management's enlarged – and unrealistic – expectations.

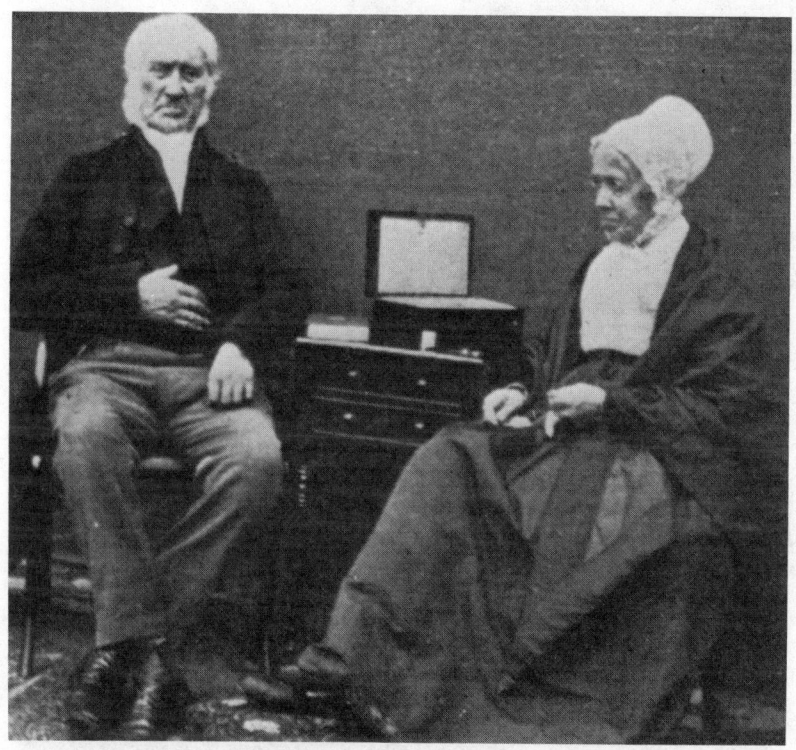

Plate 13. Thomas and Mary Allis

In appointing an ambitious young surgeon to the new post of resident medical officer, the Retreat's Committee may have anticipated some problems. Samuel Tuke, with the benefit of hindsight, wrote:

It is not perhaps very surprising that our old Superintendent, although his supervisory authority was not taken away, should feel himself a little disturbed. The Committee arranged the position of the parties as well as they could, but so it was (without venturing to say where the fault was to be placed) the plan did not work harmoniously.[21]

Thurnam came from a local Quaker family and his father had earlier served as a director to the institution. In these, and in professional qualifications, he was well suited to the post, having become a member of the Royal College of Surgeons in 1834 and served as a resident medical officer for the previous four years at

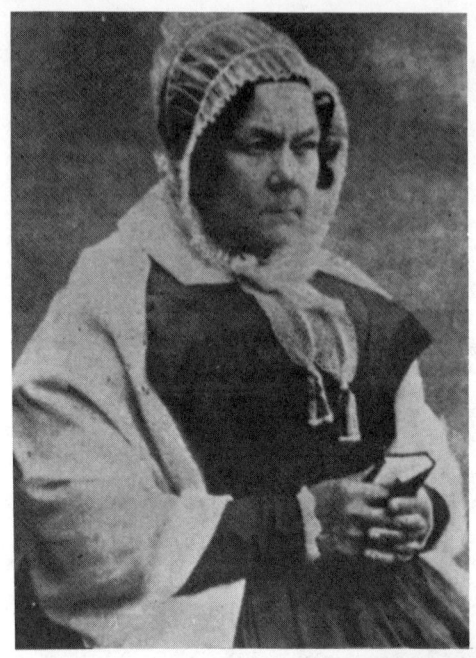

Plate 14. Hannah Ponsonby

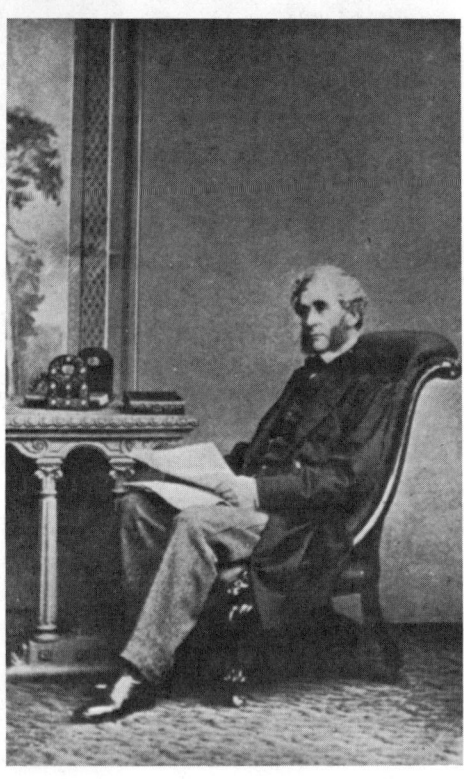

Plate 15. Dr Thurnam

Westminster Hospital.[22] His impact on the Retreat's medical treatment was immediately obvious as can be seen in the much more detailed and systematic case-records he made for each patient. Finding insufficient outlet for his energies in the day-to-day care of patients he undertook a detailed statistical analysis of most aspects of their treatment since the inception of the institution. This was published as *The Statistics of the Retreat 1796–1840* in 1841. The following year the Committee of Management sang his praises in the annual *Report* of the institution:

Experience has confirmed the Committee in its judgement as to the desirableness of having a resident Medical Officer, charged with the immediate care of the patients and their attendants, and unencumbered with the domestic and financial affairs of the establishment. They have obtained through the zeal and efficiency of their present Medical Officer, the objects they had chiefly in view in his appointment, viz: a more vigilant observation of the cases – a better record of the history and progress of the disease.

Yet this professional advance had been bought at some cost since Allis found the situation so intolerable that he had tendered his resignation and had left before the end of 1841.[23]

Allis moved a mile away to Osbaldwick, where he took on a well-established private madhouse, Hollytree House, licensed for the care of fifteen male patients. Some of his first patients had been at the Retreat[24] and Allis had acted somewhat unethically in recruiting them for his rival private establishment by soliciting their relatives to move them.[25] Not all could afford such a change,[26] but some felt that the patient might benefit. In this latter category was Robert C. His family sanctioned his removal to Osbaldwick since he was 'much attached to him [Allis], from the long period he had been under his care', and hence they 'determined to gratify RMC's wish to go with Mr. Allis'.[27] The care he was to receive at Hollytree House was good, if the comments of the Metropolitan Commissioners in Lunacy were at all accurate:

Excellent order. Clean and well ventilated. Comfortable in every respect. Good bodily health. No one under restraint. Church attended and scriptures read daily. Occupation and amusement provided.[28]

Although this comment suggested that the establishment was not formally Quaker there may have been strong echoes of the Retreat there – not only from Allis but from a later assistant, his son-in-law, William Pumphery, who had been an attendant at the Retreat.[29]

Whereas Allis was remembered as 'unpolished in appearance and manners, a hearty, vigorous man', Thurnam was seen as dapper and possessing the manner of a professional man.[30] From this description it is possible to visualise the conflict of personalities between the untutored older man and the trained young doctor. Two separate eras in the care of the mentally ill were personified in this juxtaposition. The triumph of the mad-doctor was finally realised in 1847 when Thurnam became the first medical superintendent of the Retreat. This was both a response to the Lunatics Act of 1845[31] (which demanded a medical qualification for such an office) and a formal recognition of the medical supremacy that Thurnam, as resident medical officer, had already achieved. The practical shift in power, which Thurnam had already brought about by the time of Allis's resignation, was considerable. Earlier, the superintendent was said to possess 'full authority in the house; and, in conjunction with the Medical Officers shall direct the management of the patients'.[32] But according to the advertisement for Allis's successor the superintendent's

> principal occupation will be the direction and superintendence of the general economy of the household and premises, and the keeping of the accounts of the institution. Although the immediate management of the patients and their attendants may not devolve upon the officer now to be appointed, he will, in the course of his duties, be frequently brought into contact with the patients, and will be expected to assist in their moral management by cultivating a friendly intercourse with them, and promoting their comfort and employment.[33]

The depreciation of authority and limitation of duties, from the therapeutic to the administrative, were very striking. And in choosing John and Maria Candler – retired missionaries who made it clear that they did not want a permanent situation – the Retreat Committee implicitly acknowledged their caretaker status.[34] Shortly after Thurnam had taken his M.D. at King's College, Aberdeen in 1846, the Candlers retired from the scene.

The most remarkable feature of this transition in authority from lay to medical men was the way in which moral treatment was assimilated into the area of medical expertise. This assumption of

The ascendancy of medicine

a medical monopoly over moral as well as medical treatment was a general feature of mid-nineteenth-century asylums. In 1853 the first editorial in the new *Asylum Journal,* the professional journal of asylum doctors, stated without equivocation that 'the moral system of treatment can only be properly carried out under the constant superintendence and by the continuous assistance of a physician'.[35] Scull has argued that the medical takeover of moral treatment was helped both by the generality of such early therapy that precluded the emergence of lay therapists as scientific experts and by the limited utility of medical treatment for insanity, which meant that moral management was a useful therapy for doctors to fall back on. Since they argued that moral treatment was useful solely in conjunction with medical treatment, it followed that only medical men had the necessary qualifications to manage the insane.[36] And as R. J. Cooter has suggested, doctors' interest in phrenology at this time appeared to elevate their own practice of moral therapy to that of a science. Phrenology apparently suggested that insanity could have an organic origin yet have psychological manifestations and thus need moral (i.e. psychological) treatment.[37] This study of 'lumps and bumps' on the head therefore seemed to validate the doctors' claims to expertise in moral management.

At the Retreat it was John Thurnam who began to apply phrenological assumptions to his study of patients. His early case-notes of patients, written in 1838, often contained full comments on their 'psychical state', and the physical condition and measurements of their heads. The first reference of this type was a description of case 419, whose 'forehead [is] narrow and upper part poorly developed, especially corresponding to the reflective "organs" '.[38] On 2 November 1838 Thurnam went on from measuring patients' heads to those of his medical colleagues as well as his own head. Dr Belcombe had a circumference of 21¾ inches, Caleb Williams, one of 23 inches, and Thurnam 22 inches, with 13½ inches over the vortex from ear to ear.[39] In April 1841 E. T. Craig, a lecturer on phrenology, observed some of the patients circumspectly. For example: 'this appears a well-balanced head in the moral region at least. In the absence of undue internal excitement this individual should prove amiable and tractable.'[40] No great insight into Retreat patients appears to have been derived from phrenology, either on this occasion or any other. However, Thurnam's interest in phrenology, and the help that this study seemed to give in understanding partial insanity, may go some way to explaining his enthusiasm for categorising patients as suffering from monomanias of various types. And his interest in phrenology may also have kindled his developing enthusiasm for archaeology, in which he showed particular skill in craniology. Much of this work was done in southern England, since in 1849 he was selected to become the first medical superintendent of the new Wiltshire County Asylum at Devizes.[41]

His successor as the Retreat's medical superintendent was John Kitching, who was no stranger to the establishment. A Yorkshire Friend, he had become assistant to Thomas Allis on leaving the Quaker boarding school of Ackworth in 1827. He had 'learned to dispense medicines, make pills etc., and was his pupil and assistant for 11 years', remembered Allis's daughter, Elizabeth. During this time Kitching also served a formal apprenticeship with Caleb Williams in order to qualify as a surgeon, before going to Westminster in 1838 for medical training. After graduating as a physician Kitching had run private houses for the care of the insane, along the principles established at the Retreat, at Painthorpe and Darnall Hall. Kitching was thus well qualified professionally to become the Retreat's first officer, and as an active, evangelical Friend he also embodied some of the earlier characteristics of its founders. For example, he conducted a weekly Bible reading in a poor neighbourhood of York, helped establish and manage a home for friendless local girls, and was an active supporter of the Hungate Mission, which operated in one of the most deprived areas of the city. Yet this work, which gave him close contact with members of other Christian denominations, stemmed from his own firm commitment as a Friend, and this was recognised when towards the end of his life he became a minister in the Society of Friends.[42]

Kitching had been educated in the earlier practices of the Retreat and a certain loyalty to them preserved their outward appearance, although his later professional training had given him a commitment to the medical model for an asylum. Thus, although moral therapy was continued it was in the context of Kitching's beliefs, "valuing . . . in the highest degree, the medical and physical treatment of insanity, under the conviction resulting both from theory and observation, that insanity is but the outward manifestation of a physical change in the central organs of perception and thought".[43]

Kitching's adherence to phrenology, with its localisation of mental faculties in the brain, would also have facilitated this organic view of insanity as brain disease.[44] Somaticism, with its accompanying depreciation of psychological approaches to mental disorder, was a characteristic tenet of Victorian psychiatrists by the 1870s.[45] Thus, in his claims to positivistic knowledge of insanity Kitching was typical of his generation of mad-doctors. During his time as superintendent from 1849 to 1874, patients' case-notes indicated the primacy that was given to medical diagnoses and treatment. Moral treatment was trivialised into a means of amusing or occupying patients, with no very defined therapeutic value except for melancholics. Yet its role as a tool in the moral management of patients was given increased importance. And in this concept of management Kitching was also a conformist: a new breed of superintendents was emerging whose elevated status and authoritarian attitudes gave them formidable powers within the enclosed world of the Victorian asylum.[46]

Dr Robert Baker, who succeeded the ailing Kitching in 1874, had a similar background in so far as he came from a Yorkshire Quaker family and had been educated at Ackworth. He differed crucially in not having spent his formative years at the Retreat and thus had no inhibiting loyalty to the 'old ways' when considering new ideas. Since he was relatively inexperienced both as doctor and alienist he was the more ready to listen to the views of the visiting Lunacy Commissioners on the need to update the Retreat.[47] In an age when earlier curative hopes of the asylum were seen to have been overoptimistic, contemporary interest was directed at a 'bricks and mortar humanity' that would create better alternatives to the asylum for particular groups of patients.[48] In tune with more progressive thinking at that time, Baker undertook a vigorous building programme and, by the time he left in 1892, he had instituted a hospital villa system at York. In 1875 the Gentleman's Lodge was rebuilt for thirty patients and in 1879 Belle Vue House was purchased for the use of nine ladies;[49] in the following year East Villa was built for three well-to-do patients and a Cottage Hospital provided for infectious cases, and finally in 1888 West Villa was built for twelve to fifteen acute cases (see Plates 19–21). Baker took a special pride in making this provision for the 'many patients who require isolation from home and home surroundings and special skilled treatment, but whom we dare not

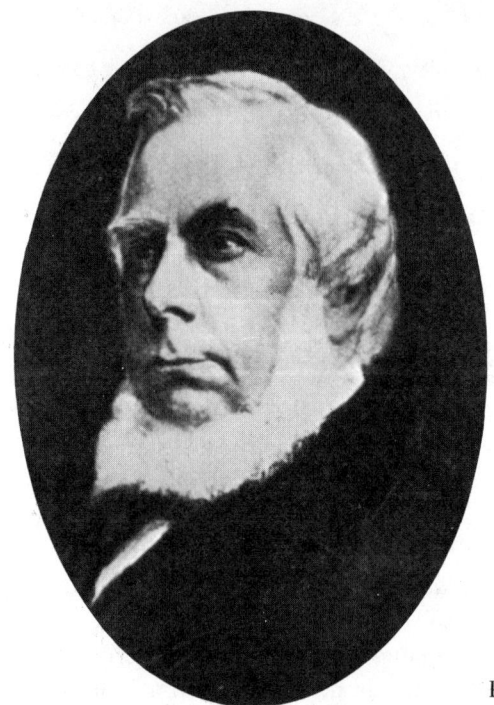

Plate 16. Dr Kitching

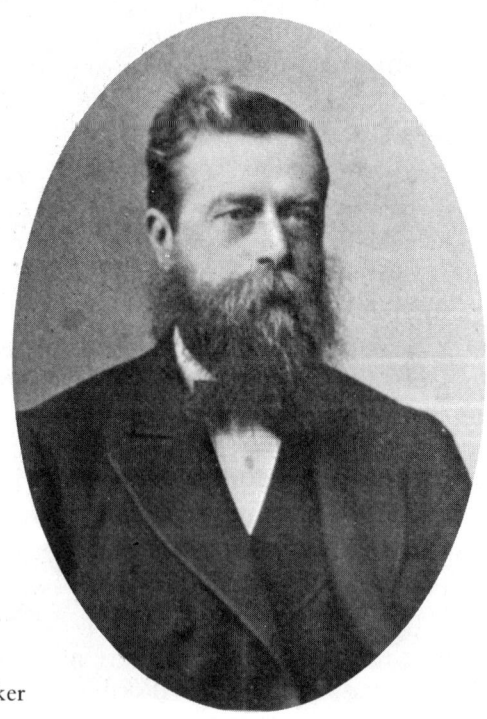

Plate 17. Dr Baker

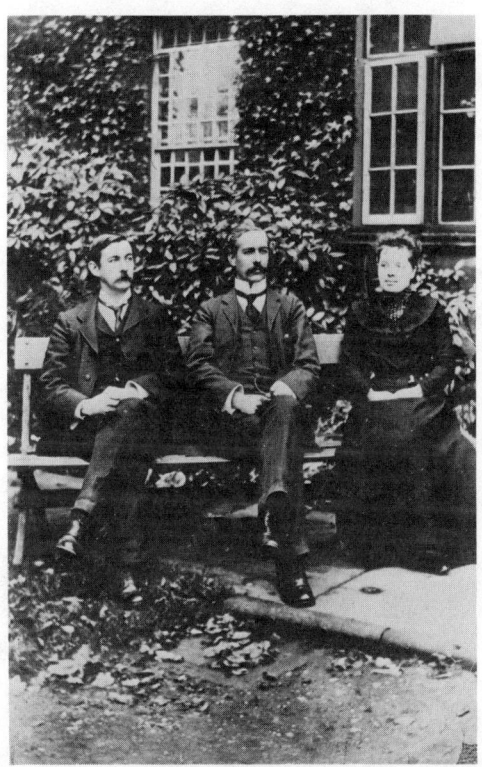

Plate 18. Drs Pierce, McKenzie (Assistant Medical Officer) and Kemp

take the responsibility of consigning to the wards of an asylum'.[50] This statement formed the key passage in Baker's lecture, delivered as president to the Medico-Psychological Association of Great Britain and Ireland at its meetings in 1892. The assembly was held at the Retreat and, as such, marked the acknowledgement of the institution's psychiatric achievement in its previous 100 years' existence.

'The founders of the Retreat had a great object of humanity before them: their knowledge of the actual capabilities of the insane . . . must have been imperfect.'[51] This informed conclusion by Samuel Tuke on the founding fathers of 1792 was also true of the inexperienced man chosen as superintendent in 1892. The Lunacy Commissioners disliked the appointment of Bedford Pierce, who 'had but very little practical experience in our asylums', and would have preferred the promotion of Dr Baker's 'excellent assistant', Dr Hind. However, the directors preferred Pierce because

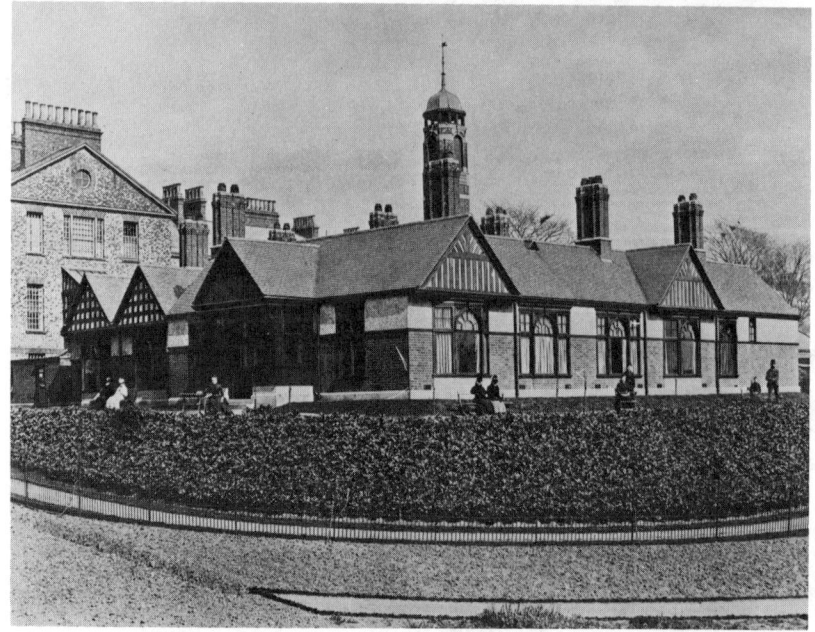

Plate 19. West Villa

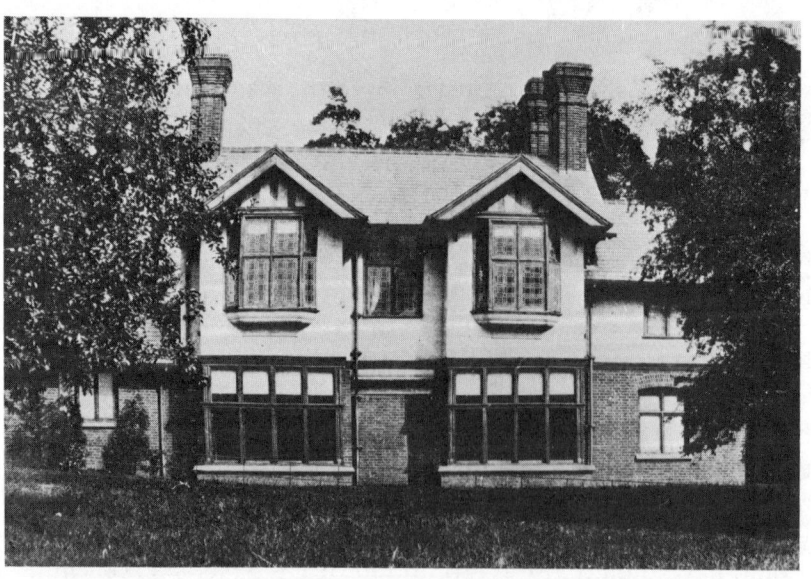

Plate 20. East Villa

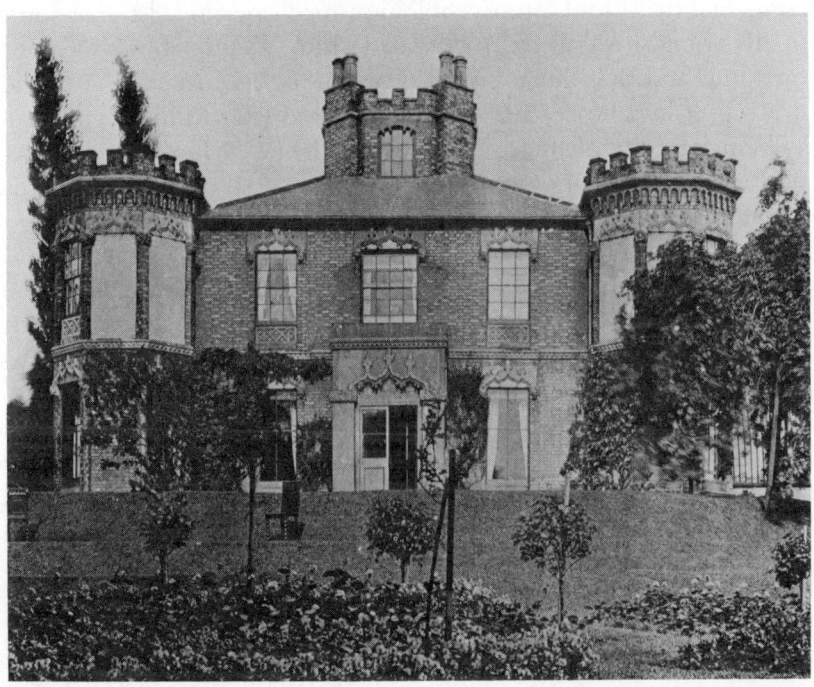

Plate 21. Belle Vue House

he was a Friend and his medical ability had impressed Dr D. H. Tuke.[52] Their choice was far-sighted since under his leadership the Retreat was again seen as a progressive institution: it was in the vanguard of the movement to transform the asylum attendant into the psychiatric nurse.[53]

Bedford Pierce's own career had lessons – the value of perseverance and hard work – that he felt his nurses could learn from. His father had died young and Bedford Pierce left school at fourteen. He served an eight-year apprenticeship with a homeopathic chemist before undertaking evening classes to obtain his London matriculation and winning scholarships that enabled him to train as a doctor at St Bartholomew's Hospital in London. At the time of his appointment to the Retreat he was a young man of thirty, working as a casualty physician at Bart's and without experience of psychological medicine. It was necessary for him to spend almost a year at Bethlem and Morningside in order to gain insight into the work of asylums.[54] He acknowledged that 'it was quite accidental that I took up psychological medicine' and also that some of his friends attempted to dissuade him, saying it was 'a poor opening' and that 'lunacy would be a hopeless career'. Pierce did not regret his choice, although he referred later to his occupation as being in 'one of the by-paths of medicine'.[55] However, he exploited to the full academic and career potential of his position: he developed an extensive private practice;[56] lectured on mental disease at the University of Leeds from 1908 to 1911; became president of the Medico-Psychological Association in 1919; and served as a commissioner on the Board of Control (which succeeded the Lunacy Commissioners in 1913). In this respect too, a Retreat superintendent reflected a more general trend in that it was noticeable during the late nineteenth century how mad-doctors extricated themselves from the routine concerns within the asylum to the more rewarding professional fields beyond its doors.[57] Yet it would be unfair to Pierce to suggest that his other interests detracted from his work at the Retreat where clarity of vision was equalled by his vigour in implementing objectives.

By 1914 the Retreat was seen by those who worked there as a hospital rather than an asylum. Dr Baker had stated, 'I strongly approve of the word hospital instead of asylum'[58] and had introduced the hospital villa system. Bedford Pierce had been 'struck with the difference between the nurses in General Hospitals and Asylums'[59] and had done his best to eliminate them. Yet in one important direction Bedford Pierce appeared to have put a brake on the medicalisation of the Retreat, since he recognised both the limitations of medication and the importance of laying 'due stress on the psychical as well as upon the physical'. And in his view that 'the attempt to separate mental and bodily factors must inevitably lead to error, since they constantly react on each other' he was implicitly acknowledging the truth of the Retreat's original philosophy of treating the insane as whole individuals.[60] That in his later years at the Retreat he was known as 'Father' also suggests that he had recreated in some sense that feeling of family that had marked the institution's earliest years.[61]

A comparison of that early establishment with the one eighty years later indicated, however, that there had been massive changes in its size and structure. In 1813 there had been only a superintendent, matron, matron's assistant and seven attendants. By 1896 there was a medical hierarchy headed by a superintendent and senior and junior assistant medical officers. On the male side of the house there was a head attendant, his deputy, three charge attendants, nineteen ordinary attendants and three night attendants. On the female side there was a nurse supervisor, two lady companions, two matrons for Belle Vue and Gainsborough House, six charge nurses, sixteen ordinary nurses, four night nurses and six nurses for Belle Vue and Gainsborough House.[62]

Before the end of our period there was also a strengthening of women's contributions to therapy at York. This was principally a reflection of wider social changes that were helping women to make a more vigorous contribution to public life, and only to a lesser extent a renewal of that egalitarian tradition in the Society of Friends, which earlier had given greater public responsibilities to Quaker women than was usual in British society. During the first half-century of the Retreat's existence it was noticeable that its matrons – Catherine Jepson and Hannah Ponsonby – were held in equal esteem, and regarded as the partners of the lay male superintendents, George Jepson and Thomas Allis. Indeed, a visitor to the Retreat in 1811 thought that Catherine Jepson was more influential than her husband:

> The mistress of the house is a good-looking, portly lady, lately married to the keeper, both Quakers. You cannot say of this couple with Molière, "Du coté de la barbe est toute la puissance", for all the consequence and the talents seem here on the side of the lady, and her husband appears merely her deputy.[63]

But with the gradual ascendancy of medical 'expertise' in the mid and late nineteenth century the untrained female — whether matron or superintendent's wife — was reduced to a subordinate role that lacked comparable status, power or influence. Female authority was not to be revived until women had themselves trained as doctors. This came with the appointment of Norah Kemp in 1898 as the Retreat's first female assistant medical officer – and indeed the first female doctor to serve in any asylum throughout Yorkshire.[64] 'An exceptionally able physician' according to Bedford Pierce, she attached great importance to the personal sensibilities of patients, recognising their need for 'congenial companionship' and 'sympathy and cheerfulness'. Her medical case-notes on female patients made an interesting contrast to some of the earlier observations made by her male colleagues with their harsh and unfeeling judgements on female hysteria and hypochondria. In perceiving that for staff 'your reward [is] in the trust your patients have in you', Dr Kemp was acknowledging one of the finest elements in the Retreat's tradition.[65]

MEDICAL TREATMENT

Traditionally the Retreat has been identified in the public mind with moral rather than medical treatment. This stemmed from Tuke's *Description* in which Dr Fowler, the first physician, reportedly reached the conclusion: 'that medicine, as yet possesses very inadequate means to relieve the most grievous of human diseases'.[66] Yet Dr Thurnam commented several decades later, after a review of the Retreat's early medical records, that it was 'not improbable that the notion of a greater neglect of pharmaceutic treatment at the Retreat than ever really existed, may have arisen from the protest which was made against all nostrums for insanity'. He also commented that later medical officers had concluded that 'more is to be effected by the judicious use of pharmaceutic means, than was thought practicable' in earlier years at the institution.[67] Although Thurnam's medical background may have caused him to emphasise what he would have regarded as scientific elements in treatment, the records of the institution confirm that medical treatment did have an important, if restricted, role even in the earliest years of the Retreat. Further, it appears that the growing ascendancy of doctors within the establishment reinforced the significance of medical methods and more especially the use of drugs.

Chemotherapy

In the early years of the Retreat Dr Fowler was said to have rejected most of the accepted pharmaceutical remedies for insanity after his own experimental trials indicated their ineffectiveness. Both he and his successors allegedly restricted medical treatment to bodily (rather than mental) disorder, and to enhancing general bodily health.[68] Thus, although it was recognised that sympathy existed between body and mind, and that medical treatments for the body might lead to improvements in the mental state of the patient, insanity does not seem to have been seen solely as an organic disease that could be relieved primarily by medical means. Dr Thurnam took a different view; since 'insanity is in truth a physical disease' he attached 'great importance to the use of physical means in the treatment of mental disorders'. He was hopeful that it would be possible eventually to 'detect those morbid conditions of the functions and of the organisation on which mental disorders depend'.[69] In addition, he recognised the validity of earlier practice at the institution in that medical treatment for physical illness might also alleviate mental symptoms.

To assess the extent to which medical practice reflected these statements is extremely difficult. It is often not possible to determine whether medical interventions recorded in patients' case histories were designed to cure physical illness, to improve general bodily health or to apply physiological remedies to treat what were seen as organic causes of mental disease. It seems inherently improbable that these theoretical distinctions assumed great importance in the minds of the doctors themselves whilst they were engaged in the routine treatment of patients. Indeed, the alienist's eclectic approach to treating disease was singled out for commendation in the standard mid-Victorian manual on psychological medicine: 'The principle advocated is that no manageable remedy ought to be excluded from the treatment of a large and diverse class of diseases.'[70] In evaluating the course of medical treatments used at the Retreat during our period it therefore seems more practicable to concentrate on subjects that can be isolated for analysis: the extent of medical intervention and the changing nature of medical remedies. Even in these two areas, however, problems of methodology and evaluation of evidence remain formidable. What follows should be taken not as definitive, but as an exploratory and necessarily tentative foray into an important but as yet under-researched area in medical history.

The extent of medical intervention increased as the assistant medical officer, D. H. Tuke, acknowledged in 1854 when he stated that there was 'very much more of medical treatment' employed at the Retreat than had been the case in the earliest years.[71] This observation is confirmed if earlier case-notes are compared with those of later patients. It is also possible to provide a crude quantitative assessment of this progression if annual apothecary's bills of the institution, published in the Retreat's *Reports,* are divided by the number of patients to give annual expenditure on drugs per patient. Although the expenditure incurred by the 'Apothecary's Shop' was included in the annual *Reports* of the institution, the exact composition of items was not recorded. It included not only drugs but leeches (an expensive item), and occasional purchases of instruments as well. However, it is not clear whether the labour component in making up the medicines varied over time, nor is it possible to express the sums in real terms because of the lack of a price index for pharmaceutical goods. Thus, no great precision can be attached to the figures summarised in series 1 of Figure 6.1. Nevertheless, in comparative terms they reveal significant differences in the institution's consumption of medical items during our period. Further, they suggest that these can be related to the predilections of individual doctors. Unless there were very large changes in either the accounting methods of the institution or in the price of drugs and other items, the figures indicate a growing reliance on medical treatments in the first half-century of the Retreat. Expenditure in the Thurnam era was twice that of the Jepson one. (To some extent the peak of expenditure under Thurnam may be accounted for by his growing use of leeches, which were becoming increasingly expensive at this time.) And the peak under Thurnam was to be attained again in the late nineteenth century under Dr Baker, who, it has been suggested earlier in this chapter, was an advocate of asylum medicalisation. The retrenchment in the intervening period of Dr Kitching might perhaps be explained by his prior training under Thomas Allis and Caleb Williams, and hence to a more even-handed commitment to moral as well as medical therapy. By the end of our period, under Dr Pierce, the average cost of drugs per patient had risen to a peak over three times the level under Jepson (see Table 6.1).

This interpretation of these trends must be qualified to some degree and an acknowledgement made of the variation within each doctor's regime. The Thurnam series is remarkably volatile and possibly reflects random elements. Fluctuations under Kitching, when expenditure fell by more than a quarter from 7s. 2d. in 1850–4 to 5s. 2d. in 1865–9 and then rose to 8s. 1d. in 1870–4, may reflect the rapid escalation of prices in these boom years. However, although no great precision can be attached to the figures of average drug cost per patient given in Table 6.1, it is clear that there were important differences in the readiness to resort to drugs in each period and that these can be related to the preferences of

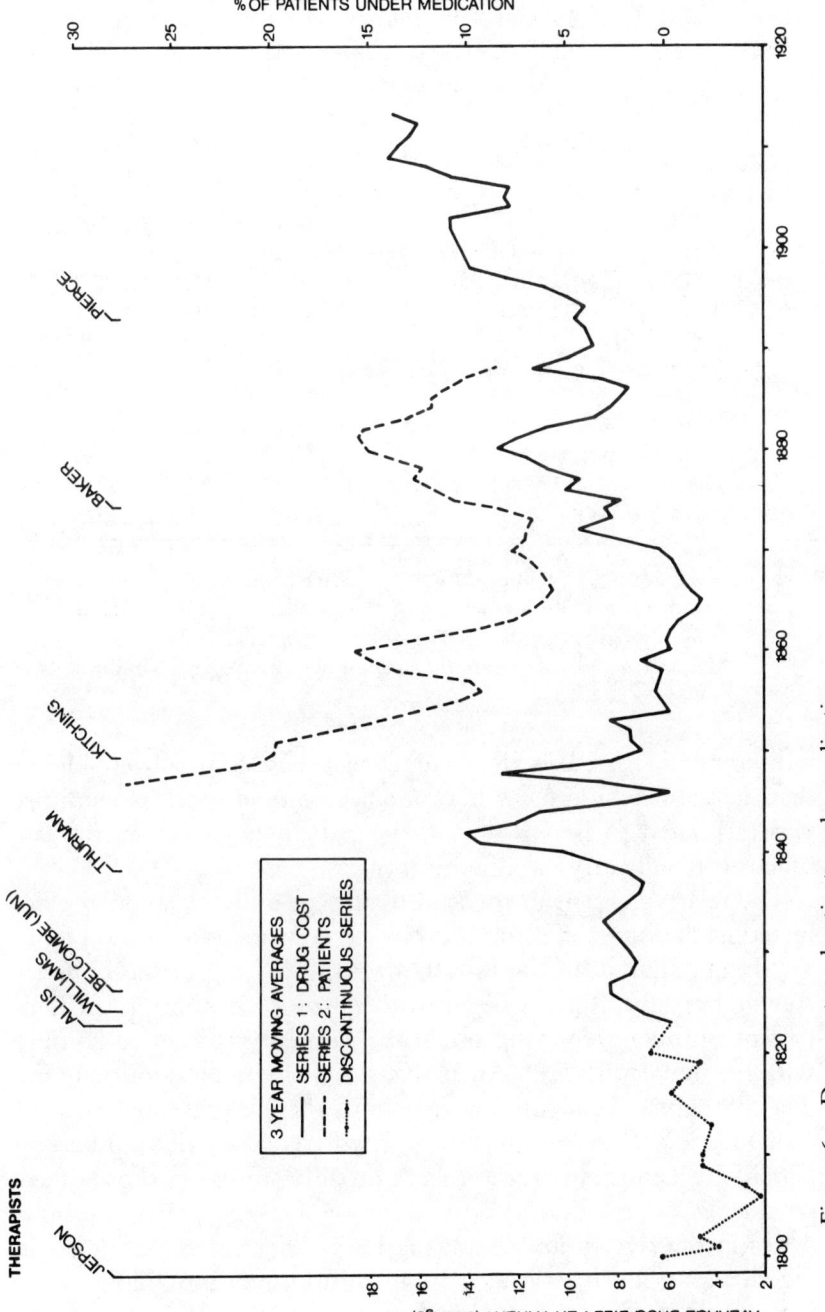

Figure 6.1. Drug costs and patients under medication

Table 6.1. *Average cost of drugs per patient, 1800–1914*

	Average cost	Index no. (1800–22=100)	Decade	Average cost	Index no. (1800–22=100)
Jepson (1800–22)	4s. 6d.	100	1800–09(6)[a]	4s. 0d.	89
			1810–19(5)[a]	4s. 6d.	100
Allis (1823–41)	8s. 0d.	178	1820–29	7s. 0d.	155
			1830–39	7s. 9d.	172
Thurnam (1842–9)	10s. 1d.	224	1840–49	10s. 1d.	224
Kitching (1850–74)	6s. 3d.	138	1850–59	6s. 6d.	144
			1860–69	5s. 4d.	119
Baker (1875–92)	9s. 8d.	215	1870–79	8s. 0d.	178
			1880–89	8s. 6d.	189
Pierce (1893–1914)	13s. 9d.	306	1890–99	10s. 11d.	243
			1900–09	14s. 2d.	315

Note: Periods of tenure shown here differ from those given in later tables because only annual figures are available in these data whereas monthly figures can be used in tables in chapters 8 and 9.
[a] Figures are available only for the number of years stated in brackets.

individual doctors. It is also evident that these figures were higher than in public asylums, where medical and surgical expenditure was estimated to be ½d. or 1d. per patient per week in the late nineteenth and early twentieth centuries.[72]

The relative extent of medical treatment under each doctor depicted in the first series in Figure 6.1 receives corroboration from a different source. In the month after the passing of the Lunatics Act of 1845 the Retreat began to keep more accurate records of patient numbers receiving medical treatment in order to comply with the new legislation. An analysis of these medical journals and weekly reports (kept continuously until 1889) is presented in series 2 of Figure 6.1. As might be expected trends in the numbers of patients receiving medication were broadly similar to those of expenditures on medicaments in series 1. This general correspondence in the two quite separate series gives greater confidence in the changing levels of drug administration over the whole of the nineteenth century depicted in the first series. The fact that the second series is independent of changes in prices is also reassuring.

The ascendancy of medicine

It is interesting that the proportion of the Retreat's patients under medication in series 2 appears to have been higher than at some other asylums.[73]

Additional evidence from the Retreat's medical case-books[74] also indicates that the extent and type of medication reflected changes in the institution's doctors. Although the data are incomplete for the early years they suggest that drug prescription was used less by Drs Fowler, Cappe and Belcombe senior than under their successors. The case-books suggest that the administration of drugs increased later, with an accelerated use first in the late 1820s (after the appointment of Dr Belcombe junior and Caleb Williams); second, at the end of the following decade with the arrival of Dr Thurnam; and third with the appointment of Dr Baker in the mid 1870s.

The first two stages of this progression can be seen clearly in relation to the increased resort to opiates in the second quarter of the nineteenth century. Opiates had been rejected in the period before this when a good supper or glass of porter was the preferred method of inducing good sleep in patients. Later, opiates were used as common sedatives for treating acute mania and for the worst cases of melancholy. Salts of morphia, tincture of opium (laudanum) and Dover's powder were administered without fear of their addictive propensities but with some concern that they induced constipation. Only in the few instances where opiates disagreed with the patient were alternatives prescribed. In its reliance on opium in its chemotherapy the Retreat was not unusual, since the drug was referred to in a standard contemporary textbook as 'the sheet anchor of the alienist physician'.[75]

Before opiates were given to patients there was concern to reduce cerebral congestion by topical bleeding or the use of counter-irritants. Cupping, for a few cases of extreme cerebral hyperaemia, was used in the early years. (A surviving bill for 1798 recorded the purchase of eleven cupping glasses at eight pence each.)[76] Less use was made of the alternative method of local depletion by leeches. This order of priority was later reversed under Dr Belcombe junior. His use of controlled bleeding at the temples or from behind the ears was more frequent than earlier Retreat practice. Thurnam abandoned cupping entirely but used leeches even more extensively. In the 1850s, under Dr Kitching, there was an occasional use of local depletion, but by this time it was becoming unfashionable and a better substitute was found in new drugs thereafter. Until the 1850s local depletion was used in conjunction with counter-irritants designed to induce suppuration. The usual method was to raise blisters on the skin by applying tartarized antimony but occasional use was made of setons or threads through the skin. In the earliest years there was a rare use of the scarifier (purchased in 1798 for £1 16s. 0d.),[77] which made a network of razor-thin skin wounds. Such interventions were justified by recourse to theoretical assumptions of sympathy between mind and body and thus to the belief that morbid action would be diverted from the centre to periphery of the body because active disease in one area was incompatible with that elsewhere. Such methods, used rarely at first, increased in later years, but were never used as frequently as was bleeding.

Close attention was paid to the amount of circulating fluids in the patient and emetics and aperients were frequently employed to control them. These agents were considered useful in restricting circular liquid flows and hence in reducing congestion in the head. In addition, the prevention of constipation, often associated with maniacal states, was thought to be beneficial in preventing nervous irritability. A variety of purgatives was employed at the Retreat: castor oil, calomel, aloes, saline mixtures, mercurials, rhubarb, and Epsom salts. Vomitives were given much more sparingly and usually in the form of a saline draught or a tartar emetic. In the 1830s a combined sedative and emetic pill gradually replaced these. This included one grain of morphia to act as a sedative, and one-eighth of a grain of tartrate of antimony that acted to quieten violence through inducing nausea. In the 1850s there was general concern that the use of nausea-inducing substances such as tartrate of antimony was being abused in lunatic asylums so that it was a method of control rather than of medication.[78] Although this theoretical distinction would appear to be an important one, available documentation of Retreat practice does not permit the historian to distinguish between the two in this instance.

By the 1870s there was greater anxiety over 'chemical restraint' in asylums because of the widespread application of new sedative drugs to patients.[79] Potassium bromide was rediscovered as a useful depressant and anodyne in 1858, and its qualities of promoting sleep, impairing sensation and relaxing the nervo-muscular system were soon seen as extremely useful for excitable, violent or epileptic patients. (Only much later did the drawback of excessive or prolonged use of bromides become apparent with the diagnosis of bromism.) From the 1860s the Retreat, in company with other mental institutions, prescribed bromides frequently as sedatives for restless patients. And in 1869 a new drug, chloral hydrate, became known: a substance that, like bromide, was a depressant and sedative. During the 1870s and 1880s the Retreat used chloral or chloral with bromide, on an extensive scale. A marked rise occurred in the number of patients who received medication at this time for what Dr Baker diagnosed as 'excitement'. The likelihood that chemical restraint was being utilised was strengthened by the evidence from a patient at that time who considered that chloral was being used to 'quench the poor sufferers into quietness'.[80]

Unfortunately, patients' reactions to medical treatment were rarely recorded. A few made their viewpoint clear in refusing to take medicine, but only two Retreat patients left written statements. Edwin R. suffered from remittent mania and had been in the Retreat on three occasions, and in other mental institutions twice, by the time he published *Madness or the Maniac's Hall* in 1841.[81]

Although the poem is itself largely concerned with a stay at Duddeston Hall near Birmingham in 1836 or 1837, the extensive notes seem to have wider application and may have been written during his third stay at the Retreat early in 1841. His verdict on doctors was uncompromising:

Oh! ye erring physicians and philosophers, who think by cupping and cathartics to dispossess the poor demented minds under your charge, of the mysterious inmate which has disturbed the current of their feelings, and deranged the powers of the intellect! Would that your folly may not some day descend upon your own pates.[82]

It is known that he had been cupped by his own doctor before his first admission to an institution and that he had certainly been purged with a variety of cathartic medicines during his three periods at the Retreat. Indeed, his third stay at York coincided with Thurnam's vigorous medical treatments when he was leeched, blistered, sedated and purged. Is it surprising to find that this patient ordered doctors to 'keep your physical nostrums to yourselves!'?

And it may be significant that Dr Thurnam deprecated his publication: 'I regret to find he is still thinking of publishing his poem on "Madness".'[83] Even after his patient had been discharged as 'Improved' in June 1841, the doctor was sufficiently sensitive about the topic to insert a critical newspaper review of the poem in the Retreat's case-book.

Thurnam was as notable for his resort to chemotherapy as was Dr Baker later in the century. And it was one of Baker's patients, Elizabeth C., who was the second patient at the Retreat to criticise its medical treatment. She was a melancholic who spent four months at York in 1876 before being discharged as 'Relieved'. Her views on chloral have already been noted and were part of a more general complaint about the Retreat's over-reliance on chemotherapy:

The general remedy appeared to be a nightly opiate. I have frequently seen 5 or 6 of these bottles in the hand of an attendant, and have good reasons for believing that they were largely dispensed. These draughts were ordered in the forenoon, and brought about 4 o'clock to the foot of the stairs, by the medical assistant, and if, during the day any patient had felt a little better and when bedtime came wished to try to sleep without the draught she had no liberty to do so. The least apparent reluctance was roughly reproved as 'insubordination'.

She disliked the chloral that was prescribed for her because of its side-effects but remonstrated in vain. Her case-notes recorded her 'nervous, anxious, morbid condition', but indicated few steps had been taken to improve it, since the only treatment recorded was of neighbourhood walks, and of course the nightly dose of chloral.[84] And the reference to insubordination was also indicative of an increasingly authoritarian medical regime that was confirmed by the experience of other patients. Whereas in the earlier years it had been possible for a patient to refuse to take medicine, under Dr Baker medicine was administered by force if other means failed. For example, Mary R. was given chloral with a gag and spoon in order to make her sleep, and Mary A. had hyoscyamine administered through a nasal tube in order to quieten her violent behaviour.[85] This increased emphasis on the necessity of chemotherapy at the Retreat contrasted with the experience of the York Asylum, where from the mid-1880s neither sedation for cases of mania nor sleeping draughts at night was utilised.

Diet and hydrotherapy

Pharmaceutical methods were only one method of treatment and were usually addressed to acute symptoms: as the patient improved so greater reliance was placed on a regimen of hydrotherapy and appropriate diet.

From its inception the Retreat had given a very liberal diet to its patients in the belief that improving general bodily health through good food, fresh air and exercise, and good sleep would aid recovery from insanity. This view contrasted with that of some contemporary medical practitioners who believed that an antiphlogistic or reducing regime, with a low diet, was beneficial to the lunatic. The general dietary, outlined in the *Description* of 1813, was as follows:

Breakfast: Milk and bread, or milk porridge.
Dinner: Pudding and animal food five days in the week; fruit pudding, and broth or soup, two days. In the afternoon, the men have bread and beer, the women tea or coffee.
Supper: Generally the same as breakfast, or bread, cheese, and beer.[86]

In fact, this gave a more austere impression than that produced by household records, which throughout our period detailed the tremendous variety of a liberal dietary. Some Friends who had relatives in the Retreat found this 'high living' objectionable: 'on my late visit . . . there was an excess of provisions supplied to the table where my brother dined . . . something like a wasteful profusion [and] a making eating and drinking almost the sole business of the day.'[87] Others, as we have seen, criticised the abundant consumption of alcohol.[88] In spite of a later adherence by some members of the staff to temperance or teetotal organisations, patients' access to alcoholic liquor continued, although on a more selective and medically defined basis. Presumably, this was because it was seen as a tonic, possessing 'medical' virtues that outweighed its 'moral' disadvantages. It may also have been seen as an essential element in the more comfortable life-style of high-fee-paying patients on whose continued patronage the Retreat depended if it was to balance its accounts.

That the dietaries adopted were the result of varied pressures was shown by the reforms of Dr Thurnam. He considered that the diet was too liberal – containing two or three times the amount of solid animal food given in public asylums – and succeeded in replacing some meat with vegetable and farinaceous food in the general dietary. He also published details of a low dietary in use by the 1830s although it is not clear whether he had also modified this:

Breakfast: Weak tea with dry toast.
Dinner: Mutton broth; and plain rice, batter or bread pudding; toast or barley water.
Tea: The same as breakfast.
Supper: Water-gruel, or boiled milk, or thin sago, or arrow root.[89]

Thurnam continued the practice of Dr Belcombe in using this low diet for isolated cases needing an antiphlogistic regime.[90] But Thurnam's interest in diet was also shown during his first three to four years at the Retreat in his specification of diets falling between the low and general dietaries. These included a regulated or restricted meatless diet without alcohol and a plain liberal diet with moderate meat.[91] Thurnam's attempt to regulate food consumption may be seen in part as the product of his more thoroughgoing medical approach to treatment that sought to *control* physical inputs, circulating fluids and evacuations in a mechanistic model of the body. Yet, like Cheyne's earlier dietary schemes, such regulation seems likely to have had an ethical dimension as well: dietary management was one way back to the moral world of sober living, and thus to health and sanity.[92]

Regulation of food included not only restrictive management to cut consumption but also various strategies to increase intake. Those suffering from melancholy were particularly prone to food aversion. Sometimes they could be tempted to eat: Benjamin W. was allowed into the kitchen to eat whatever he fancied and soon overcame his repugnance to food, and Samuel C.'s weight increased by four pounds during his first week at the Retreat.[93] But some depressive cases were more intractable and force-feeding was then begun. George Jepson described the earliest methods by which this was done in a letter of advice to a friend:

The way we have found effectual is to fasten the patient in a chair a little leaning backward with a person to hold the head and another the hands. If the patient refuses to open her mouth it becomes necessary to force it open by inserting the handle . . . of a key between the teeth in the mouth and then turning it by hold of the web so as to force the mouth open to make room for the introduction of the spoon. Then with another spoon nearly fill that between the teeth and push it forward till the point passes the ridge of the tongue, then lean the patient backwards till the liquid is poured down the throat and if she should refuse to swallow, by closing the nostrils a short time and gently stroking the throat she may be inclined to do it. A teacupful of milk and the yolk of an egg beat up [in] it and a little sugar and, if she be very reduced, a little brandy may be added.[94]

The care taken at the Retreat may be contrasted with the frequent occurrence of more brutal practices in other institutions where loss of patients' front teeth was not uncommon. Under Allis, the simple device of key and spoon was replaced by a more specialised instrument that was seen as sufficiently useful to be copied in other asylums by 1830.[95] During the 1830s the Retreat began to force-feed through a tube to the stomach, if manual compulsion with spoon or funnel failed, and this practice continued throughout the rest of the century. Usually, force-feeding was not necessary for prolonged periods, but for this patient it was considered essential:

> 24 May 1878. Edward A. died this morning at 1.10 a.m. During the past 4 years he has laboured under the delusion that he was the rightful Prince of Wales, that there was a constant conspiracy to poison him to prevent him gaining the throne. Hence he refused to take food and therefore for 2 years has thrice daily required the tubal administration of food. By this means he has been kept alive.[96]

Keeping maniacs alive during the exhausting paroxysms of acute frenzy also required careful attention to diet. 'He is fed every hour and consumes 16 eggs, 16 glasses of milk and 1 tin of Brand's Essence of Beef daily.'[97] In less extreme cases the institution was concerned to build up a patient worn down by mania: he 'was much reduced in flesh on admission and ate immoderately'.[98] Tonic supplements to diet were employed frequently for maniacs (after they had become calmer), as well as for melancholics. Until the development of proprietary products such as Easton's or Parish's Syrup, and Brand's Essence, in the late nineteenth century, the Retreat used beef tea, sago, arrowroot, milk, wine and eggs to build up such patients. In a very few cases, injections of broth (in the early years) or nutrient suppositories (in a later period) were also used.[99]

Hydrotherapy was employed continuously at the Retreat during the period under consideration. Tuke wrote with great enthusiasm of the value of warm bathing for melancholics, and even Thurnam acknowledged they were of 'great service' for this purpose.[100] They were usually administered at body heat but temperatures were prescribed in a range from 95 to 102 degrees Fahrenheit.[101] And although Tuke dismissed the utility of the warm bath for maniacs, it was later found to have value for them, if combined with cooling lotions to the head. Indeed, Dr Kitching exploited this form of combined water treatment for a variety of other cases in the 1850s and 1860s and employed not only evaporating spirit lotions to the head but also cold sprays and cold sponges.[102] Having been trained earlier at the Retreat under Allis, Kitching's enthusiasm for older forms of non-pharmaceutical treatment is perhaps not too surprising. His successor, Dr Baker, preferred to encourage use of the Turkish baths that had been installed in the New Lodge in 1877.

Yet hydrotherapy could be employed for other than the relaxing and comforting purposes so far discussed. Cold baths were occasionally used in the earliest years for cases of mania, but their effect was doubtful so they were discontinued.[103] Under Thurnam cold or tepid shower-baths or cold spongings were used for a few cases. Since these (and later cases) seem to have been cases of moral insanity or patients with a history of masturbation, the tonic effect may have involved an element of discipline as well.[104] Shower-baths were also used to subdue excited patients, as in these instances with Ellen C.:

> 23 August 1853. Being in a state of great excitement and activity . . . she was put into a shower-bath . . . until the sedative effect was produced. She was much quieter after it.
>
> 5 September 1853. A few days ago the prolonged shower-bath was again given her, and subdued her for a while, but has not had a permanent effect.[105]

In fact, this prolonged use of the shower-bath was later regulated by the Lunacy Commissioners. But a more subtle abuse of hydrotherapy was difficult to prevent as can be seen in this punitive use of the shower-bath for an incontinent patient:

> 16 September 1856. The attendant told him today that if he repeated it he would have a shower bath.

1 October 1856. The prospect of the shower bath appears to have been the means of producing this salutary effect viz. that he has not had a wet bed since the 16th.[106]

This brief review of the place of a controlled diet and of the use of hydrotherapy in the Retreat's medical treatment suggests that elements of compulsion, and of restriction of patients' autonomy, could be as evident as with the Retreat's chemotherapy. Although some compulsion might be justified as life-saving, a few instances indicated an abuse of medical power within an increasingly authoritarian regime.

THE CLASSIFICATION OF INSANITY

In preceding sections there have been frequent references to different treatments thought to be appropriate for varying forms of mental disease and it is now appropriate to turn to this nosology or classification of insanity. During its first quarter-century the Retreat's basic categories were those of mania, melancholy, mania with melancholy, and dementia. In the next quarter-century monomanias and cases of moral insanity were added.[107] There were also occasional cases of imbecility, idiocy and epilepsy not related to mental illness, although the Retreat attempted to educate the families of prospective patients to recognise the differences between those states and insanity. By 1842 the York establishment's nosology was similar to the one promulgated in that year by the Association of Medical Officers of Hospitals for the Insane. This laid down a classification of mania, melancholia, monomania, moral insanity, dementia (including imbecility) and congenital idiocy. The diagnoses of first admissions between 1796 and 1843 are depicted in Table 6.2, although its clarity is misleading. This is because the habit of reclassifying patients in the light of later perceptions made medical registers into a palimpsest of earlier and later categorisation in which interpretation of the original nosology becomes problematical. It must also be remembered that the classification analysed in Table 6.2 is static; it gives the illness diagnosed on first admission and does not therefore depict the the changes in a patient's condition. It is interesting that many of the present-day diagnostic categories were included in the table under different

Table 6.2. *Diagnoses of first admissions, June 1796–June 1843*

Disorder	Number of cases	Percentage of cases
Mania	182	36.1
Monomania	30	6.0
Mania with melancholy	53	10.5
Melancholy	162	32.1
Dementia[a]	38	7.5
Moral insanity	3	0.6
Idiocy & imbecility	29	5.8
Not mental illness[b]	7	1.4

Note: Systematic recording of diagnoses ended in June 1843.
[a] This included two described as 'stupor' and fifteen of 'incoherence'.
[b] Cases of delirium and of epilepsy unconnected with mental illness.
Source: BIHR J/1/1–2.

names: manias and melancholy approximate broadly to manic-depressive illness; moral insanity to personality disorder; idiocy and imbecility to mental handicap; and dementia to dementia.

Attempts to classify mental illness puzzle not only the later historian but also the contemporary medical man. It was said of case 470 by a perplexed Dr Thurnam:

In fact to describe his case nosologically, it would appear to be one of moral insanity, closely allied to, if not already merged in, the 'scheming insanity' of Arnold, or the 'monomania of imagination' of Browne, which state alternates with simple melancholy.[108]

Indeed, Dr Thurnam was more concerned with such matters than other Retreat doctors, who had minuted this case as one of melancholy (during an earlier stay at the institution), or (on readmission) as one of remittent mania alternating with depression.[109] A simpler classification was perhaps a more appropriate stance given the imperfect state of medical knowledge of insanity at that time. Attempts to pin-point a patient's disorder could lead to hollow, pretentious statements as in Thurnam's comment on case 702:

Mentally his state is one of incipient dementia, bordering still on chronic mania, and presenting itself in garrulous imbecility in a degree, though in more of irritable and versatile incoherence.[110]

In this context it is interesting that a systematic nosology fell into disuse at the Retreat. During much of the second half of the nineteenth century, medical labelling of patients seems to have been honoured more in the breach than in the observance. Nevertheless, additional categories were added, of which delusion and general paralysis of the insane were the most frequently employed.

In interpreting this nosology it is salutary to heed the conclusion of Dr Pierce:

It is not possible as yet to make a scientific classification of mental disorders. Were it not for this humiliating reflection, the conflict of opinions would be amusing . . . An essential point in a statistical enquiry is that the things counted under one head shall be of like nature and shall be distinct from other things placed under other heads. But when we consider the forms of mental disorder this essential point is not attained.[111]

Such professional humility was seldom evident in the public pronouncements of earlier medical men at York, although their own medical case-books gave ample evidence of the setbacks and disappointments inherent in their 'trial and error' approach. And despite the positivistic claims of nineteenth-century alienists Pierce was again both honest and incisive in his view that psychological medicine, 'in the very nature of things, is the most difficult and elusive of all branches of knowledge'.[112]

OLD AND NEW IDEAS

The positivistic aspirations of nineteenth-century doctors neither precluded a strong injection of moralistic values into their diagnoses and treatments nor inhibited recourse to older ways of viewing mental disorder. The relationship between the waxing and waning of the moon had interested Greek as well as medieval practitioners, and in the nineteenth century Esquirol had thought it merited observation.[113] At the Retreat there was some observation of this relationship in cases of both mania and melancholia, though usually when the early nineteenth-century certificates of admission suggested – on the basis of information given by others that the relationship existed for individual patients.[114] Between the

1830s and 1850s attention was also given to the humoral way of seeing individual personalities as being influenced by the four humours of earth, air, fire and water. Thus, a few patients were described in the medical case-books as having melancholic, phlegmatic, lymphatic, bilious or sanguine temperaments.[115] Categorisation of mental illness was also coloured by traditional assumptions, most noticeably in a few diagnoses of 'demonomania', or possession. Interestingly, the first diagnoses were the result of Dr Thurnam – the most positivistic of all the Retreat's doctors – reclassifying earlier cases of mania or melancholy with hallucinations.[116] The label continued to be used until at least the 1880s, since in 1885 'a lady [was] admitted to the Retreat in a typical condition of Demonomania, impulsively acting out in her conduct the directions she believed to be given her by unseen evil spirits'.[117]

The medical world at the Retreat was one of pragmatism: recourse to traditional methods for some was balanced by newer approaches for others, or an absence of medical intervention for a few. In the earlier period under Jepson or Allis, alternative approaches to medicine were used. 'No medicine is yet ordered as I am desirous of trying what control alone may do 'was the strategy adopted for Thomas H., a maniac, on his readmission in 1828. It was recognised that in some cases of mania, 'the whole brain is in a state of excitement, but of a kind over which medicine has but little power'. And for melancholics medicine might also be seen as irrelevant: Samuel D. was 'allowed to be alone and to be quiet, no medicine has been given and he seems collected and calm'.[118] Throughout our period there was an eclectic approach: if one remedy failed then another was tried. The most striking example of this was with Ellen C. When medicine, mechanical restraint, hydrotherapy and musical distraction had all failed to quieten her over a period of ten months after her admission it was decided to try animal magnetism as a last resort:

The application of mesmerism was tried for an hour and has been repeated daily since. No immediate results were apparent but she has had 3 good nights of sound sleep – a circumstance which we believe never occurred since her admission.[119]

Even the Retreat therapists' open-mindedness had a limit, however, and this was revealed at the end of our period in relation to the psychoanalytical approach. Dr Pierce admitted that although he had 'endeavoured to keep an open mind' on the subject of Freud's theories, 'I can only say that much that is written is revolting in the extreme and so far fetched as to be sometimes ludicrous, were it not so objectionable'. Although admitting that his acquaintance with psychoanalysis was 'slight', he stated dogmatically that its value was 'very limited' in comparison with alternative approaches:

I am confirmed in the opinion that the physician who studies the material factors in the cause of disease will attain greater success than he who instinctively turns to repressed complexes and other hidden psychical factors.

Pierce's conclusion was that alienists 'should be ready to listen but slow to form judgements'.[120] He might well have been thinking of his predecessors at the Retreat whose eclecticism and reluctance to formulate grand theoretical systems exemplified this cautious empiricism.

7

A hidden dimension: the asylum attendant

To them in great measure must, of necessity, be entrusted the personal charge of the patients . . . Attendants should combine in their character and disposition, firmness and gentleness; and they should be able, by their education and habits, to superintend, direct, and promote the employment and recreation of the patients.[1]

The central role of the asylum attendant was here recognised by the Lunacy Commissioners. Indeed, asylum literature in this decade – the 1850s – reached heights of rhetoric on the character and importance of the attendant unrivalled at any other time. With the general adoption of the ideals of non-restraint and of moral treatment in most asylums, there was by this time a growing appreciation of the key role of the attendant in the success or failure of its realization. But those like J. T. Arlidge, the former medical superintendent of St Luke's, who had some knowledge of asylums recognised that attendants were given duties beyond their capabilities.[2] The Lunacy Commissioners preached repetitive sermons on the need to recruit a superior class of more highly paid attendants who would be 'intelligent, judicious, industrious and active'.[3] The moral virtues that contemporaries required in the desirable attendant would probably have disqualified most asylum superintendents. Yet the counterpoint to this grandiloquent prose was that of publicity on attendants' brutality to patients, which suggested an everyday reality far removed from the ideal.[4]

This chapter will try to evaluate whether a comparable gap existed between rhetoric and reality at the Retreat by assessing the pattern of attendants' recruitment, their duties, and their performance. The historian of this institution is uniquely fortunate in that the papers of one of its Victorian attendants – William Waller – have survived to illuminate the attitudes and values an attendant brought to his work. These manuscripts form a small part of a much longer religious autobiography and hence give an overview of his vocation rather than the practical details of his daily routine. They suggest, however, that Waller had adopted a professional stance towards his work. The general emergence of the professional mental nurse from the untrained attendant was a later achievement: a discussion of the Retreat's role in this process ends this chapter.

RECRUITMENT AND WAGES

'I am so anxious to get Friends into our situations that I cannot but hope he will make the trial and that he may be a permanent valuable assistant to us.' So wrote Samuel Tuke in a fervent conclusion to a letter discussing the possibility of recruiting a young male Quaker as an attendant at the Retreat.[5] We have seen that the Committee of Management shared his view that members of the Society of Friends were most suitable in this situation and had expressed disappointment in 1827 that, owing to a dearth of such candidates previously, they had been forced to appoint non-Quakers.[6] Given the importance assigned to moral therapy at the Retreat the recruitment of attendants with the same values as their patients was obviously highly desirable. How successful was the institution in recruiting Friends to serve as attendants and how long were they prepared to stay in this difficult employment?

The earliest attempts to recruit satisfactory attendants must be seen as failures since before 1800 there had been six appointments of keepers on the male side of the house.[7] But a gradual improvement was noticeable since the first four keepers stayed under nine months, whereas the next two managed twenty-four and twenty months, respectively. However, it was in 1802 that some stability was introduced with the selection of Samuel Smith and John Binns, who each stayed in continuous employment until 1807. They then appear to have alternated work elsewhere with that of looking after single private patients at the Retreat, but both were listed as being members of the Quaker family at the Retreat in 1820. Binns was succeeded by Isaac Stansfield, who stayed until 1818, and Smith by several individuals who managed only a couple of years' tenure – John Stansfield, Thomas Wickett and Thomas Atkinson. And in 1811 the need for a male keeper at the newly opened half-way house, the Appendage, led to the engagement of Samuel Lay, who was still in service in 1820. It is interesting that those who gave the longest service can be identified as having been Quakers – Binns, Smith, Isaac Stansfield and Lay.

This was also the case for the nurses who cared for the female patients. Each of the four nurses employed in the early 1820s was listed as a Quaker member of the Retreat family in 1820. Of these Hannah Hall had been there since 1797, Hannah Woodville since 1799, Hannah Ponsonby since 1800 and Margaret Wilson since 1802. This statement is to some extent misleading as a guide to the general stability of female staff since there was apparently no clear demarcation in the early years between recruitment for work as a general servant and that of a nurse. The long service of these four individuals therefore obscured the fact that most women worked for only one or two years as general servants at the Retreat.[8]

In the early years recruitment was attempted either by notifying Quarterly or Monthly Meetings of vacancies or through the personal network of acquaintances of the Tukes and others on the Retreat's Committee of Management. By the 1840s, when the needs of a much larger institution demanded more frequent appointments, resort was had to advertisement in the York newspapers. Effectively this was an admission of failure and a recognition that the Quaker community could not supply sufficient personnel. By this time only a small minority of attendants of each sex can be identified as being members of the Society of Friends.[9]

Apart from the benefit of employing those as attendants who had similar values and attitudes to their Quaker patients, there was an advantage in recruiting those whose background and personality could be spoken for by trusted members of the Society of Friends. The utility of a sincere and reliable reference becomes extremely obvious if the testimonials are examined for those applying for the posts of two male attendants at York in March 1841.[10] (This was the only occasion for which such evidence has survived at the Retreat.) There were fifteen applicants and all were able to produce letters of recommendation that differed little from the others in attesting to their sobriety, honesty and diligence. Although neither of the successful applicants was a Friend, both regularly attended Meetings and both had good references from respected members of the Society of Friends. It is significant that they were preferred to a man with previous experience as an attendant at a

A hidden dimension: the asylum attendant

private madhouse in York. Apparently the habits developed at such an establishment were not felt to be an advantage at the Retreat where distinctive methods of treatment were pursued.

Four-fifths of the applicants lived either in York or within a fifteen-mile radius of the city. This suggests that the two young men from the Sheffield area, who were successful, had applied as a result of information disseminated through Quaker Meetings rather than through a local newspaper advertisement. Most either had worked as servants or had served an apprenticeship to a craftsman, and therefore were probably young and single. Indeed, the field of applicants was remarkably similar to that produced by advertisement two years later when William Waller was appointed. In 1841 the salary offered was £24 per annum: a sum about half way up the range of emoluments of £18 to £30 paid to ordinary male attendants. This sum was in addition to the board and lodging provided and as such compared reasonably with that available in alternative occupations. Since no perquisites were allowed to Retreat staff it was necessary to pay them a sufficiently generous sum to minimise temptation.

The standard of remuneration had not advanced significantly from the earliest years of the Retreat. The first sums offered to male keepers, of twelve and fifteen guineas,* had not proved sufficient to recruit men of good ability. It was presumably this factor, together with the rapid price inflation of the war years, that had led rapidly to an improvement to twenty guineas by the first years of the nineteenth century. There was much less difficulty in recruiting women and they continued to be paid six to seven guineas a year – the equivalent of that earned by a domestic servant. This was a natural procedure because nurses' duties straddled general domestic chores and the care of patients. It seems likely that women were usually recruited as domestic servants and then promoted to the work of nurse if they showed aptitude in that kind of duty. Of the four women described as nurses in 1820, for example, all had been recruited initially as domestic servants. The widespread tendency in the Retreat's records to label indiscriminately both male and female individuals as servant or attendant suggests that the distinction in status or duties was not a very real one to contemporaries.

* A guinea was one pound and one shilling.

Wages were slightly higher for attendants than servants and the former also received board and lodging. Salaries paid to the Retreat's male attendants in the 1840s seem to have been lower than those paid elsewhere. If we compare those paid at the Retreat in 1842–4 with those at Lancaster Asylum in 1841 we find this difference. At Lancaster the head male attendant earned £50, and at the Retreat this was £40, raised in 1844 to £50. Ordinary male attendants were paid £18 to £30 at York and £25 to £31/10s. at Lancaster. Female attendants or upper nurses received thirteen to fifteen guineas at Lancaster and less generous sums of £10 to £12 at York, where ordinary nurses or under-attendants were also paid only six to eight guineas. That attendants – although vital to the running of the institution – were lowly beings in the asylum's hierarchy is obvious, however, if we compare their salaries with those above them. The Retreat superintendent and his wife received a salary of £250 and the resident surgeon one of £200 at this time.[11]

DUTIES

Although it was easy enough to recruit personnel, the nature of an attendant's duties made it difficult to find people with sufficient physical stamina, strong stomach and good nature to perform difficult duties successfully. That ambivalence was felt to the job by even the more experienced was suggested by the history of Samuel Smith, whose tenure from 1801 was punctuated by two notices of intention to resign before his temporary departure from the Retreat in 1807. The Retreat demanded very high standards of performance and an undivided allegiance to the institution. Those who married were given notice unless they were prepared to continue to lodge at the institution.[12] That duties were onerous and needed exceptional personal qualities was recognised by Samuel Tuke in 1827 when he described, on behalf of a possible recruit, the task he would face:

> The business of an attendant requires a good deal of self command and patience. The risk of personal injury which a stranger might suppose to be considerable, I take to be *very small indeed*.
> The attendants have the charge of from seven to ten patients and have to clean their rooms and attend to the cleanliness of their persons. This is of course with some patients frequently a very disagreeable office.[13]

A hidden dimension: the asylum attendant

In order that prospective attendants should understand what they were undertaking, and also so that the establishment could know whether they could cope, they were usually taken on trial for a short period before their appointment was confirmed. Thereafter, they were on a month's notice or a month's wages.

'The business of an attendant requires him to counteract some of the strongest principles of our common nature.'[14] This observation was written by Samuel Tuke in 1815 after he had helped expose the abuse of patients by keepers (and others) at the neighbouring York Lunatic Asylum. His colleague, S. W. Nicoll, who had assisted in the exposure of conditions later wrote a book on the necessity for vigilance over asylum keepers in which he asserted:

The keeper must himself be kept. If he be not watched and punished, an asylum is likely to be little beyond an alternation of reciprocal violence between the prisoner and the gaoler.[15]

One reason for the violent ill-treatment of the York Asylum's unfortunate inmates, and for the neglect of their cleanliness and health, had been the very high numbers of patients for whom each keeper was responsible. In 1813 the ratio of attendants to patients was 1 to 28.[16] At the Retreat much better conditions prevailed for patients because it was appreciated that it was necessary to provide more generous staffing ratios.

How many patients did each Retreat attendant have to care for? The available data are summarised in Table 7.1. Column 5 of this table suggests that overall staffing ratios improved from 1 attendant for 10 patients in 1813, to 1 attendant for 3.2 patients by 1877. (The very favourable ratio for 1797 is ignored because it was distorted by the need to have attendants of each sex to care for the very small number of patients in the newly opened institution.) By 1900 the comparable figure was 1 nurse to 2.5 patients.[17] These ratios overstated the staffing available to the ordinary patient since a few high-fee-paying or difficult patients might have an attendant to themselves. Column 6 is therefore more representative of the typical care available, and this showed a smaller improvement in staffing from 1 attendant for 13.6 patients in 1813, to 1 for 5.7 patients by 1877.

The Retreat's overall ratios of attendants to patients were more generous than all but expensive private establishments as a com-

Table 7.1. *Ratio of attendants to patients*

	Attendants		Patients		Attendant to patient ratio	
	In main galleries	With special patients	Ordi-nary	Spe-cial	Overall	For ordinary patients
1797	2	—	15	—	1 : 7.5	1 : 7.5
1813	5	2	68	2	1 : 10	1 : 13.6
1823	7	3	64	6	1 : 7	1 : 9.1
1828	8	6	70	12	1 : 5.8	1 : 8.7
1840	9	9	79	12	1 : 4.5	1 : 8.7
1847	15	9	(95)	(18)	1 : 4.7	(1 : 6.3)
1863–4	16	13	(100)	(26)	1 : 4.3	(1 : 6.2)
1870–5	14	16	(104)	(32)	1 : 4.5	(1 : 7.4)
1875–7	17	23	(98)	(34)	1 : 3.2	(1 : 5.7)

Note: 'Special' means either patients with their own attendant or those with one attendant to a few high-fee-paying patients. Complete figures for selected dates are available until 1840; thereafter, estimated figures are placed in brackets. From 1847 to 1875 it has been assumed that the average ratio of attendants to special patients was 1 to 2, and in 1875–7, 1 to 1.5.
Source: See n. 18.

parison of staffing in the mid-nineteenth century indicates. In 1853 the luxurious Ticehurst employed nearly as many attendants as it had patients, and six years earlier that high-class establishment, Brislington House, had one attendant to every two patients. Rate-aided county asylums had much worse provisions. Lancaster employed one attendant to every twenty-five tranquil or convalescent patients and one to every fifteen more refractory or difficult ones. This was of the same order of magnitude as Hanwell with one to seventeen or Wakefield with one to twenty-two. Perhaps the most appropriate comparison would be that of an equivalent-sized private hospital – the York Asylum – where in 1840 each attendant had responsibility for eleven patients whereas at the Retreat it was for only eight. The Retreat's provision bettered the ideal ratio of 1 to 17 proposed by John Conolly in 1847 for pauper asylums.[19]

It was fortunate for the Retreat's attendants that they had comparatively few patients to look after because the demands the institution made of them were correspondingly high. The ideal arrangement was apparently seen as one in which the attendant had immediate responsibility for a gallery and in which the patients there formed 'a little family' who 'were interested in each other's welfare'.[20] And in looking after this group he was said in 1840 to be responsible for the

> Keeping of the day and sleeping apartments of his class in order, attending to the patients' rising, dressing, washing, and going to bed, the administration of food and medicine, and the general oversight of the whole, so that good order might be preserved in his department.[21]

Although the earliest regulations of the institution had remained conspicuously silent on the subject of its attendants, by 1828 it was enjoined on them first to be present with the patients as much as possible and second, not to employ coercion on those under their care without the permission or knowledge of the superintendent and matron.[22] Later during the 1840s – when a more bureaucratic regime was introduced – two rule books for attendants and servants were published in 1842 and 1847.[23]

The 1842 rules expressed as a code of practice the philosophy and habits that had grown up gradually during the time of the first two superintendents. Those of 1847 extended this simple pragmatism into a more elevated statement of the role of attendants in moral management that may well have been influenced by John Conolly's ideas on the subject.[24] The earlier version stated clearly the fundamental principle that should govern attendants' behaviour:

> The attendants must not regard themselves as the masters of the patients; but as the servants of *an institution founded for the relief and recovery of those* . . . *who require to be treated with the utmost kindness, patience, and forbearance.*

Attendants were to work quietly and regularly in the performance of their duties, which were to be concerned almost exclusively with the care of their patients and not with the general running of the institution. (The only exception was the female attendant who might be asked to do some needlework or starching while looking after her patients.) They were to maintain 'perfect cleanliness and ventilation' in their gallery and apartments. Wet ticking on beds was to be replaced and all ticking changed monthly. Patients' cleanliness was to be achieved through a daily combing of the hair and washing of the face and hands, and this was also supplemented by a monthly bath. All these duties were to be achieved by 11 a.m. Thereafter, attendants were to see that patients had some daily exercise and to help amuse or employ their charges. In addition, attendants were to serve breakfast at 7 a.m., dinner at 1 p.m., tea at 5 p.m. and supper at 8 p.m.[25]

The regulations of 1842 and 1847 not only specified duties but also attempted to formulate the kind of relationship that should exist between attendant and patient. Those of 1847 specified that

> they should take pains to acquire a knowledge of the character of the patients, and to obtain their confidence by friendly treatment, and by actively promoting their comfort and real enjoyment. Their requests should be complied with, within reasonable bounds; but no promises should be made, or expectations given to them, which cannot be performed. Kind and respectful, not domineering, language is to be used to the patients; and they should be asked not commanded, to do whatever may be desired of them.

Since this was the kind of relationship envisaged it is perhaps not surprising to find that the institution attempted to recruit as attendants those who had previously been in service, where they would presumably have learnt the art of shrewdly assessing the character of those employing them and also that of respectful language and demeanour. This type of recruitment was comparable to private houses with a superior class of patient[26] but formed a contrast with that of county asylums, where pauper patients were managed by keepers recruited from the working classes – as at Kent, Surrey or Lancaster.[27]

In these mid-century regulations the Retreat's attendants were also given advice on how to handle troublesome patients. This perpetuated the earliest traditions of the institution[28] in that they were not to encourage patients to express deranged ideas, or expose other weaknesses. Further, they were to 'avoid unnecessary interference' with their patients, except that in the case of excited patients they were to try 'to divert their attention to other objects', or 'to lead them to stillness'. This might mean secluding them in their own bedroom (for half an hour to an hour in the first instance), or alternatively, in the security of a secluding room. In both cases this had to be reported to the medical officer, superintendent or matron. Mechanical restraint was seen as permissible in 1842 on the initiative of the attendant so long as the prior consent of the resident surgeon or matron was obtained. By 1847, as we have seen,[29] the climate of opinion had changed sufficiently for it to be depicted as a rare event:

> No further restraint [than seclusion] is ever to be resorted to, except by the direction, or with the concurrence of the Superintendent, unless in any extra-ordinary emergency, when the attendant shall immediately inform him thereof.

When a patient had to be forcibly removed in a state of violent excitement, the regulations confirmed the earlier practice[30] of using overwhelming force through employing several attendants, so that any 'idea of resistance' on the part of the patient would be prevented. Presumably the rationale for this was that injury would be prevented.

That patients were seen as vulnerable was clear from repeated discussions on the need to safeguard them from abuses stemming from the defective personality of an attendant. At the Retreat attendants were also forbidden to threaten patients on pain of dismissal. Each attendant was exhorted to guard 'against the tendency to resent injuries, and to treat others according to their conduct towards himself' and to practise the 'strictest habits of self-government'. Whether such earnest admonitions had much impact on the attendants is open to doubt; very long working hours increased fatigue and made less likely the requisite amount of self-control necessary to surmount everyday annoyances or occasional provocation.

The amount of free time available to attendants before the 1840s is not ascertainable but the rules of 1842 specified that they were to 'be allowed occasional times of absence for the purpose of their own relaxation' so long as prior permission was obtained. Also, each attendant was to have a part of alternate Sundays off duty, or even of each Sunday. Until 1862, when there was provision of night nurses for the first time, it was expected that attendants were on call during the night, as well as on duty during the day. Indeed, the Retreat was slow to respond to the campaign by the Lunacy Commissioners during the 1850s to shame asylums into employing night staff.[31] Generally, the hours that were formally demanded of Retreat staff compared unfavourably with those attendants worked elsewhere. For example, in 1846 the rules of the Lancaster Asylum specified a thirteen-hour day, with alternate evenings off, and every other Sunday free, as well as one day off each month.[32] In demanding such long hours of duty, when ensuing fatigue would increase the likelihood of irritation and intolerance, the Retreat probably lowered its attendants' performance.

PERFORMANCE

How adequately attendants performed their duties is problematical: evidence is scarce and difficult to interpret. Much that went on in the wards must remain hidden, and the treatment of patients there is a matter of conjecture. Nevertheless, the richness of the Retreat's archives makes it possible to say rather more on the topic than is usual in historical accounts of asylums.

In the official *Reports* of the Retreat the superintendent wrote that its attendants 'could not easily be surpassed for their steadiness and moral character'. He spoke approvingly of their character, which was 'uniformly kind and forbearing'.[33] In the privacy of patients' case-notes, Dr Kitching was not always so complimentary as in this example:

> 20 February 1865. [The attendant] describes the patient as walking quietly along and by sudden impulse without any premonition, seizes his coat and splits it down, so that he almost invariably comes home in rags and tatters. I cannot give any other account of this matter, but must conclude that there is a defect in the controlling power of the attendant, who seems to have acquired no more moral influence over his patient after this long intercourse with him than he had at first.[34]

However, Kitching did recognise that the attendants' duties were 'continuous and trying':[35] other extracts from the case-books confirmed the accuracy of his perception.

Within the confined space of the patients' ward a deceitful patient could make an attendant's life unpleasant. Of one patient it was said:

> She professes great conscientiousness, candour, kindness and charity, whilst giving to circumstances and to actions distorted and malicious colouring using great exaggeration and misrepresentation, showing much quarrel-

A hidden dimension: the asylum attendant

someness, especially at intervals, so that we have found it very difficult to get attendants to stay in the ward where she is, finding by experience that they are maligned and misrepresented.[36]

Long hours were tiring and responsibility for patients at night increased fatigue. The patient 'is very restless in the night, and the nurse is beginning to feel quite worn out', commented the medical officer in worried tones.[37] Anxiety was increased when such a patient was also violent. He 'has been more unsettled lately – and a short time since he attempted in the night to throttle the attendant who sleeps in his room'.[38]

The likelihood of injury to the attendant from violent patients increased with the decline in the use of mechanical restraint, as numerous passages in patients' histories in the second half of the nineteenth century bore eloquent witness. 'This morning she [a maniac] belaboured her attendant with a tin tray – and would probably have seriously hurt her but that timely assistance was rendered.'[39] Another female maniac was said to be 'frequently very much excited. Often bruises the attendants'.[40] Cases of dementia might also cause injury. 'She is reported by the attendants to be very full of opposition and cannot be induced to do anything, and when dressed and undressed makes violent resistance, striking and kicking the attendants.'[41] It might be thought that the increased use of sedatives would have compensated for the decline in physical restraint by subduing the excitement of patients. The protection given to attendants by their use was probably substantial but the difficulty of arriving at a suitable dosage could mean that drugs were ineffectual. 'The morphia was repeated last night without benefit. The attendant reports it as the worst night he has had, being spent in shouting, tearing and fighting.'[42]

Abuse and violence were not always directed *towards* attendants. Defects in the attendant's personality, or the provocation offered by a patient, could lead to the mentally ill being harmed by those engaged to look after them. Minor ill-treatment was likely to have been unnoticed and unrecorded: harsh words, rough handling when washing or dressing a patient, unequal apportionment of food or inappropriate exaction of employment might have escaped the notice of medical officers during their daily rounds of the wards. A subterranean element of violence may also have existed. Samuel W., a long-stay patient, whose outbreaks of mania alternated with long periods of sanity, wrote a letter of complaint to the Committee of Management in 1813 in which he provided apparently well-substantiated accusations of cruel treatment of patients by a keeper, Samuel Smith.[43] This is worth quoting at some length since it gives the rarely expressed viewpoint of the patient:

> After a residence of something more than ten years at the Retreat, and having been favoured to enjoy a convalescent state of mind the principal part of the time . . . I ought to be qualified to judge a little of the conduct and motives by which the managers of this institution have been influenced . . . but having been afflicted myself at times with this grievous malady, I shall perhaps, by some be deemed *incompetent* to give an opinion . . . but I shall nevertheless state some matters *of fact* to the Committee for their investigation and consideration . . . and can bring witnesses to prove the validity of my assertions.
>
> I wish I had it in my power to say that our Governor and Governess, as well as the Men Keepers had always behaved towards the patients with Christian kindness, forbearance, and impartiality arguable to the report Lindley Murray made to me soon after I came to York, which, if I recollect right, was this. 'Samuel, our plan at the Retreat is mild and conciliatory measures, instead of that violence and coercion adopted at other Lunatic Asylums.' – But what would the *feeling* Murray say if he knew of the flogging I received at the hands of Samuel Smith? – At another time when I objected to having the straight-jacket on (which like our good, tho' affected King I have ever made resistance to having on, on account of the deprivation of sleep, wounds and pain it has occasioned me) at his throwing me down with such force as to bruise my side so bad, that I was under the necessity of having it bathed for 2 or 3 weeks, by Isaac Stansfield who was a *witness* to this act of cruelty. As was also John Binns to the former castigation of flogging. Add to this Samuel Smith's dragging Joseph G. along by the hair of his head in such manner that Joseph observed to me a few days before he left the Retreat as we were walking together in the garden (holding up his hand at Samuel Smith) 'Oh! Samuel W. I shall never forget the cruelty of that fellow' . . . I must also mention his throwing Cousin James B. down in the presence of myself and J. C. for swearing (in a fit of derangement) and eating the end of a mold [mould] candle* – after he had put him to bed supperless for three weeks together, as I was informed. And why was he put to bed supperless? – because when strapped and jacketted in bed he did his needs therein. John W. was also flogged three times by the same keeper . . . because the poor afflicted youth had not sense enough to go to the necessary to ease himself, but did his needs in his breeches – which this flogging it seems was intended to prevent.[44]

* A mould candle was one made in a mould rather than being dipped.

A hidden dimension: the asylum attendant

If we look at the case-notes for Samuel W., given in the Appendix, we can see the circumstances in which this letter was written. It is clear that the 'Governor', Jepson, felt that he was prone to malicious comments and that this letter cannot necessarily be taken at face value. On the other hand, circumstantial evidence suggests that some credence should be given to this patient's accusations. It is obvious from the names Samuel W. mentions that these incidents have occurred over a number of years because Joseph G. left the Retreat in 1804. It might be thought therefore that Samuel W. had developed a long-standing aversion to the keeper, Samuel Smith, and that his testimony was biassed against him. But there is independent evidence that Smith was *not* a satisfactory keeper. In fact, he had been given notice the previous year by the Committee of Management. It was not thought suitable for him to continue in the family, the committee's minutes cryptically stated, and the care of his private patient was given to another keeper.[45] Yet Samuel Smith continued to be re-employed at the Retreat and was still recorded as a keeper in 1820.

What then do we make of the committee's attitude in continuing to hire a man in such a post of responsibility when there were doubts about his fitness to exercise power? Was Samuel W. right to compare the Retreat to the York Lunatic Asylum in his letter's pointed conclusion, when he asked whether the committee thought it 'expedient or proper that their servants should be reprimanded for mal-treatment of the patients, as well as the keepers employed by the managers of the York Lunatic Asylum'? It may be conjectured that the managers of the Retreat might justify Smith's retention because he was an experienced attendant whose strength was a necessity for dealing with violently excited patients. Samuel W. himself needed firm action during his attacks of mania as his uncle knew well: 'when his paroxysms come on they are generally pretty violent and require control.'[46] And Smith could be deployed when others proved inadequate, as in the case of a powerful patient named Wilson S. He was a very violent patient whose attendant had to be changed to a bigger, stronger man – Samuel Smith:

15 January 1815. Samuel Smith has had the care of him, near a week, and having complete ascendancy by superior strength he steps in between [patients] when necessary to prevent affrays.

20 February 1815. Without the least provocation [Wilson S.] started up, seized his attendant by the throat and threatened to throw

> him downstairs but S. S. proved too strong for him, threw him down and held him fast until the noise was heard in the room below, and the men came to assist, which could hardly be less than 10 minutes. They then secured him with straps and shut him in his bedroom.[47]

It is significant that in this extract from the institution's case-book, implicit approval was given to actions – such as throwing the patient to the ground – that we know from Samuel W.'s letter were seen as cruelty from the patient's standpoint. Although strength was recognised as a desirable quality, both at the Retreat and at Hanwell, it was more usual to prevent the resistance of an excited or violent patient by a strong array of several keepers.[48]

The Retreat managers emphasised the crucial distinction between controlled force for a necessary objective and gratuitous violence by attendants toward patients. By its nature, however, the latter was difficult to ascertain. Patients' testimony could not be believed automatically even if it were given, and fear of reprisals by attendants, or the uncertainties of a sick mind, may have prevented accusations being formulated at all. When knowledge of unnecessary violence was obtained decisive action ensued as in this incident with a demented patient:

Last night he refused to go to bed, so the under-attendant after repeatedly trying to persuade him to go carried him upstairs – J. R. P. seized him savagely round the body so the attendant got him round the throat and threatened to strangle him if he did not leave go, which he did, and was put to bed. The attendant was this morning discharged for using this threat and using force without being authorised to do so.[49]

The Lunacy Commissioners kept a register of the dismissals and it was the statutory duty of asylums after 1853 to inform them of such cases.[50] And under the Lunacy Act of 1890 the Commissioners were prepared to prosecute attendants who ill-treated or wilfully neglected patients. They did so in the case of Fanny Onions, a Retreat nurse who was dismissed in 1894 for striking patients. Fanny Onions had been the second nurse on the Fifth Gallery for eighteen months, and although she had a sharp tongue she was seen as being cheerful and pleasant. But her temper later deteriorated so that she pushed her patients around roughly and occasionally slapped them. The Commissioners prosecuted her before the York bench on charges of common assault and ill-treatment of four patients. Evidence given against her was that other nurses had seen her strike or push her charges and that the medical officer found some bruises on the patients. But her previous exemplary character, and the relatively light charges against her, led to the minimum penalty of a forty-shillings fine being imposed.[51]

Comparing the behaviour of attendants involved in these violent actions towards patients, and the increasingly condemnatory responses by the asylum's managers during the nineteenth century, suggests that more stringent standards of self-restraint were expected of attendants by the end of our period. Moral management not only demanded high standards of conduct from the patient but also assumed that attendants would provide behavioural models for them.[52]

Attendants were also encouraged to gain their patients' confidence 'by friendly treatment, and by actively promoting their comfort and real enjoyment'.[53] Those who were skilful in doing so promoted recovery and might also quieten a patient previously agitated through insensitive handling by another attendant. Take, for example, the case of a demented patient in 1863:

14 September. The strength and size of her frame together with her violence, had so intimidated her present nurse so as to be in a great degree, incapacitating her from properly managing her.

26 October. A great improvement has taken place in the state of this patient since the change of nurse, now nearly six weeks ago. She is constantly at the nurse's side, who takes her about with her wherever she goes and when she is inclined to strike herself or tear her clothes, takes hold of her hand, and in this gentle way has succeeded in hindering her from ever injuring herself or destroying her garments. She has never been put in seclusion for this period, and there is a reasonable hope that she may be entirely broken in the course of time of her violent, destructive and dirty habits. She is generally very gentle in her manners, smiling quietly and smiling when spoken to and answering in a subdued and quiet manner.[54]

Sometimes, it was less a case of defective professional ability on the part of the attendant than a clash of personality with the patient that caused problems. A patient wrote that her nurse was 'a conscientious person, and that she has done her best in her most unenviable post, but she has a way that provokes my miserable and unsubdued spirit exceedingly'.⁵⁵ In these circumstances it was usual to allow the patient to change galleries and thus move under the care of a different attendant as in this example from 1852:

> 22 May. I have allowed him to change places with another patient in W. Waller's gallery, as he still makes heavy complaints of T. Holmes being very unkind to him, and thinks T. H. would injure him if he could. Although I consider this a delusion, it may perhaps be better to allow him to change.
>
> 21 June. He has seemed more composed and comfortable since he has been with his attendant and the more regular employment which has been required of him has been beneficial.⁵⁶

Let us now turn to the attendant, William Waller, and see how he viewed his patients. The recent discovery of his private papers allows us for the first time to gain a fuller appreciation of this hidden dimension within the asylum, although one that is still tantalisingly brief about day-to-day attitudes and feelings.

WILLIAM WALLER

> WANTED, at the Friends' Retreat, near York, a Young or Middle-aged MAN, as an ATTENDANT on the PATIENTS. One who has been in House Service will be preferred and none need apply who cannot read and write, and whose Moral Character will not bear strict enquiry.
>
> For other particulars of the situation apply to the Resident Surgeon at the Retreat. (Yorkshire Gazette, 25 November 1843)

This was the advertisement that William Waller read in the local newspaper and that led him to apply for the post in December 1843, thus beginning his employment as an attendant at the Retreat that was to last until 1856. At the time of his application he was twenty-four years old and was working as a groom near Malton some seventeen miles from York. This information, together with comparable information about the sixteen others who applied, was minuted by members of the Retreat committee who interviewed him. In Waller's case – uniquely in the history of the Victorian lunatic asylum – we can supplement this meagre record by his own personal papers.⁵⁷

William Waller had been born an illegitimate pauper in Burythorpe, a tiny hamlet between York and Malton, in 1820. He was brought up by foster-parents who ran a school and who educated him to a standard that gave him unusual powers of literate self-expression for one who had had such humble beginnings. Before working as a groom he had spent five years as a coachman to the gentry household of William Preston at Burythorpe House and had also worked for a short period at the local savings bank. His choice of job was motivated both by ambition (his private motto was 'Progress'), and by the desire to have sufficient autonomy to pursue an intensely religious style of life. On 3 May 1839 he had been converted to Wesleyan Methodism – and his religious faith now dictated his life. His journal recorded, 'My blind eyes were opened. I felt my need of a Saviour. And from that time I was determined to serve God.'[58] And his diary recorded that it was because his existing job as the groom at an inn left him insufficient time for religious thought and worship that he resolved to apply to the Retreat.[59]

Waller was determined to succeed and took the precaution on Monday, 27 November, of seeing John Thurnam at the Retreat to obtain further information about the vacancy. He set out from Malton at 3 a.m. to walk to the institution, where he recorded:

I had an interview with the resident Surgeon and was received kindly and questioned about my age and previous employment and relatives, habits of life, and many more questions.[60]

Thurnam must have been agreeably impressed as he told Waller to return on Friday to be interviewed by a committee at the Friends Meeting House.

The candidates were interviewed by six members of the Committee of Management of the Retreat – Samuel Tuke, David Priestman, Robert Walker, James Backhouse, Joseph Spence and James H. Tuke. The minutes of their meeting recorded seventeen candidates for the two vacant posts. Their ages ranged from twenty-one to forty-two years and only two were married. All but one came from York, or villages nearby, of which Waller's was the farthest from York. Seven of them, including Waller, met the advertisement's specification of being in service, seven were artisans or craftsmen and three were employed by institutions as porter or keeper. It is interesting that, as in 1841, those who had had previous work experience as keepers in an asylum were rejected. Instead, the choice fell on the oldest candidate, a forty-two-year-old butler called Richard Hammond, and on William Waller himself.[61]

Waller recorded his experience at interview in some detail. His exaggeration of certain features – increasing the number of applicants from seventeen to twenty-five – and his dramatisation of the occasion suggest the importance he attached to it:

> In my turn I appeared before the Broad-Brimmed Sages, meeting their kind but keen, searching glances. With a truthfulness which knew no artifice or mental reservation they asked me for my testimonials. I replied I had none but answered them by saying that they might write to my former employers. I then was told that I might wait half an hour. I did so. In the mean time all the other candidates except one were dismissed ... excellence of character was the test. I left the room shortly afterwards and by 3 p.m. was walking back to my lodgings beyond Malton. There I arrived at 8:30 p.m. tired and footsore having walked about 48 miles. My expenses amount to 10½d. 4 days after by post I received a letter from the resident surgeon stating that my testimonials of 6 years servitude in my two last situations had been received. I was elected.[62]

Waller was appointed to be under-attendant at the Lodge, where a few high-fee-paying patients were cared for in accommodation separate from that of the main category of patients at the Retreat.

Waller's initial elation at his appointment was soon to be deflated when he took up his duties on 8 December 1843 and

> was shown by a Friend into my new quarters, was told that I was to have board and lodgings, washing and medical attendance and £18 per annum. Well, I thought, this is going down the ladder instead of up.[63]

His confidence in himself and his high estimation of his own abilities were to be shaken still further, this time by his new social and professional situation. The Retreat evidently believed in forcing attendants to learn their job by reaction to situations rather than by prior instruction. Their prior concern to recruit candidates of good character and sense now became fully explicable. Waller recorded his first few minutes 'on the job' with his own frightened reactions in illuminating detail:

> I brought my mind down to my circumstances and was shown into a room where by the fire sat a tall gentleman, a Welshman. A law student with a suit of clothes locked on that he might not pull them off, and so destroy them. He looked at me sternly and said 'Unto me! you fiend you. What do you want here?' This he repeated twice; not liking his companionship. I backed towards the door but found to my astonishment and dismay that it fastened with a spring-lock. And the brass han-

dle was all useless – only made and placed there for the sake of appearances. I edged round the room, and standing in one corner, stood some 15 or 20 minutes ready to defend myself if needful but [the] odds were greatly against me. He came not near me but remained seated and I was relieved from my position by the appearance of the head attendant.[64]

The patient was case 669; the medical notes on his background and behaviour were remarkably similar to Waller's own comments. If Waller was indeed left alone with this patient for a quarter of an hour, it was a rude introduction to his new occupation since the doctor had commented about the patient, 'when left to himself he is not violent but becomes extremely so if approached by the attendant'.[65]

In spite of his first misgivings Waller soon settled down and did well. His salary, as under-attendant at the Lodge, was raised by two pounds after fourteen months, and then again by the same sum to twenty-two pounds in September 1845. By the following year he was felt to be sufficiently capable to become an attendant in the Second Gallery at twenty-six pounds per annum and by 1851 was earning thirty-one pounds in that situation. The next year he received further promotion to that of upper-attendant in the Men's First Gallery, and there he also received two further increments in salary. By April 1854, with a salary of thirty-five pounds, he had almost doubled his salary in a decade of service and was amongst the higher paid of the Retreat's attendants.[66] How then did he view his own progress and his duties?

He took a very conscientious view of his responsibilities and adopted a high moral tone when discussing the extent to which his own private life could impinge on his employment. In a letter explaining why he might be unable to attend a meeting held outside York he wrote:

I am a servant and as such I feel my master's interests to be identified with my own and I wish to do my duty. And when my own gratification is obtained at the expense of the neglect of known duty to my employer I lay myself open to the charge of unfaithfulness and dishonesty in the sight of both God and man.[67]

On the other hand he considered that his duties to God, as we have seen earlier, must not be forgotten because of a total commitment to earthly matters. Presumably these values help to explain why Waller was chosen by the upright and religiously inclined Quaker members of the Retreat's committee. Initially, they were sympathetic towards the exercise of his religious faith even if it was different from their own. Waller recorded in his journal:

> Here I have an opportunity of attending the Chapel every Sunday evening. And before I entered upon my duties I was determined to have Thursday evenings to myself for the especial purpose of meeting in class. Made this a part of my Agreement: one of the conditions upon which I accepted the situation.[68]

Waller's religion was not confined to his meetings and chapel but permeated his entire life, and so it was through religious spectacles that he viewed his work as an attendant. The difficulties of his work were depicted with the fervour of the Victorian evangelical who saw the commonplace happening infused with the light of its ultimate significance for his individual salvation. 'Again, hath God in his Love and infinite Compassion opened out my way: to his name be all praise. On this day I have entered upon my duties as under-attendant.'[69] The manner in which Waller chronicled his feelings about his work was that of a religious journal. This format both helps us (in illuminating how he saw his work as a religious vocation), and hinders us (in overdramatising situations as did much literature of this type). Typically, Waller abased himself before God as a 'sinful worm of the earth' and called on divine help to sustain him in the terrible tribulations that he was forced to endure. Yet if some of this exaggeration is discounted we are left with a remarkable document of self-relevation: an authentic view of the asylum from a rarely chronicled standpoint.

The strain of working as an under-attendant in the Second Gallery where, together with a fellow attendant Thomas Holmes, he had responsibility for nineteen patients, was apparent in an entry written in July 1847:

> My trials have been great while engaged as attendant on the afflicted in body and mind, and I feel I need the grace of patience, and also humility to enable me to act and think aright, and to walk as becometh the gospel.[70]

Further references indicated that he felt these trials at work were continuing. In June 1851 he became more specific about the nature of some of these problems:

A hidden dimension: the asylum attendant 161

The past three months has been a time of trial – and difficulty – so far as regards the duty of a servant placed in circumstances of danger. At times almost at a loss how to act as to best discharge my duty to my employer and those under my care. I have felt that I needed help from above.[71]

Although it is not possible to pin-point the precise nature of the danger to which Waller alludes, the circumstances were likely to have been the control of a violent patient without recourse to mechanical restraint. Earlier discussion in this chapter has emphasised the physical punishment that might be meted out to attendants by excited or deluded patients in their care.

In spite of his perplexities and adversities Waller continued to feel a profound sympathy for the insane individuals he looked after. Two verses from the long poem he wrote about his patients suggested, in lighter vein than his customary manner, the springs of his motivation:

> Let willing hearts and ready hands
> Entwine by sympathy the bands
> And all unite in the favoured plan
> And true service render his fellow man
>
> Record the truth; tis all we ask
> Whilst engaged in the task
> Which heaven hath to us assigned
> To soothe and cheer the darkened mind.[72]

In this same year of 1856, when he was thirty-six years old, he also wrote a lengthy evaluation of his work that was part of a larger stock-taking of his spiritual progress through life. This lacked the rhetoric of earlier passages in his journal and its simplicity conveyed Waller's sincerity.

I have now arrived at the noon of life – half of the journey of life is finished. And how stand my accounts? Am I progressing in the divine life? I feel that it is no easy task to faithfully discharge the duties of my position as attendant on the Insane to control the violent and unruly. By a firmness of attitude which bids [i.e. commands] defiance and disarms all provocation. And on the other hand to bend the mind down to the level of true pity and sympathy with the timid and fearful. To soothe and allay the fears of a distorted imagination. To try to guide into the right way the brother of affliction with a mind disordered (not diseased). These duties are not easily discharged if faithful to the trust reposed in me by my employers. I wish, I more than wish, I strive to do my duty and yet after all my efforts I fail to come up to the standard laid down by myself.[73]

Here Waller laid down his objectives clearly and evaluated his performance truthfully giving us for the first time the viewpoint of that most essential but hidden cog in the bureaucratic machine of asylum life.

His eventual resignation from service at the Retreat was also instructive since the circumstances that led up to it suggest the power structure of the Victorian asylum and the lowly status of the attendant within it. They also confirm the presence of certain features in his personality and the strength of his religious conviction. Waller was a proud man, as his reference to his earlier employment as '6 years servitude' had indicated. The appointment of Dr Kitching as superintendent in 1849 led to the introduction of a more authoritarian style of management that was resented by William Waller. His diary recorded 'received a check [i.e. reprimand] from John Kitching on Monday morning March 18th 1850'. Then followed a revealing addition in pencil, 'He may lead me – I wont be driven by any man.' As an attendant Waller did not have a lot of contact with the superintendent so that his antipathy could be kept within bounds. But in 1856 this situation changed, because in August he took up new duties as coachman to the institution.[74] It may be assumed that he felt this post would be more suitable when he married, as he planned to do the following month. On his marriage to Elizabeth Slee[75] (who worked as a nurse to private patients at the Retreat), the institution provided a cottage for the couple within the grounds. But within a few months Waller resigned because, as his diary explained,

one month after my marriage I found that my duties included sabbath labour and consequent deterioration of body and soul. Deprivation from the means of grace. And not a work of necessity but for mere worldly show and to increase my labour. Spoken to sometimes *like* a dog. And told by J. K. that as a servant he considered me as such. And that for no fault of my own. But having refused to tell a lie to screen him for neglect, abuse and scorn is heaped upon me, and my position made afterwards unbearable by the lordly pride and domineering manner of the man who is placed in authority over me. This treatment after a service of thirteen years and three months in an institution for the insane and after giving prompt obedience to all calls either by night or day. Keeping regular

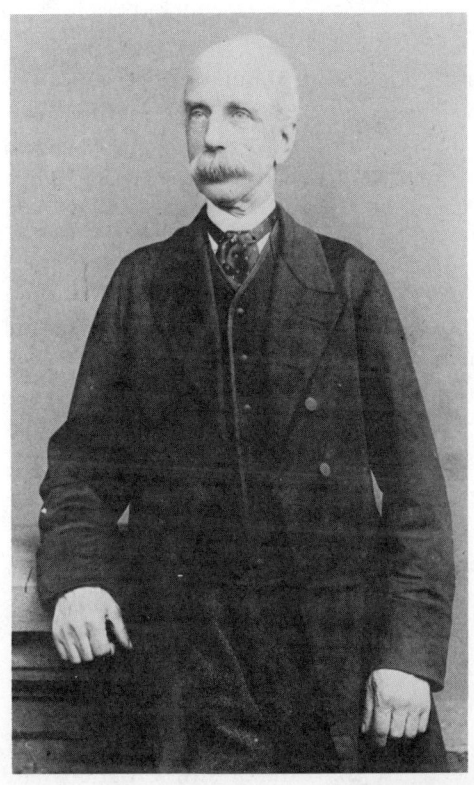

Plate 22. William Waller

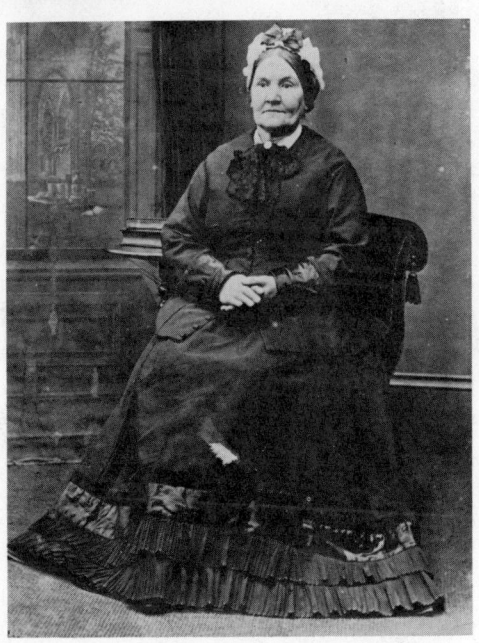

Plate 23. Elizabeth Slee

hours and serving with all sobriety and with faithfulness, honest in deed, truthful in words, striving to walk discreetly. And after all, meeting with such a reward . . . I resigned determined to trust in God and my own exertions for to obtain the bread that perisheth. Equally determined whatever I lose or gain never to forfeit my trust and hope in God. And never for any money to again work on the sabbath.[76]

The precise occasion for Waller's disagreement with the superintendent, John Kitching, remains obscure. However, it seems probable that if one incident had not led to a personal confrontation between the two men another would soon have occurred. Not only was there a conflict of personality between a peremptory master and an independent-minded subordinate but the latter's intense resentment at his Sunday duties was likely to magnify or distort any reprimand he received. In this context it is instructive to learn from his journal that he had earlier left service with a kind master, William Preston, because he felt that his brother, Thomas Preston, 'persecuted him' 'on account of my religion'.[77] Waller now acted sensibly – perhaps recognising that his unconquered will required the autonomy of self-employment – and began to act first as a free-lance mental nurse to private patients, before getting his own house licensed for the care of single patients in 1863.

In company with other working-class autobiographers Waller was obviously unusual in having an intense inner life, independent spirit and eloquent powers of self-expression. Yet precisely because of these atypical characteristics we can begin to appreciate attitudes that he may have shared in some degree with others in his occupation. Waller spoke of his job not only in terms of duty but also as a trust, and he described the qualities he saw as desirable in it. Towards his employers he tried to live up to the contemporary stereotype of faithful, obedient, honest and sober service. More interestingly, in the context of this chapter, we learn that he felt both sympathy and pity towards the insane. And he saw it not only as his function to soothe or cheer his patients, but also to allay their fears and to attempt to guide their thoughts in right channels. He tried to anticipate situations, to disarm provocation and to control unruliness or violence. In these complex tasks he was sustained both by his sense of religious vocation and by what appears to have been a genuine affection for his charges. In displaying these attitudes, values and qualities, Waller was practis-

A hidden dimension: the asylum attendant

ing many of the ideals that were later to be formulated for the profession of psychiatric nursing.

FROM ATTENDANT TO MENTAL NURSE

No subject connected with the management of the insane, either in asylums or in private practice, has received less adequate attention than the selection of proper attendants, their proper treatment, their just government, and their instruction in the various, and peculiar, and exhausting duties which necessarily devolve upon them.[78]

Writing in 1847, John Conolly was one of the few to recognise the crucial importance of the attendant if the system of non-restraint was to be successfully implemented. Although the Commissioners in Lunacy recognised the truth of this assertion and attempted in the 1850s, 1860s and 1870s to persuade asylum managers to offer better salaries in order to attract a superior class of attendant, their efforts had minimal impact. It was not until the 1880s when asylum superintendents themselves saw its importance that some progress towards training the attendant began. With the benefit of hindsight it is difficult to see why it took nearly thirty years for asylum superintendents to initiate this when so much depended on the ability of the attendant. It is possible that a lofty view from the pinnacle of the asylum hierarchy inhibited understanding of staff interdependence and that this was reinforced by Victorian society's more general undervaluation of the nursing role. Tight financial constraints within the asylum may also have made it difficult to offer higher salaries to better qualified recruits who would have been prepared to undertake such training. However, in 1885 the Medico-Psychological Association, the professional organisation for asylum doctors, published the *Handbook for the Instruction of Attendants on the Insane*. And five years later the association adopted the *Report on the Training of Nurses*, which recommended three months' probation followed by two years' theoretical and practical training in the asylum. Mental nurses were to have clinical instruction, lectures and demonstrations, as well as private study, scheduled for them in order that they could sit an examination to gain a certificate of proficiency from the association. In describing the ideal nurse the *Report* recognised that character, experience and training were requisite:

Table 7.2. *Length of attendants' service in 1896*

	Under 2 years	2–5 years	5–10 years	10–20 years	Over 20 years
Male	8	5	3	6	4
Female	11	15	4	2	2

Source: Retreat Report (1896).

The mental attributes of a really good attendant can be divided into three groups: – *Morality,* including steadiness, sobriety, trustworthiness etc.; *Suitability,* including general aptitude, firmness of purpose, control of temper, courage, intelligent and patient application of knowledge to cases, and that indescribable element of compatibility with insane people which is necessary to make control at all acceptable to patients; and lasting *proficiency,* arising from experience and careful training.[79]

Under Dr Pierce the Retreat took a lead in implementing these measures intended to transform the attendant into the professional mental nurse. In this he was undoubtedly helped by the increasing stability of staffing (see Table 7.2). By 1894 Retreat attendants were attending lectures and demonstrations given by the medical officers on anatomy, physiology and general as well as mental nursing in order to take the examination for the Medico-Psychological Association's Nursing Certificate.[80] Eight years later the York institution promoted its own four-year training scheme in which nurses who had the two-year certificate could continue with the series of lectures and also attend classes in medical gymnastics, massage and invalid cookery in order to earn the Retreat's own Certificate of Proficiency. To be considered proficient nurses needed to show 'satisfactory evidence of moral character, good health, general intelligence, and fitness of disposition'. In their fourth year nurses continuing to give evidence of meritorious service were eligible for the William Tuke Medal. The medal's motto *Cum bona voluntate servientes* (with good will doing service) encapsulated the best in the Retreat's tradition of nursing.[81] By 1907 thirty-two nurses (twenty-five women and seven men) had earned the medal and a further five long-serving members of staff had been awarded it *honoris causa*. By this time seventy-five women and seventeen men had obtained the national certificate, and thirty of them had received the Retreat's own certificate.[82]

A hidden dimension: the asylum attendant

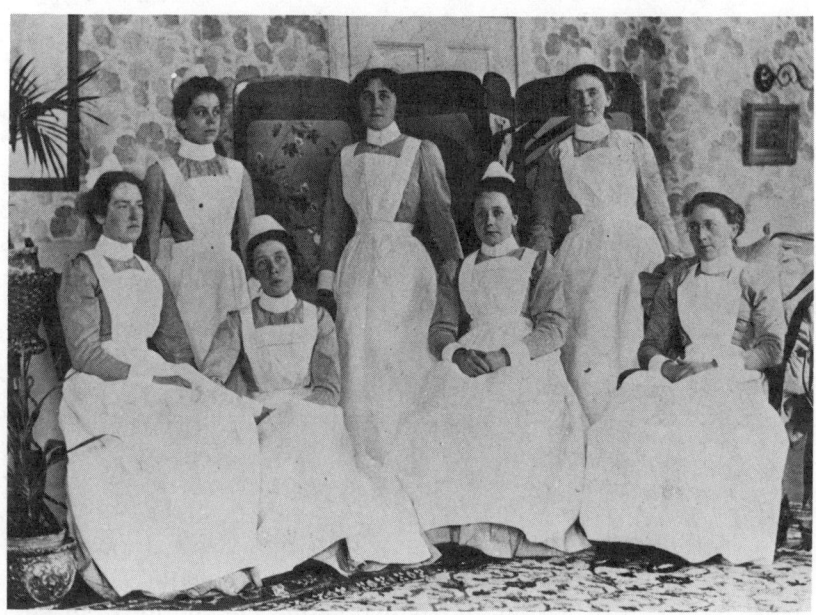

Plate 24. Nurses in c. 1900. E. Rowntree is on the left.

With approximately half its staff having been trained the Retreat found that there were more trained staff than it could promote to permanent positions.[83] In 1902 it therefore opened a private nursing department so that trained nurses could be sent out to nurse 'mental or nervous cases' in their own homes for periods of up to three months. The venture was so successful that in 1910 nurses were invited to participate in it on the basis not only of salary, but also a commission on earnings and a share of half the profits.[84]

Bedford Pierce was concerned to have not only trained nurses but a cadre of 'intelligent, high-principled women' who would see it as a 'vocation'. He argued that although such women went into ordinary nursing, they did not enter mental nursing even though their social gifts and accomplishments would be much more useful in the asylum than in the general hospital.[85] To some extent he was echoing the call of his predecessor, Dr Baker, nearly twenty years before,[86] but Pierce was sufficiently successful in improving the conditions and status of the Retreat nurses to be able to recruit some women of good family. One such was Ethelwyn Rowntree, who found enjoyment and fulfilment in nursing and was awarded the William Tuke Medal in 1905.[87]

Bedford Pierce did much to improve conditions of service for

Table 7.3. *Timetables of nurses in 1902*

	Day nurse	Night nurse
Breakfast	6.30 a.m. (7 on Sunday)	8 p.m.
On duty	7.00 a.m.	8.30 p.m.
Dinner	Noon or 1 p.m.	—
Tea	4.30 or 5 p.m.	—
Off duty	8.30 p.m.	7.50 a.m.
In bedrooms	10.00 p.m.	—
In bed and lights out	10.30 p.m.	9 a.m. (Wednesday & Saturday) 11.30 a.m. (other days)

Source: *Rules for Nurses at the Retreat*, 1902.

his mental nurses although a review of these by Edwardian times indicated just how poor they had been earlier. The Nurses Home, which had opened in 1898, provided some, but by no means all, nurses with their own bedrooms, and the remainder continued to sleep in patients' rooms. Beginning in 1894 nurses ate separately from patients, and by 1900 they also had an hour free each day away from their charges. In that same year they were given one day off each week or a half day and Sunday leave instead of two evenings (or equivalent) leave. Their hours of work remained long: beginning at 7 a.m., they did not finish work until 8.30 p.m. (see Table 7.3). In 1911 a reduction in hours brought the weekly total worked below the figure of seventy recommended by a Select Committee of the House of Commons. The amount of holiday was increased from one to two weeks in 1897, and to two or three weeks according to seniority by 1902. In 1908 the Retreat undertook to assist trained nurses with half their annual premium to the National Pension Fund for Nurses.[88]

This professionalisation of asylum staff helped to reinforce the authority of the medical superintendent since if the attendant was converted into a trained nurse she was more likely to defer to the expertise of the doctor.[89] In various ways the Retreat nurse was made to feel that she worked not in an asylum but in a hospital. Two obvious signs of this transformation were the adoption of a nurses' uniform in 1893 and the creation of a nursing hierarchy in 1901 when ward sisters were introduced on the pattern of general

A hidden dimension: the asylum attendant

hospitals.[90] In 1897 the institution's regulations emphasised the responsibility of the nursing staff for the security of drugs and the distribution of medicine to patients.

Concepts of duty and conditions of service were changing and with them the status of nurses in the staff hierarchy. This is obvious if we contrast the social links between an élite of trained nurses and doctors (which by 1905 were sufficiently fraternal for them to make up holiday parties to the Continent)[91] with the social chasm that had existed earlier between untrained attendants and doctors. An illuminating insight into this was given by Dr Pierce's private observations on his attendants, made soon after his appointment in 1892, which revealed a lofty censoriousness towards his staff. (This appears to have been similar to the attendant's book kept at Ticehurst by Hayes Newington, who was prominent in the Medico-Psychological Association's attempts to improve the quality of asylum attendance.) Pierce's comments suggested that his ideal was a reliable, teetotal, hard-working and polite subordinate. That he wanted his staff to know their place was evident from his dislike of individuals who he considered were 'opinionated' or who 'put on airs' or 'side'. Obedience was ranked highly, as in revealing comments such as 'Reliable [but] not inclined to assist officers in finding out things'.[92] Pierce demanded loyalty to the institution and this was inserted into the 1897 regulations, which stated that attendants were not to bring discredit on the institution. He expected this to be taken literally and disapproved of the behaviour of Sarah Grainger, who was called to give evidence in the Onions case. He commented that she had 'come out badly re F. Onions. Was not loyal to the Retreat then. Professes sorrow'. Since this nurse had given the key evidence that Onions had struck a patient one must wonder whether Pierce saw loyalty, and the preservation of the good name of the institution, as overriding all other considerations. We have seen from Waller's bitter remarks that Kitching also expected employees to 'fall into line' and displayed comparable authoritarianism toward his subordinates. Such domineering attitudes were acceptable within the hierarchical ordering of nineteenth-century society, and their impact was intensified in the enclosed world of the Victorian asylum. But Pierce was sufficiently enlightened to utilise his clear-sighted perception of attendants' deficiencies to try to overcome them by a positive training programme.

In the mid-nineteenth century the Retreat had recognised that patients' 'welfare, security, and comfort' were 'in great measure' the responsibility of its attendants,[93] but it had done little to lighten that responsibility until Pierce's regime. Although their duties were recognised as important, attendants' low status and poor pay were little better than those of general servants. But the Retreat did provide more generous staffing to ease the burden of long hours and exacting work, and attempted by careful recruitment and a probationary period to select and retain only those with an aptitude for the work. That they were apparently successful in this was suggested by the small number of dismissals known to be the result of violence to patients. Intemperance or lack of vigilance was a more typical cause of notice being given to attendants.[94] However, the record of hiring and dismissal was incomplete, and any minuted evidence on reasons for dismissal was so circumspect that it revealed little. For example, the minutes concerning the first attendant to be given notice stated, 'It appearing "necessary" to part with Joshua Cordingley, the Keeper of the Men Patients, he hath been informed thereof.'[95] And it was only private correspondences of the period that revealed it was Cordingley's lack of vigilance, and the ensuing suicide of his patient, that caused his dismissal.[96] Yet in spite of gaps in the evidence the general impression remains that the Retreat's record was notably better than that in the public asylums of the period, where violence to patients was much more obvious and their deaths at the hands of attendants not unknown.[97] The Retreat managers put their trust in the good character and upright values of those they selected shrewdly and continued to observe carefully. Emphasis on moral character was evident not only in the days of the untrained attendant but was also recognised as important in the later period of the mental nurse. This was an implicit recognition of the continuing truth of Esquirol's statement: 'To truly benefit the lunatic one must love him and devote oneself to him.'[98]

8

Patients

This chapter falls into two distinct but complementary sections. The first part analyses in mainly quantitative terms the changing social composition and personal characteristics of the 2,011 patients who were admitted to the Retreat in the time of six superintendents who held office from 1796 to 1910. The second part is qualitative rather than quantitative, impressionistic, not precise, and tries to evoke some of the dominant features of asylum life both as it affected and was seen by patients. As the chapter proceeds we progress from external and measurable features of the patient as seen by others to the attitudes and feelings of the patients themselves. It is perhaps a commentary on the asylum that while there is almost too much information on the first objective world of the patient, evidence on their subjectively felt experience was often absent. And although the abundance of data on the external patient world facilitated a dynamic analysis of changes in the Retreat, the relative lack of information on the patient's internal world produced a static view. It is possible that the latter presented – though inadvertently – a more authentic view for an individual patient when faced with the apparent timelessness of asylum routine within a stay of uncertain duration.

The first part of this chapter summarises and comments on some of the results of a computer-based analysis of the patients who were in the Retreat from June 1796 to December 1910. Further results are given in Chapter 9. Included in the analysis were 2,011 individuals and, since readmissions were not infrequent, these made up 2,525 cases. The Retreat's documentation was in the form of cases rather than patients, and for certain purposes the data had to be reorganised so as to reconstitute the case histories of individuals – a time-consuming and laborious process. However, in this and the succeeding chapter, most of the data are presented in the form of first admissions. This has the effect of magnifying changes that were taking place in the character of the asylum. In considering this point it is perhaps helpful to think of an analogy: the familiar distinction between the number of births and the total population. Thus, it is important to appreciate when looking at the statistical tables in this chapter that the changing nature of first admissions took a further period of time before it decisively influenced whole asylum population. This is made clear if, for example, Table 8.1 is compared with Figure 5.1; we can see that the decline in Quaker first admissions becomes evident in Table 8.1 some years before Figure 5.1 suggests that the overall religious affiliation of the asylum's population had become predominantly non-Quaker.

Evidence on the asylum's patients was unusually complete, although becoming increasingly fragmentary by the end of our period, thus making it necessary to end the analysis in 1910. One of the principal sources of information utilised for this computerised analysis was the series of admissions certificates that, except for a missing volume for 1908 and some missing individual certificates at the start of our period, provided a fairly continuous series. However, gaps in the record for the early years could be filled by the well-kept admissions registers extant for the years from 1796 to 1879. A rich source of supplementary information was the series of seventeen medical case-books, which though incomplete under the first superintendent, provided excellent detail until the 1890s. Unfortunately, the rest of the case-books have not been discovered so that data on important topics such as the outcome of treatment were missing for the late nineteenth and early twentieth centuries. Finally, a useful summary is available consisting of patients' religious background, fees paid and duration of stay in a tabulated return of admissions for the period under consideration.[1]

The data on patients are presented for six subperiods or eras in order to highlight the changing profile of the asylum under its successive superintendents. Patients are included under the superintendent in whose tenure of office they were first admitted. This means that even if the period of treatment spanned more than one therapist, or alternatively if the patient was readmitted to the asylum under a later superintendent, the patient will appear in the statistics only once. For the sake of analytical completeness George Jepson's tenure has been extended backwards to the actual opening of the asylum in June 1796, and this first era ends with his retirement in March 1823. Thomas Allis's tenure of the office of superintendent was taken from his appointment in April 1823 to his notice of resignation in September 1841. The third period has been seen as that of John Thurnam, who although not formally superintendent until 1847 had effectively gained supremacy even before Allis's retirement.[2] This third era was taken to run from October 1841 to June 1849. Thereafter, the record was straightforward: John Kitching (July 1849 to June 1874); Robert Baker (July 1874 to September 1892); and Bedford Pierce (October 1892 to the end of our analysis in December 1910).

THE CHANGING SOCIAL CHARACTER
OF PATIENTS

The most dramatic change in the social character of the Retreat is shown in Table 8.1, where the difference between an almost exclusively Quaker asylum under Jepson and a preponderantly non-Quaker one by the time of Baker or Pierce emerged clearly. (In this and succeeding tables percentages are calculated on known cases since there is no reason to think that the proportion of cases in each category differed substantially among those unknown.) Whereas only 3.9 per cent had no connection at all with the Society of Friends in the first period, 74.2 per cent had no such link by our final period. During this period too, the proportion of patients sent by Friends' Meetings declined even more markedly from one in four to one in twenty-five patients, suggesting a much more tenuous relationship between the asylum and the wider community of Friends. The growing group of patients with no religious affiliation to the Society of Friends became increasingly heterogeneous: earlier it featured Nonconformists particularly, but Anglicans later became more significant and there were also a few individuals from other sects, including a Roman Catholic nun from York and a Jewess from Bradford.[3] The watershed in the changing religious character of the Retreat's patients occurred under Dr Baker, and as we shall see later, was associated also with a change in the social class of patients and their geographical origins. A class of patients who made up a slightly more constant proportion of the whole were those connected with the Society of Friends (e.g. through regular attendance at Quaker Meetings) but without formal membership. This group was very close to that of the Quaker

Table 8.1. *Religious affiliation of first admissions (in %)*

	J	A	T	K	B	P	O[a]
Quaker	87.6	68.4	58.9	59.8	30.5	20.7	45.8
Connected with Society of Friends	8.5	15.1	14.7	9.3	8.0	5.1	8.6
Other religious affiliation	3.9	16.5	26.4	30.9	61.5	74.2	45.6
N	259	218	129	333	439	609	1,987
Affiliation unknown	1	—	—	1	1	21	24

[a] J, Jepson (1796–1823); A, Allis (1823–41); T, Thurnam (1841–9); K, Kitching (1849–74); B, Baker (1874–92); P, Pierce (1892–1910); O, Overall (1796–1910).

Table 8.2. *Gender of first admissions (in %)*

	J	A	T	K	B	P	O[a]
Male	46.2	50.9	51.2	41.9	46.6	38.7	44.1
Female	53.8	49.1	48.8	58.1	53.4	61.3	55.9
N	260	218	129	334	440	630	2,011

[a] J, Jepson (1796–1823); A, Allis (1823–41); T, Thurnam (1841–9); K, Kitching (1849–74); B, Baker (1874–92); P, Pierce (1892–1910); O, Overall (1796–1910).

patients, and in the analyses that follow Quakers and those connected with the Society of Friends will be subsumed into one group when cross-tabulations are made relating religious affiliation to other personal characteristics of patients.

Whereas religious affiliation underwent marked and cumulative changes, the gender composition of the Retreat's patients under different superintendents showed less clear-cut trends, as Table 8.2 indicates. Women usually outnumbered men although the difference in the proportions of the sexes showed a widening, if fluctuating, disparity. This trend reflected that in other mental institutions during our period, where a steadily increasing proportion of women was generally attributed to their lower mortality and

Table 8.3. *Marital status of first admissions (in %)*

	J	A	T	K	B	P	O[a]
Single	68.9	61.5	64.3	60.3	52.1	54.1	58.2
Married	21.5	28.9	27.9	30.4	37.7	37.9	32.7
Widowed	9.6	9.6	7.8	9.3	10.2	8.0	9.1
N	260	218	129	332	440	562	1,941
Marital status unknown	—	—	—	2	—	68	70

[a] J, Jepson (1796–1823); A, Allis (1823–41); T, Thurnam (1841–9); K, Kitching (1849–74); B, Baker (1874–92); P, Pierce (1892–1910); O, Overall (1796–1910).

hence longer duration of stay.[4] This reinforced the fact that in any case women outnumbered men in the general population of England and Wales by between 3 and 6 per cent during our period.[5] But the experience of the Retreat was unusual in the early nineteenth century in that men outnumbered women in most other private mental institutions, but did not do so at first at York. That the number of women exceeded men at the Retreat in these early years may perhaps be partly accounted for by the fact that women outnumbered men in the Society of Friends to a greater extent than in society generally – since male Friends were more likely to resign or be expelled from membership.[6] It is also possible that whereas in society as a whole expensive medical treatment was looked on as a form of investment particularly suited for the male bread-winner, the subsidised treatment available at the Retreat was an inducement for women to be sent there. In this context it is significant that a disproportionately large number of female patients were paid for, not by their families, but by Friends' Meetings. The growing preponderance of female over male patients towards the end of our period may well have been a response to contemporary psychiatry's stress on women's peculiar vulnerability to mental shipwreck.[7]

Table 8.3 reveals that single patients always predominated over the married or widowed. However, during our period there was an overall decline from two of three unmarried patients under Jepson to little more than one out of two under Baker and Pierce. This was the reflection of the growing numbers of non-Quaker patients. Whereas over the whole of our period 62.2 per cent of Quaker patients were unmarried, only 49.8 per cent of those of other religious affiliations unconnected with the Society of Friends were single.[8] Amongst Friends earlier restrictive regulations on 'marrying out' of the Society of Friends had led to a high level of celibacy.[9] Parallel to the declining proportion of single patients came an increase in the married, from about one in five under Jepson to more than one in three under Baker or Pierce. The widowed made up a small, but fluctuating, proportion of the total: a comparison of the marital status of Retreat patients with that revealed in the general population by census data in 1861 and 1881 indicated a similar proportion of widowed people.[10]

A study of the relation of marital status to gender in the composition of the Retreat's patients reveals that although women consistently outnumbered men among the single and the widowed (as might have been expected given the overall predominance of women over men in the asylum), there were often more married men than married women, and over the period as a whole numbers of married men and women were equal.[11] Why were married women relatively less prone to enter the asylum? It is possible that married women's responsibilities for children and the household made it less likely that treatment for a mental disorder would be considered for them at a distance from home. Evidence to support such a hypothesis comes from a number of premature removals of married women from the Retreat. For example, Jane H., who had three children of whom the youngest was only nine years old, was removed in 1829 before the satisfactory completion of her treatment because of domestic pressures.[12] This kind of case provides a thought-provoking corrective to contemporary alarmist literature on asylums, which often emphasised 'the abuses of vengeful husbands wrongfully confining sane wives'.[13]

Table 8.4 indicates that the age structure of the Retreat remained fairly constant, with the bulk of admissions being those in young adulthood and early middle age. (This 'bunching' was particularly noticeable among non-Quaker patients: over the whole period 70 per cent of them were aged between twenty-five and fifty-four on first admission compared to the 56 per cent of Quaker patients.) Retreat patients' age distribution was remarkably similar to that of other Victorian asylums for which comparable information is available – notably the York Asylum, Bowhill House in Exeter

Table 8.4. *Ages of first admissions (in %)*

	J	A	T	K	B	P	O[a]
Under 10	—	—	—	—	0.5	—	0.1
10–14	0.8	0.5	—	0.6	0.7	—	0.4
15–19	3.8	5.0	6.2	4.3	2.3	2.5	3.5
20–24	17.3	12.4	15.5	10.8	12.6	9.4	12.2
25–34	22.3	29.0	22.5	21.9	23.3	23.3	23.6
35–44	19.2	19.4	21.7	20.6	21.0	20.5	20.5
45–54	15.8	15.7	13.2	17.2	17.8	22.5	18.2
55–64	13.1	11.5	10.9	12.3	10.9	11.4	11.7
65–74	5.4	5.1	10.0	7.4	8.2	6.8	7.0
Over 75	1.5	1.4	—	4.9	2.7	3.6	2.8
N	260	217	129	325	438	561	1,930
Age unknown	—	1	—	9	2	69	81

[a] J, Jepson (1796–1823); A, Allis (1823–41); T, Thurnam (1841–9); K, Kitching (1849–74); B, Baker (1874–92); P, Pierce (1892–1910); O, Overall (1796–1910).

and the private houses at Hook Norton and Witney in Oxfordshire.[14] This age distribution contrasted markedly with that of the general population of England and Wales since whereas nearly one in two individuals was under twenty in a very youthful Victorian society, only about one in twenty-five was in this age group in the Retreat.[15] Dr Baker seems to have changed the policy of the York establishment towards the very young since he admitted two patients under the age of ten. This practice seems to have been unusual but not unprecedented: although the youngest patient recorded at Hook Norton or Witney was aged sixteen, a child of six and a half was admitted to Bowhill House. It is also evident that Drs Kitching, Baker and Pierce admitted relatively more septuagenarians than their predecessors had done. However, this growth in the proportion of the oldest patients pales into insignificance when contrasted with inpatient admissions to modern psychiatric institutions; in England during the early 1970s one in four admissions was aged sixty-five or older.[16] There was concern at the Retreat over the ageing nature of the patient body,[17] although this ageing process is not revealed by the figures in Table 8.4, which relate only to ages on admission.

The geographical origins of the Retreat's patients in the early part of our period when the asylum was predominantly Quaker were mainly a response to the distribution of members of the Society of Friends in Britain. In absolute numbers Friends were especially numerous in the mid-nineteenth century in large cities in the industrial north of England, and in London, Birmingham and Bristol. And in proportion to the rest of the population they were also relatively numerous in rural as well as urban areas in the north, and in the West Midlands, while being very thin on the ground in Wales and Scotland.[18] There were two main exceptions to this neat correlation. First, the strength of Quaker Meetings in the South Midlands (especially in Hertfordshire), and the eastern counties (particularly in Essex), might have been expected to generate more patients, and that this did not happen may have been due to successful local competition from private madhouses. Second, there were fewer patients both from the south-east and south-west than the local Quaker presence there might have been expected to produce, and this could have been because the distances involved militated against sending patients to York.

Paradoxically, Table 8.5 appears to show that in the period when the railway revolution made travelling easier, the distances that patients travelled to the Retreat for treatment became much shorter. Comparing the origins of Jepson's and Pierce's patients it is noticeable that whereas two-fifths of the former came from north of a line drawn from the Humber to the Mersey, seven-tenths of the latter came from the same area. Conversely, the proportion travelling from places south of a line from the Severn to the Wash was halved from two-fifths to one-fifth. The Retreat's shrinking hinterland suggests that its general 'pulling power' in the market for patients was declining. With the success of the non-restraint movement in the mid-nineteenth century, and the growth in the number of institutions claiming to practise the same mild methods promoted by the Retreat, families of prospective patients may have preferred to send their relatives to a nearby institution once they could see that the Retreat's therapy was no longer so distinctive. Indeed, Table 8.5 indicates that the Retreat's clientele moved overwhelmingly from being national to regional, and even, by the end of our period, local in origin. Whereas one-quarter of Jepson's patients came from Yorkshire one-half of Pierce's did so. But to some extent this is a misleading interpretation, as Table 8.6 re-

Table 8.5. *Geographical origins of first admissions (in %)*

	J	A	T	K	B	P	O[a]
London	12.0	8.3	14.7	10.8	7.0	6.7	8.9
S.E. Counties	4.2	5.0	4.7	5.1	3.4	4.3	4.3
S. Midland Counties	10.4	5.5	7.0	2.4	0.9	2.9	3.9
E. Counties	6.9	6.4	10.1	8.1	2.3	2.4	4.8
S.W. Counties	5.8	2.8	3.9	4.8	3.6	3.2	3.9
W. Midlands	13.9	9.7	10.1	8.7	3.9	2.9	6.7
N. Midlands	3.9	3.7	2.3	6.0	3.9	2.6	3.7
N.W. Counties	9.7	13.4	13.2	8.7	8.6	5.0	8.5
Yorkshire	24.3	27.2	20.1	30.5	53.4	54.0	41.0
N. Counties	7.3	13.8	6.2	12.2	11.4	13.6	11.6
Other places outside England	1.6	4.2	7.7	2.7	1.6	2.4	2.7
N	259	217	129	334	440	624	2,003
Origins unknown	1	1	—	—	—	6	8

Note: The geographical divisions are those used in the census grouping of English counties.
[a] J, Jepson (1796–1823); A, Allis (1823–41); T, Thurnam (1841–9); K, Kitching (1849–74); B, Baker (1874–92); P, Pierce (1892–1910); O, Overall (1796–1910).

veals. Quaker patients continued to be drawn nation-wide, and there was a striking similarity between the overall figures for all Quaker first admissions shown in Table 8.6, and those for the asylum in its Quaker heyday under Jepson, shown in Table 8.5. Table 8.6 shows us that the shrinking hinterland of the Retreat was due to its growing number of non-Quaker patients, 84 per cent of whom came from Yorkshire and its surrounding counties. The trend towards the recruitment of local patients who were not Quakers must have been accelerated by the growth of private practice under Dr Pierce, who attended consulting rooms in Leeds on two afternoons a week.

There was a certain irony in the fact that Friends thought it worthwhile to continue to send their relatives over not inconsiderable distances to the Retreat. Presumably, this was because its image remained that of a Quaker institution peculiarly suited for members of the Society of Friends, whereas in reality the character of the asylum was increasingly geared to the needs of growing

Table 8.6. *Geographical origins of Quaker and non-Quaker first admissions, 1796–1910 (in %)*

	Quakers[a]	Non-Quakers
London	12.1	5.0
S.E. Counties	6.2	2.2
S. Midland Counties	6.0	1.5
E. Counties	7.3	1.9
S.W. Counties	6.5	1.0
W. Midlands	10.9	1.6
N. Midlands	3.4	4.1
N.W. Counties	10.9	5.6
Yorkshire	24.0	61.1
N. Counties	10.1	13.2
Monmothshire and S. Wales	0.4	0.5
N. Wales	—	0.1
S. Scotland	0.5	1.3
N. Scotland	—	0.1
Islands	0.2	0.1
Ireland	1.2	0.4
Other places	0.3	0.3
N	1,079	902

Note: Out of 2,011 first admissions there was insufficient data on 30 patients for a cross-tabulation to be made.
[a] Includes patients connected with the Society of Friends.

numbers of non-Quaker patients. By the end of our period it was less a national institution for Friends than a Yorkshire establishment catering for an increasingly affluent clientele.

The economic circumstances of Retreat patients underwent considerable change from the late eighteenth to the early twentieth century. In 1796 William Tuke had considered that 'most of our patients are likely to be of the poorer sort', but this prediction was increasingly falsified by events.[19] We can see this by looking at both the changing social class of patients and the extent to which the Quaker community and the Retreat subsidised poorer patients' fees.

Under Jepson and Allis nearly one-third of the Retreat's patients were on subsidised terms, having either been admitted free in a few cases, or more usually on reduced rates after a recommendation by their local Meeting. William Tuke had reassured patients' relatives that 'the Committee [of Management] did not wish Friends to pay more than their circumstances would properly admit'.[20] In pursuit of this policy the lowest (or most subsidised) terms were maintained at only four shillings a week from 1796 to 1854, and the standard fee at eight shillings despite calculations in 1844 that the actual cost of maintaining such a patient was at least twelve shillings a week.[21] However, in 1854 financial expediency dictated that the very lowest terms should be raised to six shillings, in 1876 to ten shillings, and in 1890 to fourteen shillings. Some abatement came in 1898 (after economic retrenchment on household expenditure), when fees were reduced to twelve shillings, and our period ended in 1913, with a further rise to thirteen shillings. Between 1796 and 1910, 36.6 per cent of the Retreat's patients were known to have received treatment at these very low terms, and of these only 0.5 per cent were non-Quakers.

An important source of funds for the maintenance of these very reasonable terms for a substantial proportion of Quaker patients in the Retreat was the entry of high-fee-paying non-Quaker patients after 1820. In 1841 Samuel Tuke explained the rationale for their admission:

Only a limited number of patients unconnected with the Society of Friends is admitted into the Retreat, and they are all of the higher class in regard to payment. The lowest terms are two and a half guineas per week. P.S. The accommodations for patients of the highest class are very superior to what are found in private houses for the same terms.[22]

Fees for non-Quakers rose steadily and by 1910 the most affluent patients might be charged seven guineas a week. This enabled the Retreat as a non-profit-making charitable institution to subsidise a large proportion of its Quaker patients to a greater or lesser extent. In the last four decades of the nineteenth century 80 to 90 per cent of Quaker patients were treated at less than economic cost.[23] By 1893 the annual deficit on their accounts amounted to £2,000, which was met by transfers from the larger payments levied on growing numbers of non-Quaker patients.[24]

Long-term treatment for mental illness had devastating effects on the finances even of Quaker patients. For example, in 1800 a friend of Mary P., who had been receiving treatment for two years, wrote to William Tuke that the expenses attending her situation there has nearly exhausted the little property she possessed, and that her future maintenance will fall heavily on two unmarried sisters, who we believe can barely support themselves by the profit of a little shop.[25]

In such a case it was usual to have the patient nominated by her local Monthly Meeting, which because the Meeting had earlier subscribed £100 to the Retreat, enabled it under the asylum's rules to be charged only four shillings per week. Non-Quaker patients, for whom subsidy was not usually available, were removed in such circumstances and sent to a pauper asylum. It is interesting that by the 1890s local Quaker Meetings themselves began to adopt this practice. For example, a Quaker patient, Thomas R., was discharged in 1891 from the Retreat and 'taken in charge by the Relieving Officer with a view to being re-certified as a pauper patient'.[26] Three years later it was publicly disclosed that Monthly Meetings were withdrawing patients because the Retreat's lowest charges were now higher than at rate-aided pauper asylums, presumably because of the rise in the lowest terms to fourteen shillings in 1890. The Retreat's managers vainly attempted to stem this trend because

such removals to pauper asylums, however well-equipped many of these now are, seem to be especially undesirable when the mental condition of the patient is such that they are able to appreciate their surroundings.[27]

The Lunacy Commissioners had recognised the force of the charitable principle at the Retreat in 1870:

In the generally small sums that are charged for the very superior accommodation afforded here, we recognize strongly the benefits and usefulness of such an establishment as this, guided by the kindly principles of helping each other on which the Society of Friends first founded the Retreat. The principle is not so strong now as it used to be.[28]

In spite of its weakening, however, the original idea of matching accommodation to state of mind rather than social class[29] survived, as the Lunacy Commissioners acknowledged eleven years later:

Considerable difference in comfort exists between various wards but to a great extent mental condition and not the scale of payment appears to decide the distribution of payments, for instance at the Lodge which is the best furnished part of the male division, there are some cases paying only ten shillings weekly.[30]

Table 8.7. *Class of first admissions (in %)*

	J	A	T	K	B	P	O[b]
Class 1[a]	23.9	30.9	36.6	40.8	62.1	45.2	43.2
Class 2	36.6	44.2	44.6	44.1	30.8	48.7	41.3
Class 3	27.5	16.6	13.4	10.9	5.7	5.3	11.2
Class 4	12.0	8.3	5.4	4.2	1.4	0.8	4.3
N	251	217	112	311	425	493	1,809
Class unknown	9	1	17	23	15	137	202

[a]Class 1: gentlemen, bankers, merchants, landowners, professional men; class 2: retailers, craftsmen, teachers, clerks; class 3: skilled and semi-skilled workers; class 4: unskilled labourers.
[b]J, Jepson (1796–1823); A, Allis (1823–41); T, Thurnam (1841–9); K, Kitching (1849–74); B, Baker (1874–92); P, Pierce (1892–1910); O, Overall (1796–1910).

How extensively this modification of social categorisation was carried out is far from clear. It seems likely that it was the exception rather than the rule; otherwise the Retreat would have been in danger of losing the higher class of patient (on whose high fees it depended in order to balance the books), because relatives might object to such indiscriminate social mixing.

Table 8.7 indicates that the possibility of such social promiscuity diminished with time as the class distribution of patients became increasingly skewed so that upper- and middle-class patients assumed an overwhelming predominance. The categorisation has followed that used by C. Erikson and E. Isichei and is based on occupation: class 1 included gentlemen, bankers, merchants, professionals and property-owning groups; class 2, retailers, teachers, clerks and craftsmen; class 3, skilled and semi-skilled workers; and class 4, the unskilled.[31] The rationale for adopting this classification was that it enabled comparisons to be made with Isichei's work on the Society of Friends in the Victorian period. However, the neat division of Retreat patients into the four classes depicted in Tables 8.7–8.9 may conceal some ambiguity in the original data. Occupations of patients (or, in the case of women with no occupation, their husbands' or fathers') were taken from admission certificates. It is not clear to what extent the occupation given for a patient referred to current employment (in which case mental illness may have already led to some deterioration in the kind of a job an individual could do) or might refer back to what

Table 8.8. *Class of Quaker and non-Quaker first admissions, 1796–1910 (in %)*

	Quaker	Non-Quaker
Class 1[a]	24.6	66.1
Class 2	48.9	31.8
Class 3	18.9	1.9
Class 4	7.6	0.2
N	988	805

Note: Data was sufficient for cross-tabulation in only 1,793 cases of 2,011 cases.
[a] Class 1: gentlemen, bankers, merchants, landowners, professional men; class 2: retailers, craftsmen, teachers, clerks; class 3: skilled and semi-skilled workers; class 4: unskilled labourers.

was seen as the 'normal' occupational status. This very human desire to depict the prospective patient in the best possible light, together with the deterioration in family finances that often took place if the patient were the bread-winner, may explain an interesting discrepancy. Although the Retreat apparently had a growing preponderance of those whose self-categorisation put them in the upper or middle ranks of society, the institution nevertheless found it necessary to subsidise the fees of a large number of patients. In the early twentieth century between one-third and one-half of the patients were said to be paying less than the economic cost of their care.[32]

Table 8.7 shows the division of patients, where occupations were known, under six superintendents. The data presented for the last period under Dr Pierce must be treated with some caution since the larger number of patients from whom data were not available makes the end of the series less reliable. However, the growth in the proportion of patients in class 1, the fairly steady proportion in class 2 and the decline in classes 3 and 4 clearly indicated a narrowing of social intake. It is interesting that under Jepson two-fifths of the patients were skilled or unskilled workers. This suggests that the usual view of the early Retreat as a bourgeois institution needs some modification, although the stereotype is clearly apposite for later periods. But it is essential to see that, as Table

Table 8.9. *Class of Quaker first admissions in Retreat and in the Quaker community (in %)*

	Quaker first admissions in the Retreat under			Male Quakers in		
	Allis (1823–41)	Kitching (1849–74)	Pierce (1892–1910)	1840–1	1870–1	1900–1
Class 1[a]	18.8	25.7	22.7	50.0	60.8	46.1
Class 2	51.4	51.9	64.7	26.4	16.5	32.0
Class 3	19.9	16.2	10.1	15.6	15.5	14.6
Class 4	9.9	6.2	2.5	8.0	7.2	7.3
N	181	210	119	224	194	191
Class unknown	1	20	38	140	154[b]	46[b]

[a] Class 1: gentlemen, bankers, merchants, landowners, professional men; class 2: retailers, craftsmen, teachers, clerks; class 3: skilled and semi-skilled workers; class 4: unskilled labourers.
[b] Includes retired people.
Source: Figures of occupations for male Quakers, based on Digest of Deaths, are taken from E. Isichei, *Victorian Quakers* (Oxford, 1970), pp. 288–91.

8.8 reveals, the class composition of Quaker and non-Quaker patients differed considerably. Whereas virtually no non-Quaker from a skilled or unskilled working background entered the Retreat, one-quarter of Quaker patients did so. And whereas the predominance of Quakers in class 2 substantiated the 'tea merchant' image of Friends as those in trade, the dominance of class 1 among non-Quakers indicated a more exclusive clientele.

Table 8.9 suggests, however, that the social intake of Quaker patients into the Retreat may not have accurately reflected that of the Society of Friends. In this table Isichei's analysis of the occupations of male Quakers at death in 1840–1, 1870–1 and 1900–1 has been related to the occupational data for Retreat patients in comparable periods. Two factors may explain the discrepancy. First, the Retreat may have been recruiting relatively few patients from the most exclusive or wealthy Quaker homes, where families may have preferred the greater privacy of treatment at home or in a small private establishment to the 'exposure' of the more public asylum at York. Second, it is possible that the nature of the data used by Isichei skewed the distribution of occupations by recording the notable (or even enhancing the status of the less notable) within the Society of Friends, and underrepresented the more humble individual by relegating him to the large class of occupation unknown or uncertain.

This analysis of the social and personal characteristics of the Retreat's patients suggests even more striking discontinuities than continuities in the period from 1796 to 1910. The Retreat had begun in 1796 as a national institution for exclusively Quaker patients to be drawn from all social backgrounds, but with the expectation that most would be of the 'poorer sort'. The image given in Samuel Tuke's *Description of the Retreat* of 1813 reproduced this, and has been copied in books on the Retreat up to the present day. That this stereotype was increasingly misleading has been demonstrated earlier in this chapter since, by the early twentieth century, the Retreat was a regional, even local, institution, in which two-thirds of the patients were non-Quakers, and almost all were middle or upper class.

It is fascinating to see how by the end of our period there were within one building effectively two asylums, each with a quite distinctive clientele. The growing number of non-Quakers conferred a visible and changed character on the Retreat – that of an upper-class clientele drawn from the north of England. But a hidden kernel remained that retained many of the characteristics of the Retreat's original patients; this smaller number of patients were Quakers drawn from more varied social backgrounds and regions.

This diversity of the patient body is interesting. If there was a typical patient during our period it was a single woman in early adulthood from a middle-class background, belonging to the Society of Friends, and whose family lived in Yorkshire. Yet such a patient might be quite hard to locate quickly in the Retreat's records precisely because of the varied personal and social characteristics among the many individuals who were treated in the asylum. And it is this diversity within a changing asylum that presents difficulties for the attempt at synthesis that follows on the patients' world at the Retreat.

THE PATIENTS' WORLD

'As if I were a piece of furniture, an image of wood, incapable of desire or will as well as judgement' was the indelible impression left with John Perceval after his treatment at Dr Fox's madhouse near Bristol in 1832. In a well-known account Perceval spoke of the 'mysterious circumstances' in which he was committed, and the way in which 'men acted as though my body, soul and spirit were fairly given up to their control'. He complained that he 'did not find the respect given even to a child'.[33] We have no comparable statement of powerful imaginative insight from a Retreat patient to discover whether he or she experienced similar feelings of humiliation, helplessness and confusion. Personal testimonies from patients at York were fragmented, a kaleidoscope of broken images tantalisingly elusive in their incompleteness. To provide these vital fragments of evidence with greater coherence they have been set into the context of other sources of information on patients' existence in the hope that an increase in insight would outweigh any loss in immediacy or authenticity. What follows focusses on the social experience of becoming a patient, the relationships available once this status had been achieved and the accompanying feelings and attitudes of Retreat patients.

A patient's first reactions to the asylum might be those of bewilderment or fear. John T. 'was brought to York not knowing the place of his destination and thinking he was going to Scarborough',[34] despite the Retreat's requests that relatives be honest with prospective patients about the outcome of their journey. Private terrors and delusions could persist: a doctor, John A., was convinced 'that he was sent here [to the Retreat] to undergo vivisection for the benefit of science', and John D. was so frightened that 'during his medical examination he attempted to leap from a second storey window'.[35] For some other patients the mild regime and personal kindness of those at the Retreat may have soothed anxieties since it contrasted so markedly with their treatment at other institutions, and particularly so in the earlier years when mechanical restraint was more common. Deborah T. was brought to York in 1839 by her mother, 'swathed like a mummy in blankets and staircarpets, fastened with iron skewers'. On being released she commented that her relatives were 'as bad as she was', a revealing identification of madness with evil.[36] More typical of maniacal cases was that of William B., who on 21 December 1842 'was brought to the house with hands and legs bound together by cords and bands. These were immediately removed and he was allowed to sit quietly by the fireside'.[37] A good meal and warm bath followed before the patient was taken to his own room for the night.

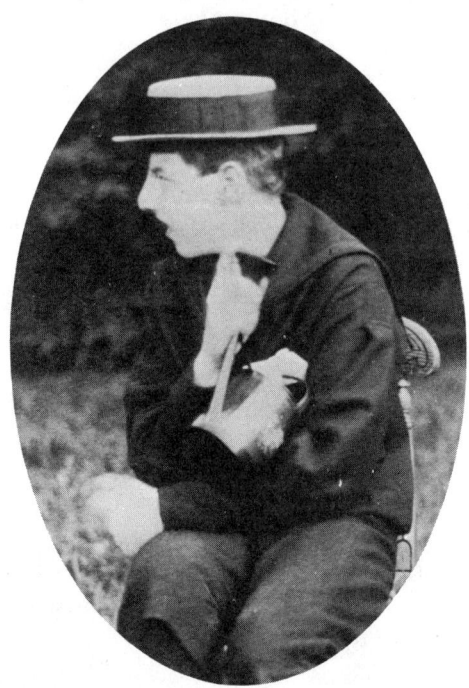

Plate 25. Thomas W (See p. 217.)

Within the space of a patient's room a limited kind of individual autonomy was possible; yet whereas others might enter the room the patient had no means to open the door from the inside and hence could only enter the gallery, or be permitted into the airing courts, under his attendant's surveillance. Therapists attempted to minimise or disguise the custodial features of the institution, as for example, by muffling bolts that might jar on patients' sensibilities, but locks and keys increased in number as the institution grew in size and complexity.[38] The loss of individual freedom involved in being a patient was intolerable to some: 'the lock and key I could not endure', wrote one ex-patient who had escaped. Despite his acknowledgement of 'thankfulness for the benefit I have derived at the Retreat' during his two months of treatment there in 1845, he was not prepared to return.[39]

The powerlessness of the inmate was particularly evident in the doctor – patient relationship, as can be seen in some of the comments made in the medical case-notes after a daily visit to the patient. Some individuals were so anxious that they were unable to talk to the doctor or to co-operate with him in taking routine measurements and observations of the pulse or state of the tongue. But more self-confident patients were also criticised by the doctor for the way in which their personal appearance or conduct did not approximate to 'medical' perceptions of normal behaviour. Individuality seems to have been increasingly constrained as we can see, for example, by the way in which orthodox forms of clothing were imposed on the individual in later years. In 1888 a young Quaker, Robert H., entered the Retreat suffering from mania, but his case-notes suggest that his 'strange garb' (see the Appendix) attracted the doctor's attention quite as much as did his mental condition. The assistant medical officer was clearly quite relieved when after several days the patient 'has now got his hair cut and a suit of ordinary clothes on and consequently looks more rational' (see Plate 26). Persuasion as to correct sartorial habits had less impact on Barnard R., in the Retreat in 1891 in his seventh attack of remittent mania. He wore what the assistant medical officer referred to as his 'grotesque fancy-costume' for almost a year, as part of his delusion that he was a military officer (see Plate 27).[40] Medical men might well have argued that dressing in normal fashion was a desirable ingredient in the progress to recovery, but the tone of denunciation betrayed the moralistic conformism that informed judgements on patients.

Social prejudices were even more obvious in male doctors' comments on female patients. Once the earlier regime of lay superintendent and matron had been overtaken by the supremacy of the male medical specialist in the mid-nineteenth century, expressions of antifeminism became overt and any troublesome female patient was likely to be categorised as 'hysterical' or 'hypochondriacal' in the medical records. A clear view of desirable feminine characteristics produced censorious comments on patients who betrayed the high moral standards expected of women in Victorian society. Predictably, Georgiana B. was reprimanded by Dr Thurnam for her 'unladylike' swearing, but the unfortunate Amelia C. was found guilty of 'a positiveness and disputatiousness hardly compatible with the feminine character'. Contemporary assumptions about the female role could also influence diagnoses

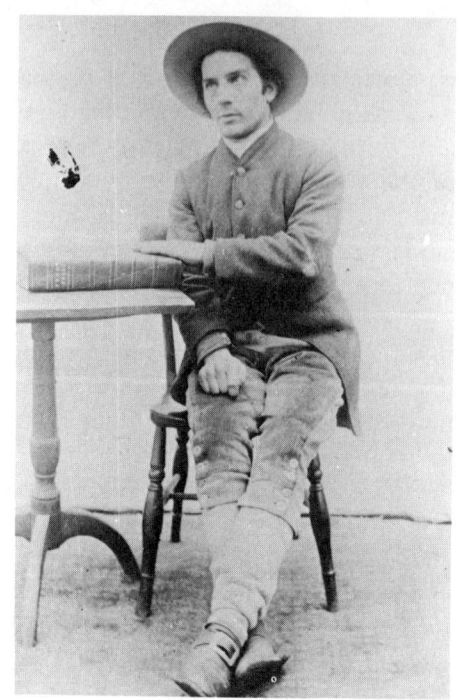

Plate 26. Robert H.

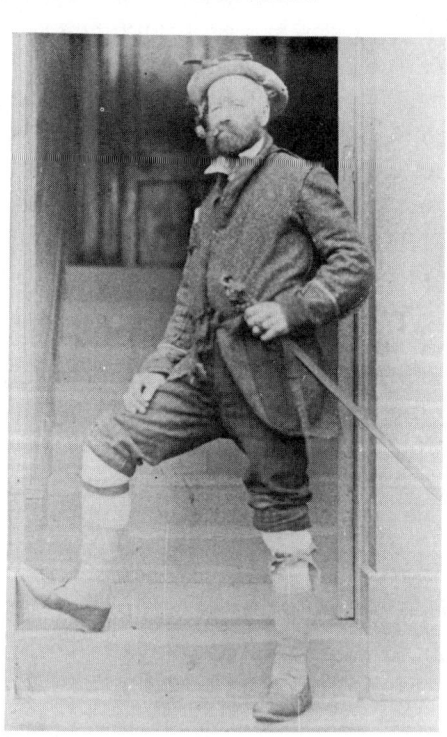

Plate 27. Barnard R.

as in several cases of 'hysterical' or 'erotic' mania.[41] Ann C. was one such patient and her case-notes stated censoriously that when the doctor approached her

> she looks up smiles or laughs loudly and talks if one does not get out of her way or look rather stern, in a manner approaching, if not actually amounting to immodesty: when feeling the pulse she often attempts to seize one's hands in hers.[42]

Culturally determined attitudes also permeated doctors' treatment of female patients as a later comment in 1891 suggests. Amelia S. was described by her therapist as

> this morning hypochondriacal and depressed. Says she has no appetite and cannot sleep. These are both facts, but largely, I fancy, dependent on her hysterical determination to appear utterly miserable and ill.[43]

He ended his observations on a note of petulant self-congratulation: 'she receives little sympathy from me and consequently does not like me.' The possibility that the rigid limitations imposed on the Victorian woman's role themselves produced either depression or rebellious nonconformity among female patients does not seem to have occurred to Victorian therapists.[44]

The increasing distance of the doctor from the patient was resented by the latter. Elizabeth C. felt that more frequent, kindly contact and a less imperiously detached attitude towards the treatment of patients would have improved her stay at the Retreat in the 1870s.[45] The situation deteriorated because of a devolution of the daily medical visitation of patients to assistant medical officers whose short tenure of office might preclude much knowledge of, or interest in, their patients. To take an extreme example, Dr Banks described Francis S. in her case-notes for 1881 as 'very pertinacious, trying to buttonhole me (at medical visits) to talk about her views of various things . . . it is very difficult to shake her off'.[46] Although it had always been Retreat practice for doctors not to converse with patients on the subject of their delusions, this reluctance to engage in conversation at all indicated the changing nature of the doctor – patient relationship. It suggests that by this time patients could be thought of more as objects to whom medicines were administered than individuals whose thoughts and feelings were vitally relevant to their moral treatment.

The doctor's judgements dictated the overall pattern of treatment, but the patient's daily activities were supervised by the attendant. Attendants played a key role in the surrogate families that therapists felt it was essential to re-create for patients within the asylum. At first all the patients in the Retreat were seen as part of 'the family' and the superintendent was described as 'the master of the family'. The recognition that the expanding size of the establishment made this increasingly a fiction led to a growing emphasis on the smaller group of patients in each ward, where 'every class seemed to form a little family'.[47] At its best under an attendant like William Waller this concept had some validity, as his affectionate poem about his patients indicated: 'Long round our table may they sit / To grace the board with mirth and wit.'[48] Yet Edwin R., who had been a patient at the Retreat on three occasions between 1820 and 1841 (as well as in other asylums), considered that there was too much stress on attendants' bodily strength and that 'till more attention be paid to their eligibility as *companions* . . . these institutions will never be conducted as they ought to be'.[49] And another patient writing thirty years later in the 1870s also criticised the calibre of attendants: the Retreat offered only inferior servants, not the care and companionship of educated Christians. Other patients, like Samuel W. in the early years of the nineteenth century, had (as we have seen) more modest aspirations in wanting attendants without brutal propensities.[50]

For some patients the ward 'family' had greater meaning. After a stay of only nine months Elizabeth B. wrote in 1819 from home to the superintendent stating that

> I shall be glad to hear good accounts of that part of the household with whom I was conversant and who are at all times in my affectionate remembrance . . . Please give my [love] to all my old friends upstairs.[51]

However, Samuel Tuke's ideal of little families where all 'were interested in each other's welfare' encountered practical problems. Some individuals' delusions made social living difficult, as was the case with the patient who thought he was 'a pillar of fire' about to set the room alight, or the woman who 'has been known to stand a whole day in one position from a belief that her feet were fixed to the floor'.[52] And social developments provided new sources of difficulty: for one 'every railway whistle seems to him to be a command to commit suicide', for another the telephone was a means to spy on her and for a third gas pipes were a means to talk to her and electricity a device to read her thoughts.[53] Others were too violent for contact to be beneficial so that scuffles broke out between patients.[54] Nevertheless, a few individuals were recorded as taking a sympathetic interest in their fellows: one patient taught another to read; another helped an infirm companion to dress each day; an octagenarian assisted a nonagenarian to walk in the garden; and a kindly individual noted of a fellow inmate that 'he had not the same binding round his mind that other people had'.[55] How much interest and contact there was between patients remains problematical since the records of the institution focussed on other topics: that they did so is in itself perhaps significant since it raised the question whether other forms of treatment were considered more important in practice.

Attitudes to the natural family of the patient revealed a comparable tension between rhetoric and reality as has been suggested existed for the surrogate one. Communication between families and patients at the Retreat was encouraged but only within a framework regulated by the therapist. 'The Superintendent reserves the right to decline to allow a patient to be visited'.[56] The passage of letters was also controlled. In this respect, the asylum shared the ambivalence with which those who ran other Victorian institutions (whether prisons, workhouses or schools) regarded the external family. They saw one of their functions as that of replacing a defective natural family and imposing greater regularity and discipline in the artificial 'family' of the institution. It is interesting to see that the rules of the Quaker boarding school at Ackworth in Yorkshire were similar to those of the Retreat in limiting contact with the external family and in encouraging inmates to adopt moral virtues of quietness, stillness, order, sobriety, moderation, decency and duty.[57] Relatives of Retreat patients seem to have accepted that restricted contact was in the best interests of the patient at certain times.[58] They were also grateful for the regular letters sent from the Retreat giving news of their members. Jane P. wrote that she had

> received thy truly acceptable letter naming that my husband had not only read my letter but had a message of love for his mother and me. It has given us great pleasure. His mother wishes to have the letter shown to all friends who call. I am very grateful for thy great kindness in so writing.[59]

Patients themselves might be less compliant. One resented 'the rigid system of surveillance and inspection of all letters [which] effectually prevents any cry of distress from reaching outside the walls'.[60] On the other hand, not all patients viewed their natural family with affection, and several showed such intense resentment against their families for having committed them to an asylum that contact with relatives was not welcome. A husband wrote despairingly to George Jepson of his wife that

> she still continues at times to run me down at a high rate, charging me with drunkenness, whoredom, hypocrisy etc . . . The last time I ordered him [a friend visiting the patient] to give my love to her but she told him she did not want it.[61]

Others viewed their treatment at a mental institution as an affliction to be concealed and hence disliked contact with friends and relatives who could themselves share, and so reinforce, these feelings. Dr Pierce recorded in 1899 that

> an intelligent lady patient recently told me that she looked upon her detention as a humiliation and a disgrace, and was now ashamed to see any of her former friends. She further said that her mother once remarked to her that whenever she heard of anyone going to an asylum, she always wished they had gone instead to the grave.[62]

Pierce had also noted that 42 of the Retreat's 148 patients in 1894 had had no visitors in the previous year, and that in only about a third of these cases had there been an adequate reason in terms of distance or poor health to explain the lack of contact. In such cases the ambivalence of the therapist to the family seems to have been equalled by the relatives' attitude to the asylum.

Visits were also encouraged, or at least facilitated, from the general public since the Retreat's Committee of Management considered that the virtues of an 'open' institution outweighed any inconvenience to patients. Regulations restricted the freedom of visitors, a necessary precaution since where they did not exist, as in the nearby York Asylum, 'some of the patients have complained that they were made a *show* of, and are occasionally . . . very much irritated'.[63] At the Retreat it had been decided that either the superintendent or matron was to accompany visitors and that the names of patients should not be mentioned to strangers.[64] The flood of visitors to the Retreat meant that these safeguards were not always adequate. John Ellis was outraged that his sister-in-law should have been subjected to a 'disgraceful transaction' when in 1821

> at least 12 young men and two or three females to all of whom poor Rachel was an entire stranger were taken thro' some of the females' apartments to hers in which at that time she was alone and in a state very unfit to be seen. It seems to me most unaccountable that these poor creatures, who have been placed in the Retreat as an institution of all others of the kind best adapted to render their situations as comfortable as the nature of their malady will admit, should thus be exhibited to gratify the idle curiosity of such as choose to see them.

Later, it emerged that it was in fact a cousin of the patient who had organised the visit.[65]

Visitors from the outside world may have reminded patients of what some undoubtedly saw as their captivity at the asylum. William F. spoke, as did others, of his 'imprisonment'. After thirteen months' treatment he summed up his own feelings as to the benefits of his stay: 'I have good meals here and that is as much as I can say.'[66] Another fellow patient, Joseph P., felt even less compliant after eight months' therapy and wrote to his sister in April 1882, 'have not received a bit of good here', signing the letter plaintively, 'what was your brother'.[67] Yet patients who were more familiar with the Retreat's regime were better disposed towards it. Elizabeth G., who had been a patient on five previous occasions, was said by her husband to be 'well aware of her situation and has strongly urged us to comply with her request to return to the Retreat'.[68] Samuel W., who was familiar with the institution because his sister was already a patient there, was said to have been 'in a state of derangement . . . [and] has for some time past been very solicitous to go to the institution at York'.[69] And even Edwin R., whose view of asylums was frequently critical, admitted that the Retreat had rapidly 'restored' his sanity on a previous occasion, and that the asylum as an institution 'was the most welcome as well as salutary, retreat from the gaze of an unsympathizing world'.[70]

It was perhaps easier to see the benefits of asylum treatment at a distance than when confined to one, as was shown by the ingenious attempts by several patients to free themselves from its care. Some patients cherished hopes that an outside agency would procure their release: one patient wrote to his father that he should get 'half a reprieve from the Quakers'; and another hoped that soldiers in the neighbouring barracks would 'annul an unlawful institution called the Retreat'.[71] A third 'got Charles Reade's *Hard Cash* after reading which he wrote a letter to the author complaining of his treatment here, and asking Reade to interfere'.[72] Some patients utilised their opportunity to complain to the visiting Commissioners in Lunacy, though few with as much skill as a solicitor who used his legal knowledge to protest that his certification had been technically irregular and hence that he should be discharged.[73]

In contrast, some patients hoped that compliance with the wishes of the Retreat's therapists and conformity to institutional rules would suggest recovery and bring about their discharge, as two cases from 1839 illustrated. John M., a maniac, 'expresses himself very anxious to get well, and with that view listens to and attends to advice'. As a druggist, with some medical experience, this patient was able to take an intelligent interest in his treatment. 'He yesterday wrote unasked an intelligent and sensible statement of his mental state and history and of the effect of moral and medical treatment here with which he presented me', recorded Dr Thurnam.[74] And a female imbecile, Mary R., attempted to gain her discharge but without the understanding to analyse her situation accurately:

> She employed herself very industriously in the kitchen and in house work, in which ever since she came, she did as much almost as a hired servant.
>
> About 2 weeks since [1839], without apparent cause, she suddenly gave over working and refused to do anything except for herself. She became very ill-tempered and dissatisfied, and petulantly demanded her discharge, saying 'she was quite well' and that 'nothing ailed her mind' and that she had 'worked hard like a slave, for seven years' thinking by doing so and conducting herself well she should get away from the Retreat. But she found it was no use, that others discharged who were idle and behaved ill, that there was no encouragement to good behaviour.[75]

Other patients used the 'open' character of the Retreat to escape from their confinement. A central dilemma of a progressive institution was that 'every step taken to increase the general sense of freedom . . . involves of necessity greater opportunities for escape'[76] and, as Dr Pierce went on to emphasise, 'considerable trouble and anxiety' (listed in that order!). Although it was comparatively simple for convalescent patients to break promises and leave the grounds, even those in a more acute phase of their illness, and with far greater restrictions, managed to gain their liberty. One individual was recaptured twenty miles away though his ankles were tied together, and another managed to escape through a window only seven inches by eleven.[77] The most eager for his freedom was Stephen S., who made ten escape attempts after 'bitterly complaining of being confined' on his arrival in October 1854. It was several years before Dr Kitching observed that he was 'not quite so persevering in his attempts to escape' and that 'he has been under such constant surveillance that escape has been rendered almost impossible'.[78]

Escaping patients' destinations varied: some went home, others merely put distance between themselves and the asylum and one enterprising individual attempted to consult another asylum doctor in order to be declared sane. This last case was that of William R., who visited Dr Charlesworth at the Lincoln Asylum on two occasions in order to consult him 'as to his fitness for liberty and business'.[79] More typical was the escape of Matthew J., who fled as far as Huddersfield, where he found his condition unsupportable, as a Friend observed:

I write to inform thee that a young man, apparently deranged has called to beg at our house this morning. He says that he is from the Retreat near York. He calls himself Matthew H. J. – and says that his father lives in Hertfordshire. He is dressed in a dark green coat, black waistcoat, brown grey trousers, white handkerchief, is nearly 6 feet high, has large hands and rather sunburnt complexion. He hangs down his head as he walks . . . At one time he says that he will return to the Retreat but he is afraid of being punished, at other times he says he will go to his father. He says he has no money and has not been to bed since he left the Retreat.[80]

Sometimes the Retreat had to resort to advertising for an escaped patient, as with Joseph Unthank in April 1871 (see Plate 28). Fifteen months after this young Quaker was admitted to the asylum suffering from delusions he took advantage of his freedom to make his way across country to Church Fenton railway station. There he took a train to Hull, a steamer from Hull to Newcastle, and from there made his way to his home in Sunderland. After a week

ESCAPED!

FROM THE RETREAT, YORK,

A Male Patient, about 35 years of age, named **JOSEPH UNTHANK**. He is a middle sized man, rather stout, round shouldered, and leans to the left side. Face round and pale; hair beard, moustache and eyes black; was dressed in a black cut-away Coat, Waistcoat and Trousers of black mixture, black silk knotted Necktie and Wellington Boots. Carried a silver lever Watch without a Guard.

The Police are requested to look out, and if they find the above described Person, to detain him, and either bring him to the Retreat or Telegraph to the Superintendent. The expenses will be Paid.

W. SESSIONS, PRINTER, LOW OUSEGATE, YORK.

Plate 28. Notice of escape

of freedom, he was recognised in the street, the Retreat was notified of his whereabouts and the patient was sent back to the safety of the asylum.[81]

Relatives' anxiety about 'his making away with himself' encouraged them to send patients to the safekeeping of an asylum. Suicidal propensities were frequently recorded but suicides themselves were rare. In earlier years patients might be physically restrained from harming themselves as was the case with Mary S., who after dinner one day in 1805 'snatched a knife from one of the servants and threatened to cut her throat, seeming quite frantic. Jacketted and held down'.[82] Later, surveillance replaced restraint, as for Captain B., who, in 1879, was stated to require 'constant watching day and night by several strong attendants or he would succeed in injuring himself'.[83] On rare occasions a patient eluded such careful watching. In 1854 Eleanor K. was stated to have been single-mindedly intent on 'self-destruction' throughout her six months' treatment. Frustrated in her attempts to pick up pieces of glass on her walks, or to use a penknife to cut her throat, she eventually found a workman's boy employed on the Retreat's new buildings, gave him money to get 'sixpennyworth of essential oil of almonds' from a chemist and then poisoned herself.[84] Patients' resort to suicide, or suicide attempts, was more a commentary on their attitude to life itself than on their treatment in an asylum, but in a few cases the latter was also a relevant consideration. Priscilla P. failed in her suicide attempt but her suicide note was eloquent on the fact that she felt asylum life worsened her condition: 'My misery is so intense and increases every day and I find it more and more difficult to submit to any rule.'[85] In contrast, Alfred K. escaped from the Retreat in order to commit suicide because he did not wish to be discharged from the institution. Dr Baker reported that he had said 'both to his father and myself that the past year had been the happiest of his life'.[86]

At the Retreat patients' freedom was curtailed, but individuality was not crushed into helpless anonymity. Goffman's generalised view of the asylum patient living within 'an enveloping tissue of constraint' had a limited applicability to conditions at York.[87] The safety of patients was thought to require some measure of compulsion, but the grey area between necessary constraint and unnecessary restriction was probably smaller than in many other mental institutions. Institutional pressures on patients certainly existed, not least from the obsessively high standards of cleanliness, neatness and decorum, and from the moral order of daily routine in which the long hours of the asylum day were punctuated into discrete forms of activity, each with their own function and value. Nevertheless, the 'curtailment of self' was limited in so far as patients had their own well-furnished rooms, kept their personal possessions and retained some freedom of choice over diet, employment and amusements. Undoubtedly, pressures for conformity squeezed this 'private space', and as the number of patients grew individual idiosyncracies became too inconvenient to be tolerated. The patient had to fit in with less fluid patterns of institutional life and increasingly to adopt approved standards of behaviour within an organised and bureaucratic regime. But this change needs to be seen within a wider context since Retreat patients numbered only one-fifth of those in the average county asylum even at the end of our period, when it housed less than one-twelfth of those in a big example like Colney Hatch.[88] It is also evident that Retreat patients had a very comfortable environment in comparison with the utilitarian standards of public asylums. They also benefitted from a more generous provision of doctors,[89] which suggests that more attention was paid to the patient as an individual than was possible in a county asylum. One patient who had previously been in a public institution commented that 'there is more of comfort, kindness and affection in the Retreat, but less of talent than in the rotten establishment at Exeter'.[90]

Mutually contradictory testimony by patients as to their attitudes and feelings on life at the Retreat means that one set of generalisations can hardly do justice to their variety of experience. In any case, evidence of patients' feelings was often filtered, refracted or destroyed by their keepers, and what remained intact was made ambiguous by the language of madness itself. In this context it is useful to reflect on a picture left by one patient depicting his view of the therapy he had received. It leaves us with a final enigmatic perspective on the patient's world at the Retreat (see Plate 29).

George S., who in about 1899 painted his view of therapy at the Retreat, was a patient from 1894 to 1912.[91] As an affluent non-Quaker with a home in the north of England, this patient was not untypical of those being admitted to the asylum at this time. His perception of the Retreat's therapy focussed on leisure pursuits: not so much those like tennis and football that were well established but those that had been introduced whilst he was a patient. His picture shows golf (introduced in 1894), bicycles (first purchased in 1897) and croquet (the first tournament was held in 1899), and interestingly, he places them all on the new cricket field of 1897. But these activities appear secondary to the patient himself, who is seen in bed in the foreground, attended by a woman who is possibly his wife and surrounded by four dogs. In a literal interpretation these could be the animals belonging to the staff: 'Topsy', the Skye terrier belonging to Dr McKenzie, is on the left; the collie dog of the head attendant, Mr Darley, is in the centre; and 'Pompey', Dr Pierce's retriever, is on the right. Symbolically, however, the patient seems to have been depicting the spirits in the form of animals whom he thought followed him around, spoke to him and occasionally fought with him. These were the delusions that

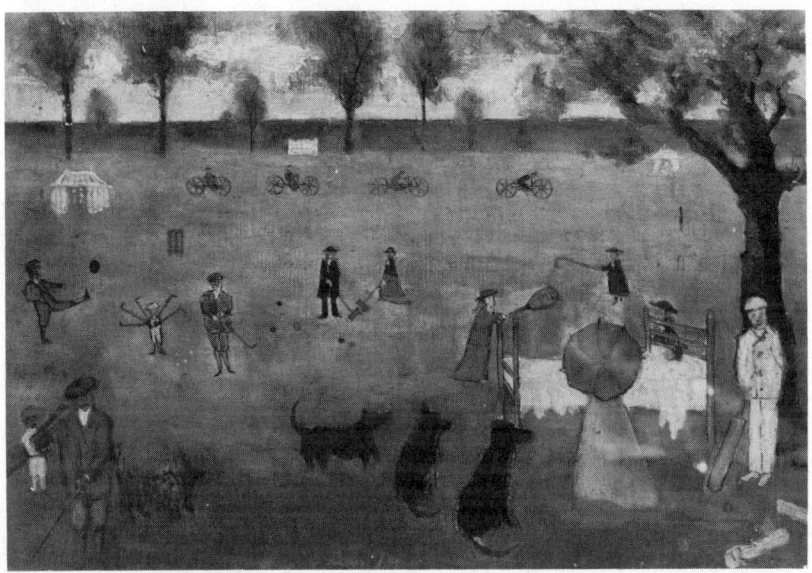

Plate 29. A patient's view of his treatment (1899)

his doctors had recorded at the time of his admission. Is it significant that the patient gave greatest prominence to his illness – threateningly symbolised by the dogs – whilst his therapy receded into the background? Or is his view more accurately seen as that of a counterpoise of forces, with the patient balanced between his illness on the one hand and enjoyable therapeutic pursuits on the other?

9

The Retreat's record

This chapter is concerned with the medical record of the Retreat's 2,011 certificated patients: the cause of their admission, their duration of stay, readmissions and the outcome of their treatment. Much of this material is quantitative and is the result of a computerised study of the patients. But other qualitative material is also introduced both to explain the data and to provide a more comprehensive picture of the medical environment. The sources used for the quantitative analyses are the same as those listed in the preceding chapter. But the failure to locate medical case-books after c. 1890 means that the analyses in this chapter of topics such as duration or outcome of treatment are less complete than were the social analyses in Chapter 8. The chapter begins with a discussion of the distinction between certificated and voluntary patients and the dilemma posed by early treatment against legal safeguards for patients. It goes on to discuss the alleged causes of insanity and the coexistence of old and new ideas on its nature. The chapter then analyses the duration of stay of the asylum's inmates, focussing on some of the long-stay patients and discussing whether their treatment was successful even if it did not lead to 'recovery'. There is a survey of the different outcomes of patients' treatment and a discussion of the meaning of terms such as 'recovery' or 'improved'. Finally, there is a consideration of readmission rates, since as we have seen, the recurrence of mental disorder meant that the 2,011 patients who were in the Retreat in our period made up 2,525 cases.

ADMISSIONS

The Retreat grew rapidly in size until the 1830s, and much more slowly thereafter. Figure 9.1, which plots annual numbers of pa-

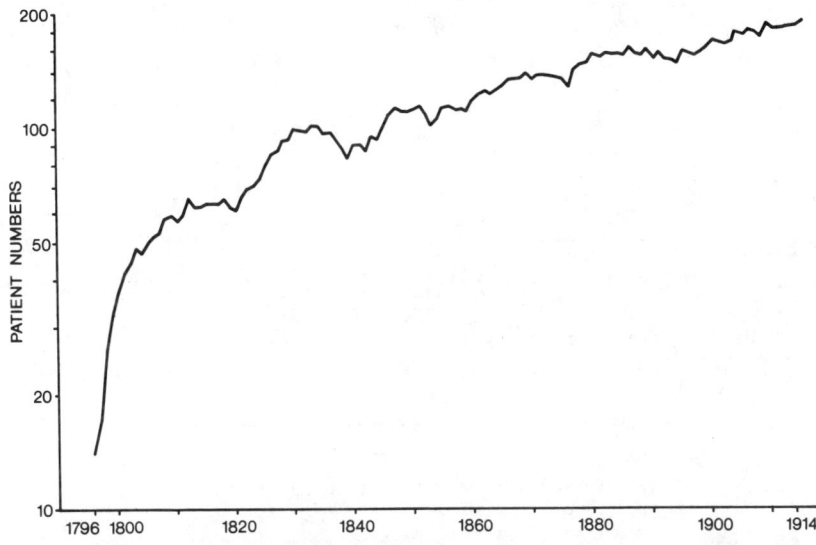

Figure 9.1. Patient numbers, 1796–1914

tients on a semi-logarithmic scale, shows this clearly since it indicates by equal intervals on the vertical scale equal proportionate changes in patient size. In 1834, after thirty-eight years of existence, the Retreat had 102 patients, but eighty years later, in 1914, it had only 190. This slowing of the rate of growth contrasted with that of public asylums so that whereas in 1827 the Retreat was three-quarters the size of the average county or borough asylum, in 1890 it had only one-fifth the average number of patients.[1] But although by this time the Retreat was a comparatively small institution, in relation to its own past, its number of annual admissions continued to show an upward trend. Indeed, an increase in the rate of admissions was particularly noticeable from the mid-1870s, under Drs Baker and Pierce (see Fig. 9.2). Under the latter an all-time high was reached with the proportion of admissions to average residents comprising one in four. Yet since, as we shall see later, the duration of patients' stay tended to decrease at this time, the growth in total numbers was relatively small.

The Retreat's admission policy was predominantly a social one in that it gave Quaker patients priority, and only secondarily was it medical. There is tantalisingly little evidence to indicate any pol-

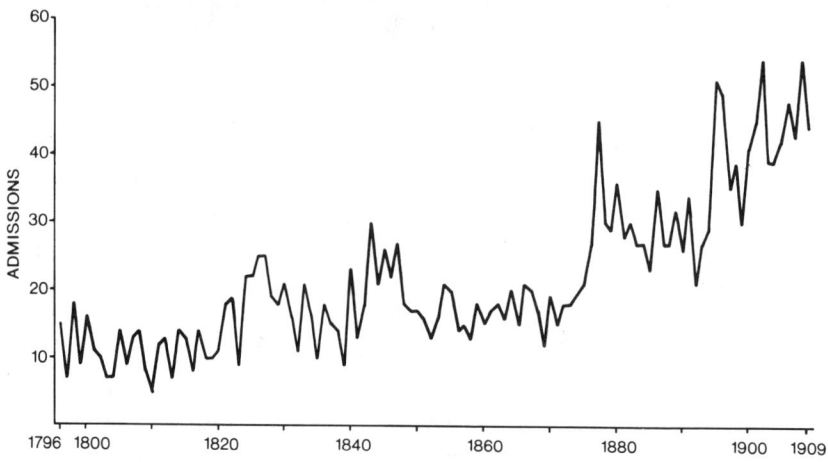

Figure 9.2. Annual admissions of patients, 1796–1909

icy of selection based on medical criteria; except for cases of mental handicap in the early years and epileptics at the end of our period it would appear that virtually all who applied were admitted. Nevertheless, a suggestion arises from a case in 1816 that the asylum preferred not to deal with very violent cases of mental illness. Shortly after they had admitted Charles L. the Committee of Management decided in April that he was

> proving more violent than the committee had reason to expect, when they consented to his coming to the Retreat. This rends it unsuitable for him to continue to occupy the only apartment which can be allotted for his accommodation.

Rejecting their first decision to send him into lodgings with an attendant, they eventually transferred this patient in July to Dr Willis's establishment in London.[2]

Emphasis was given at York – as in other contemporary asylums – to the duration of mental illness prior to a patient's admission. In 1799 Friends were encouraged to send patients earlier rather than later:

> As experience demonstrates, that the recovery of insane patients frequently depends on their being removed from their connexions, and put under proper care and treatment in the early stages of the disorder, it is earnestly recommended to their friends to remove them at an early period after the disorder appears to be fixed.[3]

Shrewdly, the Retreat's managers decided to offer a financial reduction of four shillings a week in a patient's fees during the first year of treatment if he or she had been sent to York within six months of the illness's appearance. The policy was a successful one and the managers recorded that they were 'abundantly convinced'[4] of its advantage in promoting recoveries. Periodically, they published tables in their annual *Reports* indicating the differential rates of recovery of patients in relation to the swiftness with which they had been admitted to the Retreat, and this served as a means of persuading relatives and friends to send patients promptly for treatment.

The vast majority of patients at York were certificated. From its inception the Retreat asked for a formal statement from a surgeon or physician that the individual was insane. However, it is not clear how uniformly this was adhered to since there are extant certificates for only three-quarters of Jepson's patients. In 1818 the Retreat introduced its own formal certificate in which relatives were asked to answer questions on the patient's history and a medical man was to fill in the statement: 'I do hereby certify, after personal examination of __ that I believe __ to be Insane, and a fit object for confinement in a House for the reception of Lunatics.' Ten years later its certification was brought into line with general legislation that required a separate examination and certification by two medical practitioners. The Lunatics Act of 1845 brought further changes in the Retreat's certificates in that private patients now had to have a relative or friend make a formal petition for reception and provide an outline social and medical statement of the case under a greater number of specified headings.[5] General public unease about the wrongful confinement of the sane within the Victorian asylum led to further safeguards for the patient.[6] In the Lunacy Act of 1890 judicial as well as medical authority was invoked for the detention of a lunatic. A relative or friend was required to petition a justice of the peace and to supply two medical certificates before a patient could be admitted under an ordinary reception order.

The increasing elaboration of certification posed a dilemma in that it was difficult to reconcile legal safeguards for the patient with the desirability of early treatment. A limited solution to the problem was given in legislation of 1862 and 1890 that permitted private asylums such as the Retreat to accept voluntary boarders.

To give in-patient treatment without prior certification was a course of action strongly recommended by Dr Pierce, who disliked the delays inherent in this increasingly elaborate procedure. Preventive medicine of this type meant, according to Pierce, that 'a stitch in time saves nine', a view he shared with the Committee of the Medico-Psychological Association in its report of 1913. However, this system had a restricted application since it could be used only for patients who came voluntarily and could understand what they were doing.[7]

Before 1890 the Retreat had occasional voluntary patients who were often placed in lodgings in the neighbourhood but were treated by the Retreat's doctors.[8] One such patient was Bryan S., who had been a certificated patient earlier but who on this occasion was admitted informally, presumably because his condition was giving cause for concern but was not at first thought sufficiently disordered to be committed.

> On December 16 1881 he was admitted into the Friends' Retreat as a 'voluntary patient' for three months; but he has proved since so unmanageable, so little amenable to suggestion and advice, and so incapable of controlling himself, that it is judged necessary to admit him as a certified patient. During the ten days of his 'voluntary' stay he spent money wastefully, ordered unnecessary articles, played at snowballs with common street-boys, and was dirty in his habits, and it was impossible to get him off to bed before 11 or 12 p.m.[9]

Clearly, he was not perceived as a model patient since he was not keeping his prior commitment as a voluntary boarder to abide by the rules of the institution. This extract from his case-notes also revealed the difference in the amount of control that could be exercised over a voluntary, as compared to a certificated, patient.

After 1890 numbers of voluntary boarders increased markedly: by April 1910 there had been 246 of them at the Retreat. The policy of voluntary boarding seems to have been successful since only about one in ten later had to be certificated.[10] Dr Pierce also thought it a useful innovation in reducing the penal character of the asylum and the social prejudices that surrounded insanity:

> No other disease requires a justice of the peace to be consulted before remedial measures are taken: the patient forthwith loses his civil rights; he is treated in a special institution far removed from his family, under conditions which are determined by questions of safety that concern only a small proportion of his fellow patients . . . the whole government of

the asylum emphasises the fact that the insane are not as other men but require special treatment under special conditions.[11]

That prejudices continued to be held about insanity was shown with unusual clarity by the Retreat's certificates of admission, which recorded relatives' and friends' views on the causes of the patient's illness.

ALLEGED CAUSES OF INSANITY

Causes ascribed as reason for the outbreak of mental illness were as multifarious and difficult to classify as the varied attempts by the Retreat's own doctors indicated. At first these attempted to distinguish predisposing or long-term causes from exciting or immediate causes, and each was divided into physical and moral categories. Dr Thurnam's fourfold table of this type listed among physical causes twenty-two predisposing and twenty-two exciting causes, and among moral causes he found six predisposing and sixteen exciting factors among patients admitted before 1840.[12] The overall categorisation in this computerised study was a simpler one that divided causes into physical, moral and mixed (i.e. specifying both physical and moral factors). In the numerical calculation of proportions in each category those not known were excluded. In some cases 'not known' referred to a failure to locate the documentation. In others it represented an omission on the certificate itself. Although there was a growing reluctance to speculate on the supposed cause of insanity, there is little reason to think that those filling in the certificate were much more inhibited from assigning one type of cause rather than another. Thus, exclusion of 'not knowns' from Table 9.1 should not seriously distort the analysis.

The Retreat's certificates of admission gave ample scope for patients' relatives and their doctors to speculate on the cause of their illness. As Samuel Tuke aptly commented, 'The human mind does not like uncertainty; and the relatives of the insane, are generally anxious to fix on some particular circumstance as the cause of disease.'[13] This was more evident early in our period, since under Jepson, Allis and Thurnam only one in sixteen was prepared to record 'not known' in answer to a query on the supposed cause of insanity, whereas by Pierce's time one in three certificates was of this type. A growing reluctance to speculate was also suggested by the declining proportion of patients for whom mixed causes of insanity were assigned. Mixed causes embraced both physical and moral factors and were often a rag-bag of disparate items compiled in a desperate attempt to relate incidents recollected about a patient's life history to the outbreak of insanity. As such they should be seen more as anxious attempts to come to terms with the unknown and the inexplicable rather than confident or coherent hypotheses. Two summaries of this type of mixed cause taken from the admissions register (which summarised entries on certificates) suggested the kind of conjecture involved. The first stated, 'Hereditary (partly). Always rather singular. Domestic trials (stepmother). Disappointed love (cousin).' The second read, 'Sudden subsidence of diarrhoea of 15 months duration while on a sea voyage. Preceded by scandalous accusation affecting his spirits.'[14]

The care with which such mixed causes were tabulated in this private asylum contrasted with the virtual absence of such mixed categorisation at Brookwood (the second county asylum in Surrey), or at the Lancaster Asylum for pauper patients. There, physical cases outnumbered moral ones by two to one at Lancaster and three to one at Brookwood for cases where causes were assigned in samples of patients admitted in 1879 and 1890–2, respectively. Presumably, a physical cause was more easily discerned especially when details of case histories were few.[15] At the Retreat the preponderance of physical causes was less marked as Table 9.1 indicates. Alleged physical causes of insanity among Retreat patients included head injuries (often arising from falls from horseback), alcoholism, organic deterioration arising from old age, a few cases of syphilis, and a small number whose illness was associated with the physical changes of pregnancy, childbirth and lactation. One case exhibited a peculiar irony in that the arrival of wisdom teeth was said to have produced insanity.[16]

The hereditary element in the causation of insanity (and in other social problems) provoked an increasing amount of discussion that reached a climax in the writing of Henry Maudsley in the 1870s. Those who managed the Retreat were particularly sensitive to this issue because, as we saw earlier, restrictions on marriage outside the Society of Friends resulted in much intermarriage among Quakers and gave rise to concern that this led to higher rates of insanity among Friends.[17] Tuke in his *Description* of 1813 described the 'large numbers' of cases in which there was a hereditary ele-

Table 9.1. *Alleged causes of mental disorder of first admissions (in %)*

Alleged type of cause	J	A	T	K	B	P	O[a]
Moral	20.3	20.8	30.3	32.6	45.7	44.9	34.5
Physical	54.0	32.5	30.3	41.9	45.1	44.6	42.9
Mixed	25.7	46.7	39.4	25.5	9.2	10.3	22.6
N	237	212	122	258	315	358	1502
Cause unknown	23	6	7	76	125	272[b]	509

[a] J, Jepson (1796–1823); A, Allis (1823–41); T, Thurnam (1841–9); K, Kitching (1849–74); B, Baker (1874–92); P, Pierce (1892–1910); O, Overall (1796–1910).
[b] Of these, seventy-seven certificates of admission are no longer extant.

ment but admitted that despite this, information on the subject had not been obtained 'in a great number of instances'. As we have seen, Dr Thurnam provided greater numerical precision in his view that one-third of the patients admitted since 1796 had 'laboured under a hereditary predisposition to insanity'. Significantly, he derived this estimate not merely from relatives' statements on patients' admission certificates but from other sources of information as well. He also referred to a problem encountered in any analysis of these certificates in that relatives often included collateral blood relatives in their answer to the question on whether there was a hereditary cause of insanity, thus confusing the issue by giving an affirmative answer when no direct transmission was actually involved. If these were included then the proportion of 'hereditary' cases rose to one-half in Thurnam's estimation. These may be compared with samples of patients at Lancaster and Brookwood Asylums in 1879 and 1890–2, where if individuals with a known cause of insanity only are included, comparable figures of just under one-third and one-half respectively were found.[18]

Moral causes of insanity were assigned for a growing proportion of prospective patients at the Retreat. These were infinitely varied but the most common were religious preoccupations, overstrain, business anxiety, disappointment in love, bereavement and sexual 'abuse'. Anxiety over religious salvation or an obsession with religious ideas was equally common among men and women.

But until the end of the nineteenth century it was mainly men who suffered from business anxiety or who had overtaxed the brain with intellectual work. By this time the emancipation of women led first to the entry of female students suffering from overwork, and then early in the twentieth century to business women entering the Retreat.[19] It was at this time too that the first case of female 'self-abuse' was found on an admissions certificate;[20] before this such cases of masturbation were invariably male. Contemporary thinking about masturbation as a cause of insanity undoubtedly influenced patients' own attitudes to the practice as was shown for a Quaker patient in 1863. His brother confided that he had

> been informed by the patient during a lucid interval, since the attack [of insanity], that for fourteen years he has been in the habit of self-pollution – for which he is now exceedingly penitent – and remorse for this vice has preyed upon his spirits.[21]

Men had a virtual monopoly of this type of alleged cause, and women were much more prominent where disappointment in love, family bereavement, or domestic problems was said to be the origin of mental illness.

Perceptions of the detailed causes of insanity changed within our period as Figure 9.3 indicates. This depicts the results of a comparison of Jepson's first admissions from 1796 to 1823 with those of Baker from 1874 to 1892. (Although it would have been preferable to compare Jepson's patients with those of Pierce, and thus to span our whole period, the gaps in the sources for the later dates made this inadvisable.) Fuller information on the supposed causes of mental disorder was available for Jepson's patients than for those of Baker because admissions certificates could be supplemented by information recorded in the admissions registers. All the alleged factors for each patient were included in the analysis.[22]

The most obvious difference in the way in which causation was viewed centred on the hereditary factors with a decline from 34.8 to 24.9 per cent of admissions in which this was mentioned. However, in Baker's time collaterals were frequently mentioned by relatives filling in the admissions certificates, and if these are excluded, the decline from the Jepson era is much more dramatic – falling to only 9.6 per cent of cases. Another major change between the Jepson and Baker eras came with declining references to weak-mindedness, and this decrease may be more apparent than

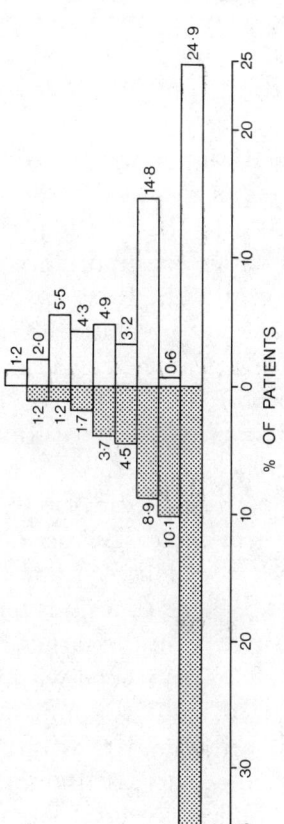

Figure 9.3. Moral and physical causes of mental disorders among first admissions

real, indicating a growing appreciation of the distinction between the causation of illness and the characteristics of the disorder itself. This distinction was clearly a matter of some perplexity to those at the Retreat who, in the earlier period, might write down the supposed cause and then minute 'cause or first symptom?' It is interesting to note that with advances in medical knowledge during our period came an increased stress in Retreat admissions on the organic causation of insanity notably through physical illness, epilepsy, old age, pregnancy and childbirth.

At this point in our analysis it is useful to pause and see how the Retreat's certificates related to those for other institutions, although this is only possible for the later period under Baker. In contrast to the figures given by the Commissioners in Lunacy for private and pauper patients admitted to asylums between 1878 and 1889, Baker's admissions showed a relatively greater importance being given to the hereditary factor (24.9 compared to 20.5 per cent) and a lesser importance to intemperance (4.9 compared to 13.4 per cent). The Retreat's admissions also suggested that more significance had been attached to moral factors in the causation of insanity than was the case elsewhere.[23]

The profile of moral or psychological reasons assigned for the origins of mental illness of Retreat patients again showed intriguing differences over time. Whereas 'disappointment in love' had been almost a ritualistic response – particularly for female patients' illnesses – in the earlier period of Jepson, 'business anxieties' or 'overwork' took on the same function – in this case for male patients – in Baker's time. It is tempting to read into this a reflection of the change from the earlier romantic age to that of the competitive problems associated with living in a mature capitalistic economy afflicted with economic depression, but this would certainly overburden fragile data with a disproportionate weight of interpretation. The increased emphasis given to domestic or professional anxieties as causal factors in the later period suggested a greater readiness to specify immediately observable features in the prospective patient's everyday life, and with it a corresponding reluctance to speculate about more distant causes. Another significant change that perhaps reflected the decline in the Quaker character of the asylum from 95 to 38 per cent of admissions, was shown in the decrease in cases of ill-regulated conduct as the perceived reason for insanity. Later suppositions about the origins of mental disorder were noticeably less moralistically disapproving, indicating perhaps a greater awareness of the extent to which aberrant behaviour was a result rather than cause of insanity.

Clearly this comparative analysis can only be suggestive, not conclusive, as to changing perceptions of insanity's causation. In the earlier period we can see that the therapists who recorded information in the admissions register had access to much personal background information on the families of their small numbers of Quaker patients, and were also prepared to speculate on both the long-term and immediate cause of insanity. In contrast, relatives who filled in admissions certificates in the later period tended to think of immediate and concrete changes in the life of the prospective patients in attempting to explain why they had become ill. Yet this change may in itself be indicative of the way in which rising numbers of patients in Victorian asylums had made insanity into a more commonplace, less mysterious, circumstance, and one that was seen increasingly as the preserve of the medical profession.

SHORT- AND LONG-STAY PATIENTS

Asylum doctors displayed great interest in the recovery rates of their asylum in relation to other institutions and seemed to take these as criteria of their success. Yet another set of statistics concerned them almost as much – those giving the proportion of patients deemed to be curable in the asylum once current recoveries had been subtracted. These must have depressed those professionally concerned: at the Retreat between 1857 and 1873 only 8.4 per cent of the patients fell into this category, a figure that differed only marginally from the 8.7 per cent at York Asylum.[24] Earlier, doctors had been more optimistic about their powers to cure the mentally ill. In 1844, when the first survey of curability had been taken, the Retreat had estimated that one in four of its patients was in this category. This was in line with the proportions returned for inmates of county and charity hospitals but was somewhat lower than those for provincial licensed houses. Unfortunately, a buoyant expectation that improved asylum facilities in mid-century would lead to a higher proportion of cures failed to materialise. Increasingly, asylum superintendents blamed their poor performance on the hopelessly chronic state of the patients who were admitted. Those running asylums felt themselves to be in a double bind since it was thought that if the asylums silted up with chronic cases, potentially curable cases of recent duration could not enter.[25] And before the end of the century the Retreat's superintendent had joined in this defensive chorus:

> We have an undoubted responsibility as regards chronic insane patients, but it is perfectly clear to me that we also have a responsibility in respect to recent and acute cases.[26]

Dr Pierce was expressing his concern in 1900 about the increasing proportion of long-stay patients at the Retreat. While rejecting a 'turning-out' system for them, Pierce felt that the number of chronic cases was preventing the admission of acute ones since the institution was so full. Earlier, he had expressed his anxiety about the way in which some long-stay patients became 'disaffected' and had an injurious effect on new arrivals. He considered – as did the Commissioners in Lunacy – that a transfer of long-stay patients between asylums was sometimes beneficial since new surroundings and fresh faces might change a patient's outlook. Clearly, a situation like that reached by the Retreat in its centenary year, when half the patients had been there for a decade or more, was not considered satisfactory by doctors who so obviously measured their success in terms of recovery rates.[27]

Was this criterion an accurate guide to the work of the asylum? In important respects it must be accounted a very partial one precisely because so many patients were in a chronic state and unlikely to recover. Humane treatment of such patients – continued whatever the disappointments, provocations and weariness – was surely an equally valid, if less quantifiable, measure of success. To care for a patient like James H., for example, from his arrival as the Retreat's fifteenth patient in 1796 until his death at the age of seventy-five in 1840 was a considerable achievement. The casenotes written at his death provided both an obituary and a testimony to those who looked after him:

> The melancholia or probably rather apathetic mania (incipient dementia) characterized as it was by sullenness, stupor and fear in this case gave way not long after his admission to very violent mania. For a long series of years, or nearly a quarter of a century, he was the terror of the place. He ran after those who approached him with stones etc. and his cries, oaths and imprecations were so loud that they were often heard at the

distance of a mile. He required nearly constant restraint with wrist straps and could only be managed by two attendants. He had no distinct lucid intervals . . . When nearly arrived at his 60th year the violence of his paroxysms of mania began to diminish, and a gradually advancing fatuity made its appearance. Little need be said of his mental state, characterised as it is by mere negatives. He is in a state of heavy, stupid dementia, harmless, tractable.[28]

Not all long-stay patients were as oblivious to their treatment or as unrewarding as patients. At the opposite extreme was Edward F., who was admitted in January 1845 and achieved the status of 'oldest inhabitant' before his death in April 1902 at the age of eighty-two. Dr Pierce described him affectionately as courteous, charming and articulate, a man who despite delusions retained a quiet sense of humour as was shown by the following story:

A well-known tradesman in York changed his business and giving up grocery opened a printing and stationery establishment. It is stated that [E. F.] called at the house and in his gentlest manner said, 'I hope your business will not be stationary but grow, Sir!'[29]

Those who looked after the chronic cases were sometimes heartened by an unexpected remission of mental illness. As one Retreat doctor observed in 1903:

The possibility of recovery in apparently hopeless cases makes the work easier and enables the staff to face much that would otherwise be profoundly discouraging. One such case compensates for a great deal of seemingly wasted labour.[30]

However, the use of the term 'wasted labour' was itself indicative of an attitude of mind that still saw cure rather than care as the criterion of success. Such ambivalence over objectives had earlier led to a general discussion on whether chronic and acute patients should reside in separate institutions in Victorian England. As the overoptimism on the curability of insanity abated, and evidence of large numbers of chronic cases in the new borough and county asylums continued to accumulate, the idea of housing the incurable in non-medical refuges was raised. This was resisted by asylum doctors who, as A. T. Scull commented, redefined 'success in terms of comfort, cleanliness, and freedom from the more obvious forms of physical maltreatment, rather than the elusive and often unattainable goal of cure'.[31] Yet this dichotomy between care and cure is probably too well defined since asylum doctors were only too aware that, as Dr Pierce observed,

> it is happily true that patients will sometimes recover who seem to be hopelessly insane, so that after years of effort success may suddenly attend us. In many cases the cause of recovery is as obscure as the original cause of the disease.[32]

Although this admission of professional ignorance was honest, it perhaps gave greater credence to the asylum as a caring than a curative institution. And the four case histories he used to illustrate his point also indicated how inexplicable the recovery of a chronic patient might be. For example, one female patient

> for seven years was profoundly depressed and agitated, and seemed to be settling down into dementia. She gradually began to interest herself in the ward work, slowly improved, her delusions cleared up and she is now taking her place amongst the family.

Such cases gave hope rather than enlightenment and provided a welcome departure from the repetitive 'no change' recorded in the infrequent case-notes of chronic patients.

Caring for patients with mental handicaps posed some of the same problems as were raised by the chronic mentally ill. Here George Fox's advice to 'walk cheerfully over the world, answering that of God in every man' may have provided the sympathy and motivation required.[33] At first, the Retreat had decided that idiots should not be admitted, but this rule was soon abandoned and the asylum accepted cases both of 'congenital idiotcy and imbecility' (as well as those in which mental disorder was also associated). But only a very small minority of idiots and imbeciles were involved: between 1796 and 1843 one in seventeen patients was in this category. There is no reason to think their numbers increased thereafter since Dr Pierce commented in 1913 that there were 'extremely few' mental defectives at York.[34] Although such patients were few in number their needs, and more especially the needs of young patients for education and training, received special attention. Dr Kitching considered that such education was 'not one purely of science . . . but it requires devotion, patience, and love'. When this attention was given over several years in an institution, then the idiot's ungainly walk is gone; the indistinct and uncouth utterance is exchanged for easy and pleasant speech; the disarrangement of the features has settled into composure and symmetry; propriety and order mark his personal habits; some mechanical skill or other productive talent has been gained.[35]

Kitching was discussing the kind of treatment available at the Idiots Asylum at Bath but his description may also serve as a kind of prospectus for the later progress of 'the idiot boy' at the Retreat (see the Appendix). Thomas W. came to York in May 1881 as the asylum's youngest-ever patient, aged only seven years and nine months. He lived with a nurse in the separate building known as the Cottage Hospital, later moving to the Gardener's Cottage. His case-notes recorded his progress:

13 August 1881. He has learnt his letters, and can pick each one out as it is named.

3 October 1881. His family considers him much improved in many respects since his admission. He is more tractable and takes his food better.

25 February 1882. Is very fond of music and can hum some tunes.

Thomas continued to prosper, as we see in his photograph taken when he was about seventeen years old (see Plate 25, p. 188). It was about this time that his nurse had to be replaced by an attendant since he was 'too animal and too manly'. His later years at the Retreat were pleasantly uneventful, but in 1898 he succumbed to a fatal attack of pneumonia.[36] The only other case where the Retreat admitted a child aged under ten was also one of 'idiocy'. Three years before Thomas W. came to York, the eight-year-old Thomas T. had been admitted. In this instance the patient was sent as a boarder with leave of absence to a private house nearby – The Poplars at Acomb – where he was systematically visited by Dr Baker.[37] Clearly, the Retreat was not designed to treat very young children, or those with mental handicap, but special establishments were few and far between until public provision was stimulated by the Mental Deficiency Act of 1913. The complement to this legislation was one dealing with defective and epileptic children in the following year.

Epilepsy affected a small minority of Retreat patients and was often combined with mental illness. No very satisfactory method of treatment was at first devised and by 1840 6 out of the 139 deaths had been from epileptic seizure.[38] Later, the Retreat adopted the standard prescription of potassium bromide and found it to be an effective method to reduce the violence of epileptic fits in some, but not all, patients. In more intractable cases mixtures of bismuth or borax were employed.[39] The impact of epileptic patients on other inmates aroused increased concern and in 1880 a special bedroom was fitted up in which to isolate them. Finally in 1897 it was decided to discourage the admission of epileptics because of their 'prejudicial influence' and hence 'the manifest evils of associating such patients with others'.[40] A contributory cause of this apparently harsh decision may have been that epileptic patients tended to be long-stay patients whereas the aim at the Retreat was to have a greater proportion of short-stay patients.

Almost half of the Retreat's first admissions stayed at York for under a year (see Table 9.2). The trend to treat patients within shorter time periods was quite marked: under Jepson, Allis and Kitching two-fifths of first admissions were treated for under one year; Thurnam and Baker had raised this to about one-half, and Pierce at the end of our period appeared to have increased this to almost two-thirds. (Quite how much Pierce had actually done so was uncertain since the medical records became increasingly defective at this time.) It is interesting that there seemed to be a positive correlation between therapists who favoured medical treatments (notably Thurnam and Baker) and shorter durations of treatment. Also striking was a continuing pattern of predominantly brief durations of patients' stays: where first admissions were concerned three-fifths of all cases were treated in under two years and with the proportion rising from over one-half under Jepson to three-quarters under Pierce. This was also true of second and third admissions where, over the whole period, 46.7 and 48.8 per cent respectively had treatment lasting under one year and a further 14.8 and 12.5 per cent respectively of between one and two years.

How did this record compare with that of other asylums? The Retreat's treatment was marginally longer than that recorded for all admissions at the Lancaster Asylum in 1849 and 1879 and the Brookwood Asylum in 1890–2 where figures of over one-half within a year, and two-thirds within two years were recorded.

Table 9.2. *Duration of stay of first admissions (in %)*

	J	A	T	K	B	P	O[a]
Less than 1 year	39.9	42.8	51.2	40.7	47.3	64.5	49.8
1 year to 1 year 11 months	15.5	17.7	10.2	13.6	16.1	13.9	14.7
2 years to 9 years 11 months	20.6	21.8	20.5	22.1	22.7	17.5	20.6
10 years and over	24.0	17.7	18.1	23.6	13.9	4.1	14.9
N	259	215	127	331	404	538	1,874
Duration unknown	1	3	2	3	36	92	137

[a] J, Jepson (1796–1823); A, Allis (1823–41); T, Thurnam (1841–9); K, Kitching (1849–74); B, Baker (1874–92); P, Pierce (1892–1910); O, Overall (1796–1910).

Even shorter periods of treatment were found at the Oxfordshire institutions at Hook Norton and Witney between 1828 and 1867 where 62 and 66 per cent respectively of all admissions were for less than twelve months and 64 and 82 per cent for under two years. The cautious attitude of Retreat therapists in evaluating the progress of their patients may have contributed to a slightly longer duration of treatment of York. But more compelling than differences between institutions was their similarity in achieving high patient turnover – a record that did not entirely support contemporary anguish over the silting up of the Victorian asylums with chronic, long-stay cases. However, a rather different impression is given if we look not at admissions (which suggest the short-stay character of the majority of patients), but at inmates. A small proportion of long-stay patients, whose numbers cumulated over the years, built up to a high proportion of patients in the Retreat at any one time. Thus, if we look at the asylum population this gives credibility to the contemporary view of asylums as filled up with chronic patients, whereas if we look at the outcomes of admissions, a more optimistic perspective on the success of therapy is possible.[41]

It is interesting to see whether one type of patient rather than another was more prone to a rapid outcome of treatment, taking the period as a whole, and examining those who were first admissions. Among married people, 55.4 per cent had an outcome within

Table 9.3. *Duration of stay of first admissions in relation to religious affiliation, 1796–1910 (in %)*

	Quaker[a]	Non-Quaker
Less than 1 year	42.6	58.2
1 year to 1 year 11 months	14.7	14.7
2 years to 9 years 11 months	22.5	18.3
10 years and over	20.2	8.8
N	1,030	821

Note: In 137 of 2,011 cases duration of stay was unknown and in a further 23 cases religious affiliation was unknown.
[a] Includes those connected with the Society of Friends.

a year compared to 35.7 per cent of single people and 33.7 per cent of the widowed. Men were slightly more likely than women to have these shorter periods of therapy – 44.6 per cent compared to 41.2 per cent. There were no very marked differences between the age groups of patients aged fifteen years or more, where a range of from 38.5 to 45.3 per cent of outcomes within a year was found, although there were slightly higher proportions in the middle range of twenty-five to fifty-five year olds. The very few individuals admitted as free patients were most likely to have a rapid outcome, with 61.5 per cent within one year compared with 50.4 per cent of those paying normal fees, and 40.6 per cent of those on subsidised terms – the latter were almost invariably Quakers. Table 9.3 indicates that a rapid outcome of treatment was much less likely for Quakers, with only 42.6 per cent within a year, compared to 58.2 per cent for non-Quakers. Financial pressures on non-Quaker pateints may well have been a significant cause of this differentiation. And since the proportion of non-Quaker patients increased rapidly under Drs Baker and Pierce this could have been important in the shortening of periods of treatment that we have noted occurred at this time.

The relationship between outcome and types of mental disorder can only be studied for a smaller number of cases with first admissions before June 1843. Melancholics were more likely than maniacs to have outcomes within two years – three out of five compared to two out of five. The mentally handicapped were particularly likely to become long-stay inmates and half of these patients had periods of treatment of ten years or more.

Dr Thurnam's analysis of periods spent at the Retreat in relation to outcome between 1796 and 1840 was useful in suggesting that the most successful outcomes followed the shortest period of residence, with a mean of 1.32 years for recovery, 2.25 for improved cases, 3.06 for the unimproved and 8.83 for those who died.[42]

OUTCOME OF TREATMENT

Since the Retreat classified the outcome of its patients' treatment under five headings (discharged recovered, discharged improved or relieved, discharged but not improved, died, or remained in the institution), it will be helpful to clarify how the asylum defined the first three categories before discussing a statistical analysis of the outcome of treatment.

Given the importance attached by asylums to their results in comparative tables of patients' recoveries it is perhaps surprising that there was so little discussion of what 'recovery' meant. Samuel Tuke defined it as, 'where the patient is fully competent to fulfil his common duties, or is restored to the state he was in previously to the attack'.[43] Dr Thurnam merely paraphrased this in his analysis of 1840:

The term *recovered,* has been applied only to those cases where the patient has been so far restored as to appear fully capable of performing, with propriety, the duties belonging to his station in the world.[44]

Yet he immediately went on to clarify this clear-cut definition by cautiously admitting that sometimes 'upon a minute examination, traces of mental disorder might still be detected'. Seventy years later Dr Pierce was even more circumspect when he commented on

the extreme difficulty in deciding what is meant by the term recovery . . . In many cases, however, there remains an instability, a latent tendency to mental disorder, although at the moment [of discharge] no sign of insanity can be discovered.[45]

The increased wariness discerned was probably induced by additional experience gained by the asylum in readmissions of patients previously discharged as recoveries.

For practical purposes, however, the Retreat's doctors, who decided whether patients had recovered, took as their criterion the readiness of an individual to resume normal life, as did doctors at other mental institutions.⁴⁶ They proceeded carefully in their evaluations, soberly assessing a patient's behaviour during a prolonged convalescent period before deciding 'recovered after a long period of trial' or 'after a long time of probation'. For some, this convalescent period was spent at the Retreat but with more frequent forays into the outside world through attendance at York Meeting, or through social visits to local Friends. This was true of an early patient like Mary S., who in 1809, after seven years of treatment, was discharged. Her case-notes explained that

> having been a long time slowly mending she became sociable and comfortable; and after a few months of trial amongst us in the family return'd home with her sister this day.⁴⁷

For some male patients there was preparation for a resumption of the business of earning a living by 'day-release' while at the Retreat. In 1814, for example, it was planned to send Samuel T. to 'Joseph King's, Grocer, in Walmgate on days and to return to Retreat on nights for a while'.⁴⁸ And between 1811 and 1822 convalescent patients could live in the Appendage, a 'half-way house' just outside the gates of the city.

A period of convalescence was likely to have been more prolonged at the Retreat than at most other mental institutions since at York financial pressures to remove patients prematurely were reduced by charitable assistance given to many patients' families. As Thurnam explained, this period of 'probation' was extremely valuable since it revealed the full extent of the patient's recovery and might suggest that a further period of treatment was necessary.⁴⁹ This was illustrated in 1854 by Ann B., who

> had her sister staying in York for about a week and frequently visited her at her lodgings – in addition to seeing her here. This slight trial of strength proved to her, she said, that she was much less equal to the world than she expected. She accompanied her sister home, and stayed 3 days. She enjoyed her visit and appears to have exercised self-control, but she does not feel more disposed in consequence to leave the shelter of the Retreat.⁵⁰

So what might seem to constitute a convalescent state within the asylum might not be sufficiently robust to withstand the problems of an unprotected existence in the world outside the asylum gates. In an interesting discussion of the condition of Elizabeth W., who suffered from partial dementia, Dr Kitching highlighted the doctor's dilemma in deciding whether discharge was in a patient's best interests:

> She remains at present in a state approaching convalescence. She is evidently of feeble mind and unable to bear the trials and contingencies of an independent life without great risk to that degree of mental soundness which she now enjoys; and therefore so long as she is content to remain in her present position, it appears best to take no steps for her removal from the Retreat. In case she become, without relapse, urgent for her removal, it would seem proper to arrange with her friends for that purpose.[51]

Both women remained in the asylum until their deaths, apparently less as a result of illness than of what today would be called 'institutional neurosis', or an atrophy of personal initiative.

For some patients in the borderland between convalescence and recovery there was another option to the restricted life of the certificated patient in the status of voluntary boarder. Although our earlier discussion indicated that this was not legally defined until 1862, the Retreat used the device before this in a few cases. Shortly after his second discharge as 'recovered' in 1829, Thomas T. wrote from his home 'begging to be received as a boarder in the house, stating that he could not live comfortably at home'.[52] He resided at the Retreat for the two next decades although in 1849 his condition had deteriorated to a point where he was readmitted as a certificated patient. It is interesting to compare this patient with Thomas B., who, although a certificated patient for much the same period (from 1829 to 1845), spent several of these years boarding with a farmer's family nine miles from York, returning to the Retreat only when he had paroxysms.[53] It was probably not coincidental that this patient was discharged as recovered in September 1845 only a month after the passage of the Lunatics Act had made the process of certification more rigorous and given powers to an external body – the Lunacy Commissioners – to inspect the Retreat. Yet his swift readmission in 1847 for treatment lasting five months, and again in 1850 for a further period of three months, does not necessarily suggest that the increased rigidities of certification coped better with remittent cases such as this than had the Retreat's earlier, more flexible, system.[54] Indeed, the opportunities given by the system of voluntary boarding, made more generally available under legislation of 1890, reintroduced this element of flexibility. The Retreat used this device as a means to prolong convalescence for certain of its patients. For example, in 1905,

> Three patients formerly under certificates on their recovery remained as voluntary boarders for several months until they felt equal to face the world and it is satisfactory that they all have kept well.[55]

With these kind of pliable definitions of what constituted recovery it becomes more problematic to decide what differentiated those who had recovered from those in the second category who were stated to have been merely improved or relieved. Thurnam, again paraphrasing Samuel Tuke, attempted to grasp the nettle:

> In cases which, upon discharge, still required the particular care of their friends, though so far benefitted by treatment, that further residence in the institution was thought unnecessary, patients have been considered as discharged improved.[56]

However, in view of what has been said previously on the fragile state of those classified as having recovered, his statement begged as many questions as it answered. Dr Pierce was probably more realistic when he spoke of patients who had been improved as still possessing 'some signs of mental peculiarity'.[57] Patients discharged as improved or relieved usually left at the request of their relatives or friends and presumably before their doctors viewed their treatment as having been successfully completed. In addition, a few patients who escaped and were retained by their friends were placed in this category, as were patients who, although not completely without signs of their illness, had 'appeared calm for a considerable time' and therefore were thought fit to be discharged by their doctor.[58]

The third category of patients – those discharged as 'not improved' – was more readily distinguishable from those who had recovered or improved. Patients in the non-improved class were either those taken away by relatives against the advice of doctors, patients who were removed to other asylums (generally for financial reasons) or, more rarely, individuals who escaped early in their treatment and did not return.

Most patients in the fourth category died from natural causes since suicides were rare: only five were recorded before 1840 and they were even more infrequent thereafter.[59] Patients in this fourth category had usually had a long period of treatment at the institution as we have seen, and were also advancing in years: between 1796 and 1840 the mean age at death was fifty-six for Quakers and forty-seven for non-Quakers. In Dr Thurnam's estimation only a very small minority of the 139 deaths in this period were attributable either to brain disease or to epilepsy.[60] This connection between insanity and pathological changes interested alienists: autopsies began at the Retreat in the 1820s to investigate it and to analyse any brain lesions discovered in dissection. From this perspective most autopsies seem to have produced disappointing results. However, in 1855 it was found that a patient previously diagnosed as a congenital imbecile had a brain of only half the normal weight.[61]

Mortality at the Retreat was low in comparison with that in other asylums. Thurnam's research concluded that between 1796 and 1840 the asylum had a mean mortality of those annually resident of only 4.6 per cent whereas at the West Riding Asylum at Wakefield it was as high as 16.2 per cent for the period 1818–41.[62] A few years later John Conolly estimated that the percentage of deaths based on the average numbers of patients in public asylums between 1835 and 1845 had been 9.6 per cent whereas at the Retreat it was only 5.3 per cent.[63] And if we compare the Retreat with the neighbouring York Lunatic Asylum for the period 1855–70, we find that the former had 5.1 per cent deaths on average numbers of patients whereas the latter had a rate of 7.3 per cent.[64] A major reason for this difference between the Retreat and other asylums was that the Retreat had a mainly middle-class clientele whereas most other public institutions, including the York Asylum, took at least some pauper patients, whose physical condition on admission was frequently poor. Over the whole of our period the Retreat's death rate, on average numbers of inmates, remained low (see Fig. 9.4). Probable contributory causes for this low mortality were good standards of care for patients; the relatively affluent circumstances of its admissions; and high material standards within the asylum. But this stability contrasted with the death rate of the general population of England and Wales, which showed a substantial decline during the same period.[65] This divergence may

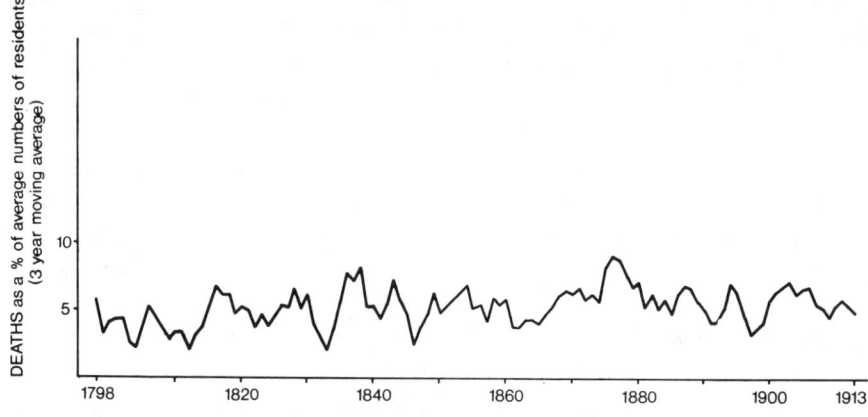

Figure 9.4. Deaths as a percentage of average numbers of residents, 1798–1913

perhaps be explained both by the patients' different age structure on admission and, in the latter part of our period, by the ageing nature of the Retreat population.

What was the achievement of the Retreat in relation to the criterion seen as more important by therapists and patients alike – that of rates of recovery? Table 9.4 indicates that, as the managers of the asylum argued, duration of illness prior to admission was related to its outcome. Four-fifths of the 615 patients admitted before 1840 recovered when the illness prior to admission had lasted less than three months and the illness was the first attack of insanity, whereas only one-fifth of cases of over a year's duration subsequently recovered in the Retreat. Table 9.5 suggests that duration of stay of patients at the Retreat was also related to the outcome of treatment. Of those who were known to have recovered, 70.1 per cent of first admissions recovered within a year, whereas only 2.0 per cent of recoveries were among patients whose treatment had lasted ten years or more. The proportion of those who had improved or been relieved also showed a steady decrease over time, whereas that of those who died tended to increase with duration of stay. Looking at the data in another way, Table 9.6 suggests that of first admissions known to have been discharged within one year 58.2 per cent recovered and a further 20.6 per cent had been discharged as relieved or improved. The proportion of those recovering or improving then decreased as duration of treatment

Table 9.4. *Duration of mental illness prior to admission in relation to outcome, 1796–1840 (in %)*

	Class 1[a]	Class 2	Class 3	Class 4
Recovered	79.2	46.1	62.1	19.4
Improved or relieved	4.2	12.1	11.4	12.0
Not improved	1.0	2.2	3.8	8.3
Died	10.4	20.9	13.7	37.3
Remained in 1840	5.2	18.7	9.0	23.0
N	96	91	211	217

[a] Class 1 were cases of first attack and not more than 3 months' duration; class 2 were those of first attack and between 3 and 12 months' duration; class 3 were cases not of first attack and of under 12 months' duration; class 4 were cases where duration of illness had been over 12 months.
Source: Thurnam, *Statistics of Insanity*, table 17.

Table 9.5. *Outcome of treatment of first admissions in relation to duration of stay, 1796–1910 (in %)*

Duration of stay	Recovered	Relieved or improved	Not improved	Died	Remained
Less than 1 year	70.1	56.2	38.5	20.3	—
1 year to 1 year 11 months	16.8	20.3	17.5	11.4	11.8
2 years to 9 years 11 months	11.1	20.3	38.5	28.7	37.2
10 years and over	2.0	3.2	5.5	39.6	51.0
N	505	222	109	429	51

Note: Of 2,011 first admissions the outcome and duration are known for only 1,316 cases; in 558 patients outcome is unknown, and in 137 cases duration of stay is unknown. Among the latter, outcome is also unknown in 113 cases.

rose, whereas the proportion of those whose treatment was terminated by death increased with the length of their stay in the asylum. The Retreat's figures indicated a fairly rapid outcome for 61.7 per cent of first admissions within two years, but with 21.7 per cent staying between two and ten years, and a residuum of 16.6 per cent who remained for ten years or more. It was the pa-

Table 9.6. *Duration of stay in relation to outcome of first admissions, 1796–1910 (in %)*

	Less than 1 year	1 year to 1 year 11 months	2 years to 9 years 11 months	10 years and over
Recovered	58.2	41.7	19.6	4.6
Improved or relieved	20.6	22.1	15.8	3.2
Not improved	6.9	9.3	14.7	2.7
Died	14.3	24.0	43.2	77.6
Remained in 1910	—	2.9	6.7	11.9
N	608	204	285	219
Outcome unknown	325	72	100	61

Note: Of 2,011 first admissions, the outcome is unknown in 558 cases and duration unknown in 137 cases. Among the latter outcome is also unknown in 113 cases.

Table 9.7. *Gender in relation to outcome of treatment in first admissions, 1796–1910 (in %)*

	Male	Female
Recovered	35.9	39.4
Improved or relieved	17.4	16.0
Not improved	9.1	8.5
Died	35.3	31.0
Remained in 1910	2.3	5.1
N	607	733
Outcome unknown	280	391

Note: Of 2,011 first admissions the outcome was unknown in 671 instances.

tients in the last two categories whose chronic state so depressed contemporaries.

Cross-tabulations of the known outcome of treatment for first admissions with the social and personal characteristics of these patients suggest some differences in the likelihood of recovery. Table 9.7 indicates that recovery was slightly more likely for women,

Table 9.8. *Marital status in relation to outcome of treatment of first admissions, 1796–1910 (in %)*

	Single	Married	Widowed
Recovered	39.6	37.3	28.5
Improved or relieved	14.1	21.7	13.0
Not improved	8.9	8.6	8.9
Died	33.7	29.2	48.0
Remained in 1910	3.7	3.2	1.6
N	778	410	123
Outcome unknown	352	225	54

Note: Of 2,011 first admissions, the outcome of treatment was unknown in 631 instances, and marital status unknown in a further 69. Among the latter, outcome was also unknown in 40 cases.

with 39.4 per cent of cases, than for men, with 35.9 per cent of cases. Single patients were slightly more likely than married people, and substantially more likely than the widowed, to achieve recovery (see Table 9.8). However, the larger proportion of the married in the improved or relieved category, when compared to the single, suggests that a desire by families to have wives or husbands home, before the doctors were prepared to signify that treatment had reached an entirely satisfactory conclusion, may have depressed the proportion of married individuals among the recovered. The lower recovery rate of the widowed was probably accounted for by their greater average age and hence their higher age-specific mortality rate. Much more significant differences are found when the ages of patients are related to their outcome of treatment. Table 9.9 indicates a marked downward trend in the proportion of recoveries for older age ranges: from 52.5 per cent for those under nineteen to 13.9 per cent for those over seventy-five years. Table 9.10 indicates that Quaker first admissions had a higher recovery rate than did non-Quakers, with 41.2 per cent against 31.2 per cent. A major cause of this difference was that Quakers predominated in the earlier period when general recovery rates were higher. It is also likely that recovery rates of non-Quakers were lower, and their improvement rates higher than those of Quakers, because non-Quaker families were prone to terminate expensive treatment prematurely. In contrast, Quaker patients who

Table 9.9. *Age in relation to outcome of treatment of first admissions, 1796–1910 (in %)*

	Under 19	20–4	25–34	35–44	45–54	55–64	65–74	Over 75
Recovered	52.5	51.2	46.0	35.2	32.2	32.9	17.6	13.9
Improved or relieved	13.5	12.8	19.8	16.9	20.5	11.2	14.4	8.3
Not improved	5.1	12.8	7.7	11.5	8.5	7.5	7.2	—
Died	27.2	20.8	22.5	33.7	35.7	42.8	57.7	75.0
Remained in 1910	1.7	2.4	4.0	2.7	3.1	5.6	3.1	2.8
N	59	164	298	261	224	161	97	36
Outcome unknown	18	71	157	133	128	64	39	19

Note: Of 2,011 first admissions 629 outcomes are unknown and age was unknown in a further 82 instances. Among the latter, outcome was also unknown for 42 cases.

Table 9.10. *Religious affiliation in relation to outcome of treatment of first admissions, 1796–1910 (in %)*

	Quaker[a]	Non-Quaker
Recovered	41.2	31.2
Improved or relieved	12.3	25.3
Not improved	5.0	15.7
Died	38.5	22.3
Remained in 1910	3.0	5.5
N	878	458
Outcome unknown	204	448

Note: Of 2,011 first admissions outcome was unknown in 652 cases where religious affiliation was known, in 3 cases outcome was known but not religion, and in a further 20 neither was recorded.

[a] Includes those connected with the Society of Friends.

benefitted from subsidised terms tended to stay longer in the asylum to complete their treatment, and hence were more likely to be labelled as recovered rather than improved. It is also possible that Quaker therapists felt a greater responsibility towards Quaker patients and, because of shared values, were better placed to treat them successfully.

Table 9.11. *Outcome of treatment of first admissions under different superintendents between 1796 and 1910 (in %)*

	J	A	T	K	B	P	O[a]
Recovery	45.0	44.7	38.4	35.7	32.7	25.9	37.8
Improved or relieved	11.9	13.5	13.6	16.6	24.0	15.3	16.7
Not improved	4.2	10.2	10.4	5.5	13.0	10.6	8.8
Died	38.9	31.6	37.6	41.2	27.7	2.4	32.9
Remained	—	—	—	1.0	2.6	45.8	3.8
N	260	215	125	308	346	85	1,339
Outcome unknown	—	3	4	26	94	545	672

[a] J, Jepson (1796–1823); A, Allis (1823–41); T, Thurnam (1841–9); K, Kitching (1849–74); B, Baker (1874–92); P, Pierce (1892–1910); O, Overall (1796–1910).

The outcome of treatment under different superintendents is shown in Table 9.11. The number of patients whose outcome was unknown was so large under Dr Pierce (because of a failure to find the medical case-books for this period) that we should ignore the results for this subperiod. Taking the recovery rate from Jepson to Baker we can see a steady decline in the proportion of patients in this category from the late eighteenth to the late nineteenth century. The rate of recovery shown in Table 9.11 refers to the percentage of recoveries based on total numbers of first admissions. By 1870, however, asylum doctors were dissatisfied with this type of measurement and preferred to express recoveries as a percentage of annual admissions. This decision may well have been motivated by a desire to show the work of asylums in a more favourable light since computing the outcome in this way produced a higher recovery rate. Figure 9.5 shows the record of the Retreat in achieving recovery rates as determined by this alternative method of calculation. It is based on the figures published in the Retreat's *Reports* after 1870 (series 2) and on a reconstitution of the data in admissions registers and medical case-books for earlier years (series 1). It is significant that the two independently calculated series in Table 9.11 and Figure 9.5 show a downward trend in recovery rates.

Jepson and Allis would appear at first sight to have been much more successful than their successors in bringing about the recovery of their patients, although it is an open question whether this

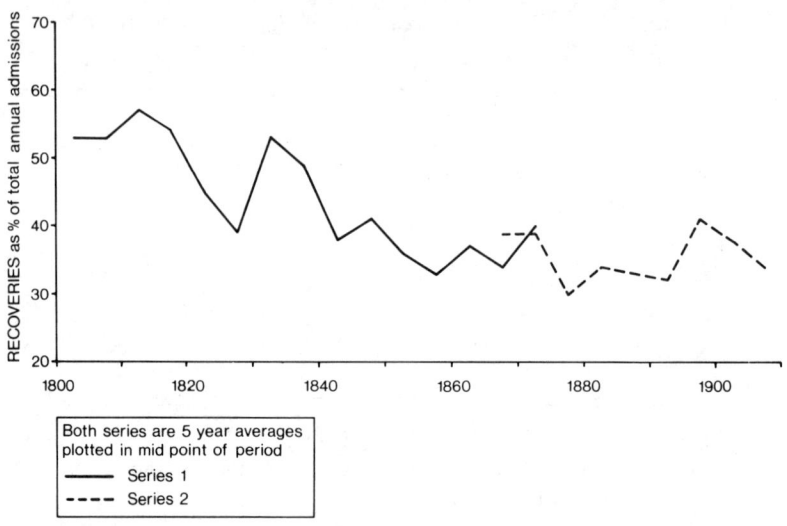

Figure 9.5. Recoveries as a percentage of annual admissions: five-year averages, 1801–1910

might have been due to the primacy of moral treatment, the overwhelmingly Quaker character of the asylum or the skills of lay therapists. But comparisons over time also raise difficult issues on the equivalence of the criteria. An alternative explanation might suggest that with growing experience, asylum doctors became more cautious and hence more reluctant to specify 'recovery' rather than 'improvement'. That there was a doubling in the proportion of patients discharged as improved or relieved between Jepson's and Baker's eras – from one in eight to one in four patients – gives some substance to this argument. And if the percentages of patients in the recovered and improved categories are taken together, there is almost no difference in the outcomes over time (see Table 9.11). Unfortunately, we have insufficient evidence on how therapists arrived at their decisions to decide which interpretation is more appropriate.

The long-term record of the Retreat between 1796 and 1910 shown in Table 9.11 suggests a 'recovered' rate of 37.8 per cent and an 'improved' rate of 16.7 per cent for first admissions. Given that the outcomes of one-third of the total first admissions were unknown, we might be inclined to regard them with some reservations. However, the Retreat doctors took the data for all admissions for a slightly longer period from 1796 to 1913 and arrived at very similar figures. Out of 2,651 cases, 1,041 recovered (39.2 per cent); 429 were improved or relieved (16.2 per cent); 264 were not improved (10.0 per cent); 729 died (27.5 per cent); and 188 remained in the asylum (7.1 per cent).[66] How did this record compare with that of other asylums? Thurnam's table of relative recovery rates compiled in 1840 suggested that the Retreat's achievement was comparatively good, although Conolly's researches five years later came to the opposite conclusion.[67] Given the problems we have already discussed in relation to a comparison of recovery rates even within one institution, it hardly seems a profitable exercise to attempt extended comparisons between different asylums, when variations in the type of patient admitted, and in the way in which some establishments restricted the admission or duration of stay of incurables, further compound the difficulties of comparative evaluation.

READMISSIONS

The doctors' verdict on the outcome of treatment apparently bore little relation to the likelihood of later admission.[68] The problem of relating states of recovery with later relapses or recurrences of mental illness was an intractable one and much professional as well as semantic ingenuity was applied to it. Samuel Tuke's footnote on this subject was characteristic of much discussion:

> Patients who have recovered, and have returned to the institution *relapsed,* are not noticed in this summary as being recovered; unless they have finally been discharged in that state.[69]

This appeared to put the emphasis on the period of time between recovery and relapse, and this point was also emphasised by Dr Thurnam in his analysis of readmissions:

> In some of these cases the re-admission has not been the consequence of a distinct *recurrence* of the disorder, but has been rendered necessary by a *relapse,* which has occurred shortly after a too speedy removal from the institution, on the appearance of amendment.

In part this seemed to contradict parallel statements on the unusual length of the convalescent period at the Retreat, which had been instituted precisely to prevent this type of situation occurring.

Thurnam admitted that case histories of readmitted patients were usually too imprecise 'to distinguish relapses from distinct recurrences'.[70]

For the purposes of our statistical analysis, however, a readmission is defined as an instance in which the Retreat doctors thought fit to give the patient a new case number. It is interesting to try to see why these were given in some instances but not in others. Some patients presented no difficulties, like Ann B., who suffered from mania with melancholy and was in the Retreat in 1805–6 and again in 1824–6. Her friend wrote to Samuel Tuke about her second attack of mental disorder:

> Thou will probably recollect Ann B. who left the Retreat about 18 years ago in a state of perfect recovery from her malady. I am sorry to say that without showing any sign of a return during all that time it has again returned in a most decided, unequivocal manner.[71]

Yet a comparison of other cases raises questions. Why was Samuel W., who suffered from remittent mania, kept as a patient at the Retreat throughout his periods of illness and remissions between 1803 and 1824 whereas Margaret B., who suffered from the same complaint, was discharged recovered and then readmitted nine times between 1807 and 1846?[72] Here, as in other cases, the reason seemed to be found in the different social circumstances of the patients rather than in their medical condition, but clearly the difference in policy adopted for them made a difference to the asylum's rates of readmission.

Patients with remittent mania were those who reappeared most frequently and who were therefore most prominent in tables of readmissions. It will be interesting to discuss the course of treatment of the three patients who were readmitted most frequently. The patient with the highest rate was Sarah G., who entered the Retreat on twenty separate occasions between 1814 and 1860. Aged only twenty-four on her first admission, she withstood the ravages of her disorder to die in 1871, still in the Retreat, at the ripe old age of eighty. Apart from an interval of eight and a half years between her first and second attacks, and the eleven years of more continuous illness during her final period in the asylum, this patient's illness took a fairly regular pattern. The intervals between her illness were generally about a year to eighteen months (although in three instances they were of two and a half to three years), and her periods of treatment were short, averaging between three and eight months. Elizabeth G., also a sufferer from remittent mania, entered the Retreat ten times between 1823 and her death in 1842 although she had had many previous attacks even before coming to York. Her pattern of illness appears to have been more irregular than Sarah's with intervals of two to eighteen months between attacks and longer periods of eight to eleven months in the asylum. Elizabeth W., who entered the Retreat fourteen times between 1891 and her death in 1915, also suffered from remittent mania, although in her case this was associated with weak-mindedness. Her illness took a fairly predictable pattern with between three and nine months of remission between treatment periods of one to five months, except that the last three periods in the asylum lengthened from one, to two, to ten years respectively. The histories of patients suffering from remittent mania obviously increased the rates of readmission and qualified the meaning of 'recovery', highlighting the fact that it was not synonymous with cure. For the first two of these patients (whose outcome of treatment is known, unlike the third, each period of treatment ended with a verdict of 'recovered'.[73] In this context it is not surprising that Samuel Tuke (probably after talking with George Jepson) should comment, 'I know not what degree of sanity is generally thought sufficient to warrant the application of the term "*cured.*"[74]

Yet this note of agnosticism should not obscure the fact, shown in Table 9.12, that 83.9 per cent of the patients had only one period of treatment at York and a further 11.6 per cent had two periods of therapy over the period 1796–1910. It is interesting to see that an increasing proportion of patients had only one period of treatment, from 76.9 per cent under Jepson to 89.2 per cent under Pierce. A downward trend was evident in the proportion of patients readmitted for two or more occasions, during successive superintendents, although within this trend the proportion of second admissions rose for a time under Allis and Thurnam. The readmission rates at the Retreat were higher than in some other contemporary mental institutions: at Hook Norton and Witney madhouses in Oxfordshire, 86.4 per cent of patients were admitted only once between 1828 and 1867,[75] and 86.3 per cent fell into this category at Bowhill House, Exeter, between 1801 and 1869.[76] That the Retreat's readmissions were more frequent was probably

Table 9.12. *Total number of stays of patients (in %)*

Number of admissions	J	A	T	K	B	P	O[a]
1	76.9	73.8	75.9	85.3	86.6	89.2	83.9
2	12.3	19.3	20.2	11.1	9.3	8.8	11.6
3	6.5	4.1	2.3	2.1	2.1	1.6	2.7
4	2.3	1.4	—	0.6	1.2	0.2	0.8
5	0.8	0.9	1.6	0.3	—	0.2	0.4
6	—	0.5	—	0.3	0.2	0.2	
7	—	—	—	—	0.2	—	
8	0.4	—	—	0.3	0.2	—	0.6
10	0.4	—	—	—	—	—	
14	—	—	—	—	0.2	—	
20	0.4	—	—	—	—	—	
N	260	218	129	334	440	630	2,011

[a] J, Jepson (1796–1823); A, Allis (1823–41); T, Thurnam (1841–9); K, Kitching (1849–74); B, Baker (1874–92); P, Pierce (1892–1910); O, Overall (1796–1910).

because Quaker patients were more likely to be sent back to the same institution than were mental patients at other asylums. The declining rates of readmission towards the end of our period may be a response to a number of interrelated factors: a declining proportion of Quaker patients; the omission of readmission figures after 1910 so that Pierce's figures are understated; and the use of voluntary boarding as an alternative to certification. It is likely that declining rates of readmission also reflected the decreasing attraction of the Retreat as its distinctiveness in therapy abated and its influence lessened.

10

The Retreat's influence

That a small institution for the care of mentally ill Quakers should during the early nineteenth century attract almost as many notable visitors as the famed Gothic magnificence of York Minster would not have been predicted by the Retreat's founders. However, the publication in 1813 of *A Description of the Retreat* by Samuel Tuke, the grandson of the founder, was to transform an obscure establishment into a Mecca for the enlightened. The *Description* was the first full-length account of asylum practice; it crystallised many of the ideas concerning the insane and their care current at that time, and presented them in non-technical, easily assimilated prose. Thus it aroused the interest not only of 'professionals' engaged in the care of the insane but also of well-meaning individuals concerned about contemporary social problems. For them the humanity and efficiency with which institutions were run appeared to be an index of their country's level of civilisation. Visits to institutions such as the Retreat became a virtually obligatory element in a tour undertaken by a responsible citizen.[1] And since some members of this educated public were involved as governors, trustees or visiting justices in the practical oversight of institutions in their own locality, their interest in visiting a model establishment like the Retreat was also utilitarian. For those unable to visit York, the *Description* itself became a progressive handbook or guide to the newly emerging world of asylumdom.

Why did Tuke's *Description* have such an impact? Tuke broke new ground in describing a particular institution and the therapy pursued there, rather than writing a more abstract analysis of insanity and its treatment as had earlier writers on madness. Tuke's diary[2] informs us that he had read many of the standard medical works on the subject by Haslam, Pinel, Ferriar, Arnold and others but he did not follow their method of presentation. It is possible that this stemmed from the fact that although he had wished to pursue a medical career, he had been prevented from doing so and hence felt that he lacked expertise in this area. A more important reason may also have been that he had no intention of writing a lengthy theoretical book but instead aimed at a shorter and more practical work. Even before his father, Henry Tuke, had requested him to write his account in 1811, Samuel Tuke had expressed his determination 'to collect all the knowledge I can on the theory of insanity, the treatment of the insane, and the construction of lunatic asylums'.[3] And in the *Description,* abstract views on the nature of insanity or the character of the insane were integrated in similar vein into a series of commonsensical observations on treatment. Theoretical speculation in isolation was virtually absent. What general observations there were appeared to stem from an account of pragmatically determined courses of treatment. Indeed, the character of the text was a mirror image of Tuke's own preparations for writing since this alternated conversations with the Retreat superintendent, George Jepson, a study of Retreat cases and more general reading in psychology, philosophy and medicine.[4]

The *Description of the Retreat* was written simply in language that was intelligible to the lay public (instead of being addressed solely to a specialist audience). Only one of its six chapters was devoted to medicine, and even this was as much concerned with such everyday matters as diet, exercise and bathing as with technical subjects like drugs. Elsewhere the emphasis was on the concrete: the location, plan and living arrangements of the Retreat; the reception, routine and occupations of patients; and the methods of restraint together with the occasions when it was used. Readers were able to build in their own mind – through a gradual accretion of detail – both a firm image of the Retreat's pattern of living and an understanding of what moral treatment involved for its patients. They were introduced to George Jepson with his judicious and humane methods of treating the mentally ill. And through case-studies they partook of vicarious drama as when a manacled patient of Herculean size arrived, was freed from his chains, and through mild treatment was brought swiftly back to sanity. Or they might empathise with the individual who on being brought from a harsher establishment run on more traditional lines exclaimed that the Retreat was 'Eden, Eden, Eden'.[5]

With a beguiling simplicity Tuke had taken his readers on an intellectual tour in which the subject of insanity had emerged from the dark shadows of traditional usage into the full light of public debate:

> When once its practicability is demonstrated there is an end to reasoning on the subject . . .
> This was my secret view in the History [i.e. the *Description*] of the Retreat and its success has proved the omnipotence of facts.[6]

Through demonstrating that a milder therapy was a workable, successful way to treat the mentally ill, the *Description of the Retreat* provided reformers with valuable ammunition for their campaign to improve conditions for the mentally ill. 'By the weight and importance of . . . facts' one can 'almost force the general introduction of a better system' was Tuke's own belief and programme of action.[7]

The *Description* forced those who practised older methods of treatment for the insane on the defensive. Nowhere was this more obvious than in York itself where the fifth English asylum for the insane had been founded in 1777. The physician to the York Asylum, Dr Best (writing under the pseudonym Evigilator), protested in the local press against the illiberal and grossly unfounded comments made in the *Description* about other institutions.[8] From Best's point of view even more damaging than Tuke's book in publicising the mild methods used at the Retreat was a contemporary advertisement for a private madhouse to be run along the same lines by the Retreat's physician, Dr Belcombe. This provided direct rivalry for patients not only with the York Asylum but with Best's own private house as well. Best felt that this advertisement was both unprofessional and incorrect in claiming superiority of treatment. The intemperate nature of his response hardened a long-standing local suspicion that the asylum's patients were being ill treated. In his reply, Tuke stated that although the *Description* had not been concerned with particular institutions he was interested to know what reasons had caused 'this extreme tenderness' in Best's mind.[9] Dr Best hastily tried to end the public discussion he had aroused, and to dampen heightened interest in the affairs of the Asylum.[10] But to no avail.

Those who had been concerned about the nature of this closed institution now began a public interrogation of its physician, reminding him that the 'proper management of lunatics is no mere private concern'. One authoritative letter acknowledged the importance of Samuel Tuke's book in opening up the state of the asylums to public scrutiny. 'It seems as if he [Best] were conscious, that the readers [of the *Description*] . . . would necessarily be led to compare the Retreat with the Asylum, and to draw conclusions by no means favourable to the latter.'[11] Those at the Retreat in fact played a much more important part in the reform of the York Asylum than is usually thought. But because of earlier unsuccessful attempts by a Retreat party to stimulate reform at the asylum these efforts were at first taken unobtrusively, and others – notably Godfrey Higgins – thus automatically moved into the limelight. So although three generations of Tukes joined in the war of words in the local press, only the founder of the Retreat, William Tuke, did not follow the custom of writing under a pseudonym. Henry asserted that 'the asylum has been wrested from its original design . . . instead of being a public charity it has become a source of private emolument'.[12] Samuel stated that 'the means of preventing, detecting, and correcting abuses which are provided in most other similar institutions are not found provided' at the asylum.[13] And in a magisterial letter William Tuke reminded the Asylum's governors of the regulations that in other institutions safeguarded patients' interests.[14]

That the asylum's poorer patients desperately needed the kind of safeguards that operated in the Retreat and elsewhere was soon revealed. Godfrey Higgins, a West Yorkshire magistrate who had sent a pauper patient (William Vicars, or Vickers) to the asylum the previous spring, published the details of Vicar's filthy, lousy, bruised and half-starved condition on being discharged in October 1813. Other cases of neglect and ill-treatment were brought forward at the Asylum Governors' Quarterly Court in December 1813: among them was Martha Kidd, who had wounds to her head and a dislocated hip, and the Reverend Mr Schorey, whose ill-usage by his keeper included being kicked down stairs. However, the governors' complacency over the state of the asylum was stiffened by Best's resistance to an investigation. It took vigorous action by Samuel Tuke – in encouraging local gentlemen to subscribe twenty pounds to the asylum to constitute themselves as new governors – before the reforming process was initiated early in 1814. What remained intractable was the problem of discovering the full extent of the problems in an institution where governors had ceased regular inspection twenty years earlier and patients' relatives and friends had been denied access even longer. The day after the investigating committee began its work a fire destroyed part of the asylum and killed four patients. Although this dramatic blaze was probably accidental it heightened the feeling that vital evidence was being concealed. So too did the burning some days later of many of the asylum's records by the steward after his accidental disclosure of systematic peculation by Best and his predecessor, Hunter. But the key that opened the door to reform came in March 1814 with the discovery by Higgins of four secret cells or 'low grates' at the asylum that were horrifying in their overcrowded and excremental conditions. This provided decisive proof that only root-and-branch reform would suffice.[15]

The Retreat's influence on that reform was highly significant. One of the new reforming governors of the York Asylum, S. W. Nicoll, concluded that 'The "Description of the Retreat" was unquestionably the prime mover' of its reform.[16] The book provided a model for reform both in delineating a mild therapy for patients and in suggesting that an asylum should be an open institution with an adequate system of inspection to check performance against objectives. When two members of the York Asylum's newly appointed Committee on Rules and Management visited the Retreat in January 1814 they were 'much struck with the contrast' between the two institutions.[17] And the committee's suggestions on new rules and regulations for the asylum, which were adopted at the Annual Court of Governors in August 1814, were clearly influenced by those of the other psychiatric institution in the city. Those associated with the Retreat were also in the forefront of reform: Samuel Tuke, as a new governor, gave his advice on the asylum's new buildings and was active on the Committee of Management set up under the new regulations. William Tuke, also one of the new governors, was one of the first visitors appointed to inspect the asylum at regular intervals.[18] After nearly all the existing staff had been dismissed from their posts at the York Asylum, George Jepson helped the new officers to organise the institution on new lines.[19] By December 1815 Samuel Tuke could conclude 'I believe the *system* of one is as mild as the other' when comparing these two psychiatric institutions in York.[20]

To see this reform of the York Asylum only as a swift triumph of mild methods over harsh ones, or as the victory of enlightened reformers over cruel, misguided or greedy individuals, would be an over-simplification.[21] The asylum's officers were obviously trying to discredit the reformers when they depicted them as motivated by personality or party rather than by principle.[22] Yet the reformers themselves may have given some credibility to this interpretation of events since in the heat of the battle they concentrated on specific instances of abuse by particular individuals. But since there was no consensus on the nature of mental illness or on methods of treatment, their focus on obvious cases of cruelty was probably strategically correct. It was only gradually that the more important underlying issue of the relationship between the public and such an institution was emphasised. As Higgins explained:

If the misconduct of the York Asylum is to be palliated, softened, and excused so may that of every other institution . . . if we permit it to be said that the charges of abuse are a mere cry of faction, – that personal hostility, and not public principle, is at the bottom, – every keeper of every lunatic receptacle may have his personal enemies too, and the whole question may be resolved into party spleen or professional envy. As an example, the York Asylum stands alone. Instituted by persons of the first character, conducted by those who founded it, and their no less respectable successors, the vigilant attention of the public at large . . . could alone rectify the abuses which existed.[23]

And it was urging this necessity for public inspection of asylums and madhouses that was to be the main outcome of the Select Committee on Madhouses of 1814–16 after its review of abuses at York and also at Bethlem. Evidence to this committee by William Tuke on the mild therapy practised by York Friends at their establishment gave further publicity to the Retreat.[24] When included in the same volume as evidence on abuses at other establishments, the simplicity and humanity of his testimony stood out in dramatic contrast. In this context it must have appeared doubly compelling to contemporaries and been one factor in the growing influence of the York Retreat.

The public spotlight on the Retreat came at a time when the typical establishment for the care of the mentally ill was the small private madhouse. Although other private establishments – such as Laverstock House or Brislington House – were as advanced in their humane methods of treatment, only the York Retreat gained sufficient publicity to act as a model for others.[25] One crude indication of the extent of its influence was the adoption of the name

Retreat by a minority of private houses. These were found in ten counties stretching from Gloucestershire to Lancashire on the western side of England, and from Sussex to County Durham on the east. Not surprisingly, most were located in Yorkshire itself where there were eleven other Retreats scattered from Leeds in the west to Hull in the east.[26] Most, however, were in the countryside around York and thus in conscious imitation of the rural surroundings of the Friends' Retreat. Although adoption of the name indicated that the proprietors recognised the popularity of 'mild methods' practised at the original Retreat, and hence its pulling power in recruiting patients, the use of the name 'Retreat' did not necessarily guarantee that this mild therapy was actually implemented.

In some instances private houses advertised explicitly that they would employ the same methods used at the Retreat:

At Clifton, near York, a private establishment has been formed under the direction of the Physician to the Retreat, or Quaker's Asylum, for the reception and cure of persons afflicted with nervous complaints and insanity, with a view to introduce, on a small scale, the mild methods of treatment in use at that institution.[27]

Dr Belcombe's close contact with both establishments would have ensured that there was a reasonable degree of congruity. This should also have been the case at Hollytree House, Osbaldwick, a private madhouse taken over by Thomas Allis on his retirement from the post of Retreat superintendent in 1841.[28] It is perhaps more doubtful whether Joseph Taylor had picked up sufficient insight on the York Retreat's methods, from his brief three months' employment as an attendant there in 1798, to run his own private house on these lines. Yet he ran successive 'Retreats' at Southcoates (1823–5), Cottingham (1825–34) and then Hessle (1835–48), all in East Yorkshire.[29] Other Yorkshire madhouses apparently had no direct contact with the Retreat but still claimed, as did Dunnington House, to 'follow the system so successfully observed at the Friends' Retreat, York'.[30]

An institution that spelt out in more detail what it understood such a system to mean for its own practice was Sculcoates Refuge in Hull. At its opening in May 1814 it stated:

In this institution every attempt consistent with humanity will be made to restore the patient. No coercion, no restraint, but what is absolutely necessary to protect the attendant and to prevent self-destruction will ever be employed. Those moral means which are so well pointed out in the late publications on this subject, and so well exemplified in a neighbouring institution, will be had recourse to in order to bring about that desirable object, health of mind.[31]

One of the founders of the Sculcoates Refuge was William Ellis.[32] He was to become the first medical superintendent of the West Riding Asylum, one of a cluster of county asylums created as a result of legislation in 1808. Ellis visited the York Retreat on four occasions: the first in 1816 was some eighteen months before his new appointment was made; the second occurred in May 1818 when he and his wife were actually journeying from Hull to visit the almost completed asylum at Wakefield; the third visit was only a month before he took up his duties in November 1818, and the fourth in July 1822.[33] Indeed, the intimate connection between these two institutions justified D. H. Tuke's verdict that the asylum at Wakefield was 'the legitimate child' of the Retreat.[34]

A visit to Wakefield today might appear to disprove such a statement since the complex of asylum buildings erected there is so huge and multifarious that it seems to be rather a cuckoo's offspring than a genuine descendant of the small-scale domestic buildings of the York Retreat. However, Samuel Tuke's ideas substantially shaped the new asylum. This came about through Tuke's friendship with Godfrey Higgins, the magistrate who in October 1814 moved at a meeting of West Riding justices that a new asylum be built for the Riding. Higgins had worked closely with Tuke to reform abuses at the York Asylum, and their lengthy correspondence indicated the mutual respect and trust that had sprung up between them. It was because Higgins had been so horrified that pauper lunatics from the West Riding had been sent into the inhumane conditions of the old York Asylum that he determined that a better asylum should be built in the western part of the county.[35] Who better to consult on its design than his friend Samuel Tuke, whose *Description of the Retreat* had made him an authority on the subject? Accordingly, Tuke was invited to the early meetings of the committee supervising the erection of the new asylum. He wrote 'Instructions for the Architects who prepared designs for the West Riding Asylum', and in 1815 addressed to the justices a more detailed pamphlet for their guidance, *Practical Hints on the Construction and Economy of Pauper Lunatic Asy-*

lums.³⁶ Characteristically, Tuke said that he had been 'much surprised' to have been consulted and was also diffident about his pamphlet.³⁷ The justices were, however, in no doubt as to their debt to Tuke and gave him an inscribed piece of plate to show their appreciation.³⁸ When the plans and elevations of the asylum were published in 1819, it was deemed appropriate to reprint Tuke's 'Instructions' and *Practical Hints* as a fitting introduction to the volume.³⁹

The plans indicated how substantially the architects had been influenced by Samuel Tuke's ideas, although the declivity of the site made it more suitable to construct a three-storey building rather than the one of two storeys envisaged by Tuke.⁴⁰ However, it is interesting to see how far Tuke's ideas on the ideal asylum had in turn progressed beyond those of the Retreat. By 1815 Tuke regarded the Retreat buildings as in important respects old fashioned and inconvenient.⁴¹ At Wakefield he stressed features that were lacking at the Retreat such as the importance of seeing the asylum as a whole so that patients could be classified according to their state of mind, each class being given interconnecting day-rooms, galleries and courtyards. Having recently been engaged in the reform of the York Asylum he also emphasised the necessity of a building where superintendence of patients by attendants, and of attendants by superior officers, was easily attained:

> The regulations of an asylum should establish a species of espionage, terminating in the PUBLIC: this cannot be effected in an ill-constructed building. One servant and one officer should be so placed as to watch over another. All should be vigilantly observed by well-selected and interested visitors.⁴²

In spite of this sombre passage, Tuke's tone in his introduction was more buoyant than in any of his other writings on insanity. 'Happily, however, ignorance and indifference on this subject have greatly lessened', he wrote; '. . . under proper moral and medical treatment a large majority of lunatics do certainly recover.'⁴³

Tuke's optimistic tone was perhaps conditioned by the increasing amount of contact between those administering the Retreat and others engaged in the care of lunatics who sought to learn from their experience. This can be seen in the growing number of visitors to the Retreat, an area in which the impact of Tuke's *Description* was readily discernible (see Fig. 10.1). English visitors who

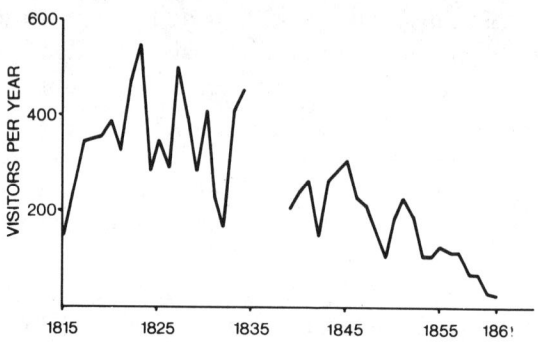

Figure 10.1. Visitors to the Retreat, 1815–61.
(*Source:* BIHR D/3/1–3, Visitors Books [1798–1861]. The series is broken because figures for 1835–8 are incomplete. Before 1815 the books were not utilised systematically.)

were professionally interested in the Retreat came from all kinds of establishments: from four of the seven voluntary hospitals created before 1800 (Bethlem, Liverpool, Manchester and York), and five of the nine county asylums established before 1830 (Nottingham, Bedford, Lancaster, West Riding and Cornwall), as well as from small private madhouses. Among later visitors from private houses was George Bompas of Fishponds in 1841 and Samuel Newington of Ticehurst in 1859. Some of the visitors' comments suggested that a visit was rather akin to a pilgrimage. Dr Robert Moody of Tamworth, 'who has an establishment for the reception of insane patients, . . . was induced to visit the Retreat from the high character he had received of it in a variety of ways and is happy to say he has been very highly gratified in every respect'.[44]

The frequency with which visitors from Ireland came to the York Retreat indicated the strength of its influence there. Two Quaker Retreats had been created, at Loughall (near Armagh) and at Donnybrook (near Dublin); the latter was set up on similar lines to the York establishment in 1810. In that same year the achievements of the York Retreat were also publicised in the *Belfast Monthly Magazine* by Thomas Hancock, a Quaker doctor from Antrim, whose interest in the Retreat had begun during his schooldays at Ackworth and was deepened by his correspondence with his schoolfellow there – Samuel Tuke. But it was Tuke's book rather than Hancock's articles that roused concern for the Irish insane.

The Richmond Asylum, which opened in 1815 as the first progressive asylum in Ireland, had adopted moral treatment following 'a publication of a Mr. Took, manager of the York Asylum'. The duties of the asylum's moral governor were modelled on those of the York Retreat's superintendent as were some of the asylum's devices for restraint. And when legislation of 1817 and 1820 had created a national system of district asylums it was noticeable that visitors to the York Retreat came from towns where these institutions had been established.[45]

The extent to which the Retreat could shape the character of other asylums was exemplified most clearly in its relationship with one of the first English county asylums, the Nottingham Asylum, which opened in 1811. 'This affords a prospect of our doing some good beyond our own sphere', confided Samuel Tuke to his diary in October 1811 on learning that Thomas Morris and his wife were staying at the Retreat. Having 'undertaken the superintendence of an institution for the insane at Nottingham', Tuke recorded happily, '[they] are now studying the proper mode of treatment at the Retreat.'[46] Morris later told Jepson that this experience had been 'of the greatest use to him', and the physician of the Asylum, Dr. Pennington, informed Tuke that the Morrises had imitated 'closely the admirable system' of 'mild and humane management practised at the Retreat'. Dr Pennington concluded that it was to the Retreat's influence that 'the favourable report of the Nottingham Asylum is principally to be referred'.[47] The impact of his visit to the Retreat was reinforced by the *Description,* as Morris fulsomely acknowledged:

Mr. Tuke's publication [I] am glad to say has been by the governors here generally read and much approved and admired; it is replete with good practical influence, and shows most clearly the deep research, and goodness of heart of the author. In short your establishment I sincerely believe is considered the best in the kingdom, or the whole world.[48]

The Retreat's influence was greatest in the second and third decades of the nineteenth century. At a time when nine county asylums were opened in England and four asylums were founded in Scotland it was natural that those responsible for these new institutions would turn to older, well-known asylums as exemplars. In this new world of asylumdom there was neither a set of practical manuals to provide blueprints nor a cadre of trained professionals to realise them. Visits to other asylums, such as the Retreat, provided in-service training for asylum architects, newly appointed officers and conscientious governors.[49] Within this fluid and expanding institutional network there was much cross-fertilisation of ideas and practices. Thus, although the Retreat was a seminal influence there was only a selective and piecemeal assimilation of its ideas. In the case of the West Riding Asylum, for example, where Tuke's influence was direct and incontestable, it is obvious that practices at other asylums – notably those at Derby and Glasgow – were also imitated.[50] Pragmatism and a concern for the practicable, rather than ideology, dictated an eclectic absorption of ideas by inexperienced asylum officers. Within this melting pot of concepts and practices the Retreat's moral treatment may have appeared attractive because of its well-proven character. And for asylum governors and visiting justices its mild therapy accorded with the newly fashionable orthodoxy (promoted by the Select Committee on Madhouses) that prescribed a humanitarian regime for asylum inmates.

Asylums in Scotland were amongst those significantly affected by the Retreat: four of the five asylums created between 1800 and 1830 acknowledged its influence. The managers of the Aberdeen Infirmary and Lunatic Asylum (founded in 1800 as the second such institution in Scotland) sent their new superintendent to York in 1813 'to learn what happens at the Retreat'. They also requested a copy of the rules and regulations of the establishment that they referred to as 'one of the most perfect in the island'.[51] At Edinburgh where the next Scottish asylum was created thirteen years later, Robert Reid, its architect, visited York to see how the Friends' Retreat was fitted up. It was also planned to send the newly appointed superintendent to learn from George Jepson, and to try to recruit keepers who had worked at the Retreat. The physician to this asylum, Dr Duncan, had visited York in 1812 when he decided that the Retreat was 'the best-regulated establishment in Europe' and had 'set an example which claims the imitation' of every nation. In his report on the new asylum of Edinburgh Duncan suggested that it should be modelled on the York Retreat.[52] This was not to be the case in every respect at the next Scottish asylum, that of Glasgow, whose architect, W. Stark, had visited the Retreat and been very favourably impressed, but whose eventual panopticon building owed nothing to the York institution.[53] But at the Dundee Asylum, founded six years later in 1820, the Retreat was again a formative influence and its regulations lay 'constantly in the apartment of the superintendent as the guide of his conduct'.[54]

Ironically, one of the most discernible changes made by the Retreat in Scottish asylums' practices appeared to be in showing them how mechanical restraint could be effected along more humane lines using straps rather than strait-waistcoats or other devices. In 1813 Jepson was asked to send to Edinburgh 'two of the leather strap machines which they use in confining patients, and which still allow them to employ their hands to a certain degree'.[55] Some time later the Glasgow Asylum requested 'half a dozen of your spring buckles for straps' as they wished 'to apply them at those times, when the patient can have an opportunity of unbuckling the common ones'.[56] And the superintendent of the Dundee Asylum asked for a replica of the instrument 'employed in administering food to those who persist in refusing to take it'.[57] This kind of correspondence was not confined to Scottish asylums since both English[58] and American institutions made comparable requests.

In March 1818 Caleb Cresson, a Quaker from Philadelphia who had visited the Retreat, wrote to thank Jepson for sending him straps with buckles and keys used 'for confining patients to beds'. These were now in use not only at the Friends' Retreat in Philadelphia but also in other American asylums.[59] Cresson had asked Jepson to send an export order of a gross of such devices via Liverpool to Philadelphia. This transaction gives a vivid glimpse not only into the cohesive world of asylumdom (where such far-flung exchanges were so readily accomplished) but also the almost familial network that operated within the Atlantic community of Quakers. American Quakers were prominent in the foundation of about half the American asylums created before 1824 and looked to the York Retreat as a model. The scope for its influence was very considerable since by 1800 there were only three hospitals – in Pennsylvania, Williamsburg and New York – that catered for the mentally ill in the United States.[60]

In 1811 Samuel Tuke recorded in his diary that he had 'sent off some remarks for his American Friends, who propose establishing a house for the insane drawn from the experience of the Retreat'.[61] This was published as an unsigned contribution to the *Eclectic Repertory and Analytical Review*, a journal run by a group of physicians in Philadelphia.[62] Tuke's article, 'Hints on the Treatment of Insane Persons', showed a close similarity in its ideas to his full-length exposition of moral treatment in the *Description,* published two years later. And the *Description* was soon brought out in an American edition that – as the New York Quaker, John Griscom, commented – was 'much read in America'.[63] It was in Philadelphia, with the foundation of the Friends' Asylum for the Insane at Frankford in 1817, that the practices described in this volume first took root. Thomas Scattergood, a travelling minister in the Society of Friends who had visited the York Retreat, was in the forefront of the move to build this asylum in 1813. An abridged copy of Tuke's *Description* was made for circulation among committee members and contributors and this provided the inspiration for their evolving institution.[64] Close contact was maintained between the English and American Friends' Retreats: many Quakers from Pennsylvania continued to visit the York institution.

A much larger and non-sectarian institution – the Bloomingdale Asylum – was also a direct descendant of the Retreat. The New York Quaker, Lindley Murray, had settled in York and had become both friend and guide to the Tukes in their creation of the Retreat. Murray corresponded with Thomas Eddy, who was prominent amongst the governors of the New York Hospital and who championed the need for that hospital to set up an asylum solely for the care of its mentally ill patients.[65] It was as a result of this fortunate set of circumstances that Samuel Tuke was prompted to address a letter, through Eddy, to his fellow governors, laying down the principles that guided the York Retreat.[66] Eddy also lectured them, stating that 'Tuke's Description impressed him the most of all the works on insanity he had consulted. No work contains so many excellent and appropriate observations.'[67] It was largely as a result of Eddy's championing of the concept of a 'Rural Retreat' that thirty-eight acres were purchased for a second hospital, this time exclusively for the insane, at Bloomingdale on the outskirts of New York.[68] At its opening in 1821 the governors declared that the asylum was opened

> with the express design to carry into effect that system of management of the insane, happily termed *moral treatment,* the superior efficacy of which has been demonstrated in several of the hospitals of Europe, and especially in that admirable establishment of the Society of Friends called 'THE RETREAT', near York in England.[69]

Samuel Tuke, on learning of their plans 'to rival the Retreat' wished 'with all my heart they may surpass it for I am persuaded we have not reached the *ne plus ultra*'.[70] That those at Bloomingdale continued to see the York Retreat as in some sense an alma mater is suggested by the comment in 1863 of its physician, Dr Brown, who after a visit there wrote that 'the genius and the earnestness of Tuke still abide among his successors'. The lasting influence of the Retreat on Bloomingdale, as at the Frankford Retreat, was seen in the way both had imitated the York Retreat in their architecture, and in giving supreme authority to a lay superintendent.[71]

The third asylum to be strongly influenced by the York Retreat was less committed to the supremacy of moral treatment that lay superintendence implied. The Hartford Retreat in Connecticut was unusual in being founded in 1824, not by laymen, as had been the case with other early American asylums, but by doctors. And its first superintendent, Eli Todd, was a physician. The ideas of the York institution, faithfully recorded in Tuke's *Description,* were very influential at Hartford. Its name and the model of organisation adopted were those of its English counterpart. Eli Todd's analysis of the principles guiding the new asylum was apparently strongly influenced by those given in Tuke's *Description* with their concern to treat patients 'with the tenderness of genuine sympathy', their stress on a simple environment and their desire to provide a genteel range of amusements and occupations for inmates.[72] But a rival influence was the writing of Pinel with his greater stress on medical treatment. Eli Todd emphasised that moral therapy needed to go hand in hand with medical treatment since 'the mind and body are so connected that there can scarcely be a disease of either in which the other is not involved, and in which medical and moral treatment may not be advantageously combined'.[73]

Like the Hartford Retreat the McLean Asylum (which had opened six years earlier at Charlestown near Boston) had a medical superintendent. Before undertaking his duties Dr Morrill Wyman had visited the asylums at Hartford and Bloomingdale. In New York he met Thomas Eddy, who personally conducted him round the new asylum and gave him Tuke's *Description* as a memento of his visit. In spite of his medical training Wyman was sufficiently convinced by the example given by the York Retreat and its imitators to give moral treatment the principal role in curing mental disease. The Retreat's influence was reinforced under a successor, Thomas

G. Lee (previously one of Eli Todd's young doctors at the Frankford Asylum), who introduced many other features of the Retreat to the McLean.[74]

The clear imprint that the York Retreat had made on America's early corporate asylums was evident only in a more indirect and diffused form in the next generation of state asylums in New England and New York. Samuel B. Woodward, who had been active in promoting the Hartford Retreat and knew this institution intimately, was appointed in 1833 the first superintendent of Massachusetts's asylum – the Worcester State Hospital. He continued to consult Dr Eli Todd, the head of the Frankford Retreat, in order to learn 'this novel business'.[75] And one of his successors, Dr Merrick Bemis, was sufficiently interested in the York Retreat to visit it in 1856.[76] At the asylum in Brattleborough, Vermont, another of the early state asylums, William H. Rockwell, a young physician from the Hartford Retreat, was appointed in 1836 as the first superintendent. Predictably, perhaps, the asylum was known as the Brattleboro Retreat.[77] Seven years later, Amariah Brigham went from his post as superintendent at Hartford to a comparable position in the new asylum at Utica in New York.[78] However, it was not merely through the indirect channel of the Hartford Retreat that the York Retreat's ideals were transmitted to American institutions. A steady stream of American visitors came to York; amongst them were that redoubtable reformer Dorothea Dix, and in 1845, Dr Isaac Ray, formerly superintendent of the Maine Insane Hospital and arguably the most influential psychiatrist in the United States.[79]

That Tuke's ideas had assumed a compelling relevance was mainly due to the leading role taken by Quakers in promoting the early corporate asylums. But the considerable intellectual impact made by the writings of Benjamin Rush and Philippe Pinel meant that these ideas did not go unchallenged. The greater importance they gave to medical treatment in the relief of insanity was reflected in the more even significance of medical as well as moral therapy in American asylum practice.[80] In their moral treatment, however, American asylums showed a remarkable fidelity to the principles Tuke had publicised. This can be seen, for example, in the statement by Woodward who, in spite of his belief in medication, outlined in 1841 the philosophy of moral treatment used at the Worcester Asylum in words that Tuke could have subscribed to:

> By our whole moral treatment, as well as our religious services, we inculcate all the habits and obligations of rational society. We think the insane should never be deceived . . . They may be held responsible for their conduct so far as they are capable of regulating it. By encouraging self-control and respect for themselves we make them better men.[81]

And six years later Dr Amariah Brigham, superintendent of Utica Hospital, gave a definition of moral treatment that suggested the *Description's* ideas provided a shorthand currency to describe contemporary practices in American asylums:

> The removal of the insane from home and former associations, with respectful and kind treatment under all circumstances, and in most cases manual labour, attendance on religious worship on Sundays, the establishment of regular habits of self-control, diversion of the mind from morbid trains of thought, are now generally considered as essential in the moral treatment of the insane.[82]

In the Old World the influence of the York Retreat was more circumscribed than in the New: continental Europe had no comparable body of organised Friends through which the lessons of the Retreat could be disseminated, and alternative domestic models of reformed treatment for the insane existed in France and Italy in the work of Pinel, Daquin, Esquirol and Chiarugi. However, this did not entirely preclude interest in the Retreat's work. Among several French visitors to York was Dr Ferrus (1784–1861), Pinel's successor at the Bicêtre.[83] Contact between the two institutions was maintained by Samuel Tuke, who visited asylums in Paris in 1824. Interestingly, he thought that 'they might certainly take some useful lessons from *us,* but I think there is also a good deal to be learnt from *them*' in medical treatment.[84] Conversely, it was in the Retreat's practice of moral treatment that French interest was greatest. The penetrating character of remarks on the inner significance of the Retreat's practices made by the Genevan doctor, Delarive, after a visit to the Retreat in 1798 have been discussed in an earlier chapter.[85] More typical was the kind of concrete, external description given by the distinguished French economist, Jerome Blanqui, after a visit in 1823. He concluded that 'tenderness and healthy living are the two main bases of treatment'.[86] It was this aspect of the Retreat that also struck the Italian visitors, who were more numerous than the French. Count Pecchio of Milan wrote one of the fullest descriptions of the Retreat and commended its 'simplicity, cordiality, order and quietness'.[87]

It was these moral attributes that also attracted Maximilian Jacobi, who translated Tuke's *Description* into German in 1822. Significantly, Jacobi took as his epigraph for this translation, 'And truly only his heart, the veritable faculty of ideas, elevates man above himself.' Jacobi, a prominent institutional psychiatrist whom D. H. Tuke described as the 'Nestor' amongst German asylum superintendents, forged a close connection with the York Retreat. A founder of the Siegburg Asylum near Bonn (which he directed from its opening in 1825 until his death in 1858), Jacobi approached his work from a humanitarian and philosophical standpoint that saw foreign experience such as that at the York Retreat as relevant to his own somaticist position. He visited York in 1834 and his relationship with those who ran the Retreat was sufficiently close for John Kitching to translate Jacobi's *On the Construction and Management of Hospitals for the Insane* and for Samuel Tuke to write a lengthy introduction to it. Although Jacobi's own work was challenged within his own country, the publicity that his translation of the *Description* had given to the Retreat contributed to an increased number of German visitors to York.[88] Among them in 1842 was J. G. Kohl, who praised the Retreat's 'admirable order' and the 'beneficial and tranquillising influence' of work on the insane. He thought that the institution had 'led the way in the march of improvement, and has served as an invaluable model in the reform of other English madhouses'.[89]

On receiving the first copies of the *Description* from the publisher, Samuel Tuke had hoped God would 'prosper this imperfect effort to awaken the public sympathy' towards the 'afflictions' and 'sufferings' of the insane.[90] The publicity that the book gave to the Retreat was reinforced by the accounts of visitors there, whose interest had in many cases first been aroused by reading either the *Description* or reviews of it. The most notable of these reviews was that of Sydney Smith in the *Edinburgh Review* who captured the reading public's imagination with his views on 'Mad Quakers'. 'It does not appear to them that because a man is mad upon one subject, that he is to be considered in a state of complete mental degradation, or insensible to feelings of gratitude.'[91] Knowledge of these milder methods – used successfully with the insane at the York Retreat – was a major factor in changing the climate of public opinion and thus facilitating their diffusion elsewhere. In a private letter written in July 1825, Samuel Tuke described how a few years earlier

> there was then a struggle between the two systems – that of gentleness and that of brute force. – Now, happily, I think the question, theoretically, may be said to be determined in the public mind, and magistrates and other persons concerned in the public establishments for lunatics, are, almost without exception *anxious* to introduce the best mode of treatment.[92]

Although Tuke, with characteristic modesty, made no reference to the role played by the Retreat in this revolution, two years later a select committee paid the institution an appropriate compliment. In making enquiries on the conditions of the insane its question about moral treatment merely paraphrased Tuke's *Description:*

> In the moral treatment of the Patients, it is considered an object of importance to encourage their own efforts of self-restraint in every possible way, by exciting and cherishing in them feelings of self-respect, by treating them with delicacy, more especially in avoiding any improper exposure of their cases before strangers in their own presence, and generally by maintaining towards them a treatment uniformly judicious and kind, sympathising with them, and at the same time diverting their minds from painful and injudicious associations.[93]

This period marked the zenith of the Retreat's influence, as was also indicated by numbers of visitors to the asylum. The annual average in the two decades 1815–34 was 350 and 353, whereas that from 1839–48 was 234 and from 1849–58 only 137. Other institutions were now to extend the potential of moral treatment through the practice of non-restraint and thus to be the new focus of public interest.

If the Retreat had shown the possibility that mechanical restraint could be restricted, the Lincoln Asylum laid down as a principle that it should be discontinued.[94] Charlesworth and Hill at Lincoln steadily reduced the extent to which restraint was used until in 1837 non-restraint was implemented as a principle.[95] John Conolly introduced the system successfully in the much larger asylum at Hanwell, after his appointment there two years later. Conolly had read Tuke's *Description* while a medical student in Edinburgh and had visited the Retreat in 1839.[96] He commented later:

All of us who have followed in the path of William and Samuel Tuke, at however great a distance, must ever gratefully acknowledge the extent of our debt to them. It is true that neither they nor Pinel ventured wholly to abolish mechanical coercion; this was left for Charlesworth to attempt, and for Gardiner Hill to carry out, at Lincoln, and for Hanwell to confirm on the largest scale . . . every historian of these establishments must point to Pinel and Tuke as the men who led the way for the more complete system of non-restraint.[97]

With the almost universal adoption (or at least a nominal lip-service paid to) the system of non-restraint in mid-century English asylums, the Retreat's refusal to adopt the principle proclaimed its 'conservative' rather than 'progressive' nature. It underlined the extent to which, by the second half of the nineteenth century, this asylum was less a blueprint for current imitation that a historical inspiration.

That the Retreat was considered the alma mater of moral treatment was indicated by the constant stream of visitors there, whether to consult Jepson or Tuke, or visit the institution. It was to be expected that Friends should be prominent amongst them, whether notable individuals like Elizabeth Fry or J. J. Gurney, or more obscure members who felt it their duty to visit such a 'painfully interesting establishment'.[98] It was also predictable that amongst its visitors should be social reformers (such as Robert Owen), those in public life (including several MPs and the Duke of Wellington), or those professionally concerned with the insane (who came from nearly every country in Europe and from many parts of the United States). However, the majority of its visitors fell into none of these categories. Some of these visitors' reactions are known: Grand Duke Nicholas of Russia exclaimed frequently, 'c'est parfait! c'est admirable!'[99] Others left signatures only, amongst them the skilful drawings of the seven Senecan Indians from North America who visited in 1818 (see Plate 30). That ordinary members of the public continued to come in such numbers suggested the Retreat's enormous reputation. This reputation was acknowledged more formally by the Medico-Psychological Association when it met at York in 1892 to honour the Retreat's centenary and desired

> to place on record its admiration of the spirit which animated William Tuke and his fellow workers a hundred years ago, its appreciation of the mighty revolution which they inaugurated, and its thankfulness for the beneficent result which their example has secured in the humane and enlightened treatment of the insane throughout the world.[100]

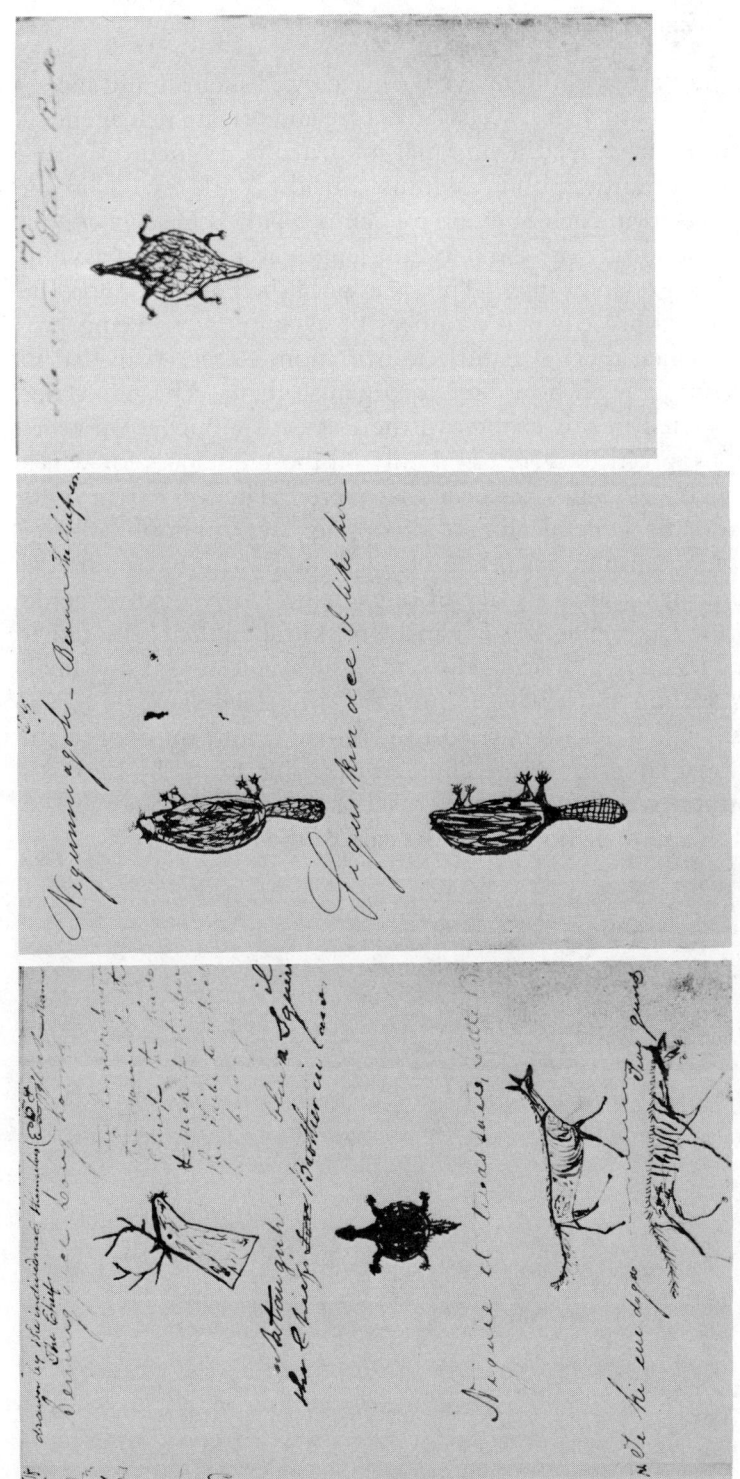

Plate 30. Signatures in the Visitors Book of six Senecan Indians and their chief who visited the Retreat in 1818

That the Retreat should have been accorded such significance is paradoxical. Its tiny size, sectarian nature and private management might have guaranteed it minimal influence in a nineteenth-century world of large, public asylums. But the York establishment was rescued from such oblivion by Samuel Tuke's *Description*, the first and for some time the only full-length account of an asylum run on 'progressive' lines. This was published at an opportune time when unprecedented numbers of asylums were being created, but when there was little information – other than that in the *Description* – on how best to organise them. The numerous examples cited in this chapter of the Retreat's influence on other institutions' practices were based only on those instances for which documentary evidence has been discovered. The full extent of its impact on the general climate of opinion was undoubtedly far greater. Contemporaries acknowledged the Retreat to be a model institution: it became a place of pilgrimage where visitors could see that the *Description* was not an act of skilful publicity but rather mirrored its early practices. However, the atypicality of this small Quaker asylum must have limited the effectiveness of its moral treatment when admirers tried to translate it into quite different institutional environments. Thus, in the long term, the Retreat's contribution was not so much to act as a model as to serve as a symbol of a new orthodoxy in the care of the insane.

Appendix:
Selected case-notes of patients

Case histories are a neglected but rich source, not only for the history of medicine, but for a variety of other areas in social history including that of the family. However, they raise difficult problems of interpretation, including the central issue of how far the historian can generalise from a particular example.

Four case histories have been chosen here to illustrate changing methods of treatment and distinctive attitudes to Retreat patients during the nineteenth century. Such a small sample cannot be said to be representative of the range of mental disorders treated at the Retreat although the first case (one of mania) and the last (one of melancholia with mania) present very common mental disorders. The second example is one of only a small number of cases of moral insanity and has been picked because it exemplified with unusual clarity the moralistic attitudes of therapists. And the third example is included because its rarity gives it exceptional interest. It is the case history of the youngest patient to be admitted to the Retreat, a boy who was an 'idiot' and whose case-notes illuminate a little-known historical area – the care of the mentally handicapped.

The first case history – that of Samuel W. – is of importance since it is by far the longest and most detailed record kept of any patient's treatment during the time of the Retreat's first superintendent, George Jepson. In these early days detailed observations were made about approximately only one-third of the patients, and presumably these were chosen because they were of particular interest to Jepson. In addition, a short summary was compiled for all patients, and this is also reproduced for Samuel W. to enable a comparison to be made between the two types of records. The fuller case-notes on this case of remittent mania are richly suggestive both of the treatment given and the attitudes to the mentally ill from 1804 to 1823. They demonstrate the continued use of medical methods (cupping, scarification, purgatives, emetics and sleeping draughts); the recognition of the importance of good diet and sleep in restoring health; and the reluctance to use restraint to control mania except as a last resort, when a strait-jacket was put on with sufficient show of force to prevent resistance. The careful record made of recurrent symptoms of impending illness was used to try to anticipate, prevent or control a fresh 'paroxysm'. It is significant that social methods were seen as important in doing this, first through seclusion from company during the disorder, and then through a phased reintegration into the communal life of the Retreat 'company', when the patient was seen as ready for it. During Samuel W.'s periods of remission it is interesting to see how permeable the Retreat was in relation to the outside world with attendance at Quaker Meeting in York on First Day, social visits to local Friends and outings with relatives when they came to York. Samuel W.'s case-notes also make explicit the moralistic attitude inherent in the therapist's view of the insane and the moral values imposed on the patient through a code of conduct: at various times this Quaker patient is recorded as making 'promises of good behaviour', asking 'pardon for his misconduct' and regretting his 'pride and haughtiness'.

The second selected case – that of Lucy F. – exemplifies these moral values even more clearly, although with the significant difference that the 'perversity' of the patient's moral feelings themselves constitute in the eyes of her therapists an important part of her mental disorder. Her case-notes deal with three separate periods of treatment and cover the years from 1842 to 1846, 1846 to 1853 and 1855 to 1856. Their fuller, if episodic, character typified those made by Dr Thurnam before 1849, and Dr Kitching thereafter: the former's interest in medical treatment and the latter's concern for moral management were obvious, although details of medication for physical illness have had to be omitted for reasons of space. In addition, the careful recording of the young woman's life gives us an interesting insight into the relationship between the Quaker community and the Retreat, and the implicit expectations and assumptions Quakers made about its role.

By the time the next selected patient entered the Retreat the nature of the asylum had changed with the recruitment from the locality of increasing numbers of non-Quaker, upper-class patients. Thomas W. illustrated this trend although the nature of his disorder – epilepsy and mental handicap – remained that of a small minority. His initial case-notes suggest Dr Baker's unfamiliarity in dealing with such a young, mentally handicapped child but also his interest in promoting Thomas's development. The slowness of that development has led to a shortening of the case-notes reproduced here so that those that record either 'no change' or purely physical ailments have been omitted. It is interesting to see in the doctor's observations on the patient's growing cleanliness, tractability, regularity in habits and obedience the same preoccupations that were seen in those on adult patients (see Plate 25). Some deterioration in the quality of observation, and in the sensitivity and compassion shown towards the patient, seems evident in the gradual switch during 1884 to 1885 from Dr Baker's notes to those of a succession of assistant medical officers.

The lack of sympathy inherent in the late nineteenth-century case-notes made by assistant medical officers on Robert H. is manifest in their comments on the 'rigmarole' he talks, the 'great nuisance' he is said to be in the ward, and the 'strange garb' he wears. The contrast in the tone of these case-notes and those on Samuel W. eighty years earlier is very striking. So too is the change from mechanical to chemical means of restraining violence and subduing excitement. Robert H.'s case history also reveals a characteristic obsession of Victorian alienists with masturbation – termed 'self-abuse' – as a cause of mental illness. The continuing concern of Retreat therapists to convert their patients into industrious, well-behaved conformists is typified here – not least by the anxieties displayed by the therapist towards this patient's unconventional attire (see Plate 26).

CASE 85: SAMUEL W.

(Admitted) 1803 12 month 3. Samuel W.* late of Alton, Hampshire, a widower aged 43 became first deranged about 12 years ago. After the first paroxysm had an interval of 4 years – has since had intervals of from 12 months to half a year or less. Is noisy and violent, sometimes strikes his attendants and during his paroxysms which are only of two or three weeks continuance the inter-

---

* Brother of two sisters, cases 67 and 110.

vals between [are] very uncertain. The paroxysms coming on may be perceived by his becoming inquisitive, repeating verses, and imitating preaching, and a peculiar cast, and winking with one eye, and they are preceded by sleepless nights. All medicine has been given up for some time except some opening pills occasionally. The disorder is hereditary in an uncommon degree. Has been confined at different times at a House kept by Dr. Brown at Eggemount near Staines from whence he was removed to this place in a calm state and with his own approbation. The paroxysms generally lasted about 6 weeks and occurred with much regularity, once in 12 or 15 months.

1824 8 month 30. Died from a decay of nature, in a very calm and quiet manner, having declined in health for some months

SAMUEL W.

(Admitted) 12 month 3. Noisy and violent during the paroxysms of his disorder. Quite calm during the intervals which have been of very uncertain duration. Has had maniacal paroxysms of 2 or 3 weeks duration at uncertain intervals for 12 years past, during the intervals calm and rational.

1804 12 month 16. Has had no paroxysms of the disorder since his admittance though frequently symptoms such as used formerly to precede them – stomach disorder, a sense of tightness about his head, costiveness – unusual inquisitiveness, a certain earnestness in making remarks, and over-anxiousness about trifles. He has occasionally taken emetics, been several times cupped between the shoulders and on the neck with scarifications, taken opening pills – saline mixture etc.* He has gone much out on visits etc.; his health and strength have gradually improved, he is considerably increased in flesh – He this morning went from here on a visit to his relations at London – Alton etc. and to return in 5 or 6 weeks.

1805 1 month 20. Returned.

4 month 13. He seemed in unusual spirits, unsettled and full of projects for going hither and thither all the day yesterday, and in evening up with G. J[epson] from market, today was suddenly affected with a dimness of sight succeeded by headache, a sense of

---

* See chap. 6, 'Medical Treatment', for a description of these early medical methods.

tightness about the head, and in the region of the hypochondriasis which felt hard to the touch. His spirits seemed considerably affected and said he felt unable to connect his ideas so as to answer to any question that was asked him. After dinner about 7 oz. of blood was drawn by cupping from the shoulders over the spine and back of his neck. A cathartic mixture was administered which operated well in the evening and procured another stool in the night. Ess[ence] Cephalic* was applied to the forehead. He had a tolerable night. Next morning felt much relieved from all the symptoms and this morning – 4 mo. 16 – appears to have regained his usual state of health and spirits.

4 month 18. At n[oon] took 4 grains of calomel [?]. Next morning a cathartic mixture.

4 month 20. Last night was affected with the headache: stomach disordered. Weak and debilitated today.

6 month 24. After having been discharged and living at H. T[uke's] (who very humanely took him as a visitor on trial) 16 days he suddenly became deranged and returned to the Retreat. Seemed to have lost the government of himself in a great degree – extremely noisy in a preaching way repeating verses etc; censorious to the last degree; daring threatening and insulting when opposed; violent; talks ribaldry, swears etc. etc. The 22nd by Dr. B[elcombe]'s direction he had 23 oz. of blood taken from the temporal artery. Took twice in the space of one hour 11 gr[ains] of tartarized antimony which operated fully both ways. During the operation he was calmer, but presently after more violent than before. Has been since of necessity kept under close restraint.

8 month 19. In the space of 5 weeks he began to sleep well which he had not done during the paroxysm, gone gradually calmer and has been about 2 weeks clothed and in his right mind. Yesterday was at York Meeting in the evening.

11 month 6. Something more than a fortnight ago he manifested an unsettled discontented state of mind and was very full of complaining talk calling me aside about something which he spoke of as of the greatest importance tho' in themselves merely trifling and there seemed likely to be no end of his discourse had I not left him abruptly – [He complained of] want of attention from friends and want of invitations to their houses. His room not to his mind

---

* A medicine said to be good for 'distempers of the head'.

etc. etc. Next morning was cupped with scarifications presently after which he was calm and like another man. [On the] 3rd and 4th instant he again manifested an anxious complaining disposition. [On the] 5th cupping was proposed but he would not comply. The disorder has gradually increased and this morning (on 6th) he is quite gone. Has slept less than usual 2 nights.

11 month 20. On the 6th instant near night he became extremely noisy in the yard, got up to the window pulled down the sash and attempted to force himself through into the parlour but was prevented by a keeper. Became noisy, vociferous, and abusive. Became more calm after promised amendment and was suffered on this condition to lie in bed loose and he gradually grew better without any restraint save keeping mostly in the Gallery. Has been 3 times at Meeting and is at present pretty well composed.

11 month 26. Last first day (24th) he went to Meeting as usual (his face seemed sunk or thinner than usual), sat there quietly till the conclusion and when Friends were ready to go out he took off his hat and wished to express a few words by way of caution that all might be cautious of in any manner contributing to the support of war, then began to ramble on to another subject in a raised tone of voice. Upon which he was led out into the yard where he knelt down all the while continuing to speak aloud. He was got into a house, a chaise sent for in which he was brought to the Retreat, speaking aloud with very little intermission all the way. He asked for wine with egg to recruit his exhausted spirits which being denied he refused to take his dinner. Took very little. After had an unquiet night, became extremely noisy towards morning, had the strait waistcoat put on and confined in the low room during the day. Refused his food with a view to conquer us. Near bedtime was calmer, took his supper, was liberated from the straight waistcoat, took 2 asafetida pills,* had a quiet night, slept well, and is quiet this morning tho' not quite himself.

11 month 29. Blood was drawn from the shoulders and neck by cupping which took away a tightness which he said he had felt in his temples for 2 weeks and afterward appeared quite calm.

11 month 30. Had a tooth taken out which had interrupted his sleep.

12 month 2. Remains calm.

---

* Asafetida was a gum resin used as an antispasmodic.

Appendix

12 month 13. This evening was much agitated, exhibited a charge against one of the keepers, which upon full investigation on the 14th proved unfounded or a mistake, and then he fell under [?] and seemed to weep.

12 month 16. Yesterday he wrote an almost incomprehensible letter to H. T[uke], was very talkative finding many faults, looked wild with his eyes, in short had all the symptoms of a paroxysm, except preaching and fury. Had a hearty supper and slept well. Has been repeating the Universal prayer as he says 'to make believe'.

12 month 18. Last night noisy nearly the whole of it. This forenoon broke the window of his room, 11 squares, [and] was then removed into the new back room where he pulled the bed up and with a piece of wood it was fastened with, broke a hole through the wall. Did other damage and it would seem had an intention to maim or kill one of the keepers but was overpowered and well secured. Our intention was to have got through the paroxysm without irritation or restraint but this seems impracticable. He manifests an artful and malicious disposition.

12 month 30. He continued raving without apparent amendment to the 26th, he appeared calmer [on the] 27th, still more so [on the] 28th. In the morning seemed to converse so much like himself had his usual clothes put on and has since passed his time in the dining room with the company, and today for the first time since the commencement of the paroxysm dined with the Company in the Committee Room – behaved well.

1806 1 month 22. Continued pretty well till about this time, has been several times at Meeting. And today [although] there appeared some difference in him we ventured him to meeting. On [the] 26th first day his cousin, H. C. and S. H. being returned to York he was at meeting in the forenoon and with the Friends dined at H. Tuke's where he appeared somewhat agitated, his eyelids quivering. [He] whispered with his cousin and after dinner proposed leaving [before] the evening meeting and coming home. 27th with G. J[epson] next day tho' he said he had slept well was evidently fast bordering on a paroxysm. Wrote a letter to his uncle consisting of 4 sheets prose and verse, the last sheet most extravagant. In reading which he raised his voice to an unusual pitch and went off quite distracted and was removed into one of the arched rooms so that he would not do any mischief.

2 month 8. He has spent his time since the above mostly by himself in a small room without being tied and done no material mischief. The 6th instant he was a little calmer, smoked his pipe in the upper dining room in the evening very quietly. Yesterday and today at liberty and quiet.

3 month 18. Was cupped on the shoulders and neck with scarifications about a week ago. Last night had an Emetic Ipecarar* 20 grains, Tartar emetic 4 grains. This morning cupped and scarified and took a cathartic mixture.

5 month 24. Has since last report been several times indisposed both in body and mind for which he has taken opening pills, saline mixture and been cupped [at] different times, which relieved him apparently – relieved and saved from going to extremes. Has been very well for about the week last past.

7 month 29. Last first day but one, the 20th instant, he was just on the edge of a paroxysm (having been for nearly two weeks previously extremely prying, inquisitive, and frequently whispering and finding fault with the servants in the family). He was prevented from reading and speechifying in the family and enjoined to keep himself still and quiet. Took some opening medicine, had a good supper at night with strong malt liquor, after which he slept well and was next morning calm and saw into the state of mind he had been in the day before, acknowledged his errors and asked pardon for his misconduct. He was cupped the same forenoon with scarifications since which time he has conducted himself in an orderly manner.

8 month 13. Having been a few days previously very busy about other people's affairs, finding fault with the conduct of one, vilifying another, prying and watching. On the 10th in the evening he began in the usual way of preaching and became quite noisy and frantic, and being shut in a room pulled off his shirt and threw it out of the room. He remains shut up.

9 month 1. During this paroxysm he has been frequently very noisy and sometimes dirty but has offered no violence to any one tho' near all the time even in a room. 3 days ago he was dressed in his usual clothes, came out into the mens' sitting room and has since dined with the Company in the Committee Room, behaving well, but has a wildness in his eyes.

11 month 11. Has continued pretty free from insanity, but has

* Probably a colloquial rendering of ipecacuanha, used as emetic, purgative and diaphoretic.

had various bodily complaints for which he has been twice cupped and taken various medicines.

1807 1 month 14. For about the last 2 weeks his spirits have frequently been flat and unsettled with headache and feeble pulse. Aperients were administered and two nights ago he took an emetic, Antimony 4 grains Ipecac[uanha] 20 grains p.v. which in the space of 3 hours produced a full operation, brought up a considerable quantity of bile, relieved him much and he had been much better since.

1 month 22. On the 17th his Cousin E. W. came to York, on the 18th they dined and drank tea and supped together at H. Tuke's in York, on the 19th they went to see the Minster, were on the top, and drank tea at Littlemore at Charlotte Richardson's etc. etc. On the 20th he discovered considerable hurry and elevation of spirits, nevertheless his cousin coming up, and this being the last day of his stay S. W. was permitted to accompany him again to the city where they dined at H. T[uke]'s, visited Catherine Cappe,* C. Richardson etc. etc. drank tea at the school. During the course of the day, he was talkative frequently whispering to people, showing scraps of poetry, a certain wildness in the eyes, and flushing of the face. He accompanied his cousin as far as Ouse Bridge, late in the evening retired to bed near midnight, and about 2 o'clock next morning – 1 month 23 – broke out in a paroxysm with loud exclamations in a preaching tone. As usual is very curious about his victuals and if not gratified with just such as he asks for will sometimes refuse to take a meal.

2 month 27. During this paroxysm he has been noisy as in former ones but less irritable; for about 2 weeks at latter end of it he was pretty calm but full of talk. The 24th instant he came out to his meals and has behaved well since.

1808 1 month 28. Since the last report has with great attention and frequently taking medicines, losing blood by cupping etc. been preserved pretty steady and conducted himself more peaceably in the family than formerly, till within the last 5 days, that [i.e. when] he has manifested a great hurry on his spirits – by many projects, great loquacity, from alteration in his voice, and a certain wildness discoverable in his eyes.

* Catherine Cappe, philanthropist and author (whose stepson had been physician to the Retreat), was a friend of the poetess Charlotte Richardson and edited her poems.

1 month 29. Repeated verses and etc. in bed and arose early in the morning, manifested great hurry of spirits during the day.

1 month 30. This morning after being very noisy in bed got up and dressed himself about 3 in the morning, spent the day in great activity until ten at night, became quite outrageous and was of necessity removed into another lodging room for safety, but not fastened. Has been, as formerly, very fond of reading, writing etc.

1 month 31. During the night he did all the mischief and made all the noise he could, broke a wooden lid, and tore his bed clothes.

2 month 22. During this paroxysm he was some days indulged with liberty and much indulged in other respects, but at whatever point we stopped in complying with his numerous claims, like a petulant child, he flew out and became frantic. It seemed therefore necessary to lay him under restraint and on account of his mischievous tongue to seclude him from company under which treatment he became calm and governable and this day was admitted into the parlour in his usual dress. (N.B Has several times broke his promises. Broke S[amuel] S[mith]'s shin by striking with his foot.)

2 month 29. Has remained since very calm, sensible and humble.

3 month 18. Frequently has complained of depression of spirits and sometimes wept – walking out and exercise in the garden and suitable company relieve him.

6 month 25. Has been extremely talkative and fond of writing and reading verses quite in the extreme – full of projects respecting Charlotte Richardson's publication and this afternoon I heard him reading in the strain of voice peculiar to his paroxysms.

6 month 26. I was called up at half past 3 this morning, he having got up, dressed himself in his gown, and vociferating in his usual maniacal strain. Upon promise of good behaviour was permitted to remain in the first mens gallery 'til 10. I returned from Meeting when I found he had broke his promise and said many insolent and mischievous things; about 4 p.m. therefore he was put in the low back room. N.B. is as formerly artful in currying favour with *one* of the keepers whilst he quarrels with the rest.

7 month 31. Having slept well 2 nights and become calm and rational he was permitted to come out this morning and behave well. During this paroxysm he was only waistcoated 3 days and

Appendix

nights at the first, the rest of the time loose – frequently noisy but not so mischievous as formerly. Made frequent use of the cold bath.

9 month 3.   Has been a few days very full of talk and projects, much employed about verses and C. Richardson's poems.

9 month 6.   He went to C. R.'s lodging at Ackham, called at L[indley] M[urray]'s* and then at H. Tuke's without the knowledge of any of the family, returned peacably with G. J[epson].

9 month 8.   Noisy last night.

9 month 9.   Again so extremely noisy that he was removed this morning into the low room but loose.

9 month 12.   Had the short waistcoat put on at his own request; he fell down with it on and hurt his head – has an affection on the right side of his face apparently paralytic as his mouth is drawn to the opposite side and his hearing impaired and eye distorted on the same side.

10 month 1.   Having slept several nights and become gradually quieter he was admitted into the mens sitting room and his usual lodging room. The paroxysm has left him low spirited and more feeble than former ones.

11 month 29.   His uncle J. Crowley his brother Edward and his son came to York to see him. They stayed three or four days his uncle and son came up to the Retreat. Samuel accompanied them to several friends houses and did not discover any improper affection of mind till after they were gone – but on first day at Meeting he felt overwhelmed as it were with sorrow and incidentally went out – the next day discovered signs of approaching disorder – on third day wrote a long letter part verse – on fourth day began to be noisy and in his preaching way.

12 month 9.   As he had never fully recovered from the debilitating effects of his former paroxysm he was put into one of the beds in a room in the upper stor[e]y of the gallery where he was fastened to it with the bed-straps – the consequence is that he has rested quietlier than when loose and says this morning he has slept eight hours last night – he is however still much deranged.

1809 1 month 13.   After having been fastened for four nights he was let go at liberty in the galleries and yard – he was frequently very noisy incessant in his demands so much so as would require

---

* The famous grammarian from New York who had settled at Holgate, York.

if they were all complied with several persons to attend him and as we wished if possible to keep him quiet we indulged him very much yet found it impossible to please him. As usual he reckoned up and repeated all the spiteful things true or false he had heard or invented against those who had anything to do with him. Two or three days ago he discovered signs of amendment and has now become calm and pretty much himself. This paroxysm of six weeks duration.

1 month 22. He went to Meeting for the first time since this paroxysm.

4 month 9. Since the end of the last paroxysm he has been subject to frequent attacks of low spirits and reflected with regret on his former conduct, feeling as he said judgement for his pride and haughtiness. The seventh inst. he said he was exceedingly sleepy and went to bed at 8 in the evening without supper. Yesterday morning he got up about 5 went downstairs opened the front door went down to York in his nightcap and a scotch plaid. He crossed the river in a boat then returned went to the Minster Prayers at 6 – when over, knelt down, prayed (as he told me) for the man who was executed two days before – preached – then began to repeat Pope's Universal Prayer. He was then led out and two of our men found him in College Street and brought him home. Was very noisy great part of the day Lodged in the large S.E. upper room has this morning broken seven squares of glass and pulled his mattress to pieces. He was now put in the gloomy back room.

4 month 10. Has slept in one of the arched rooms, loose, but has torn his blankets and it was deemed necessary to put the strait waistcoat on to prevent him from doing more mischief.

4 month 15. This afternoon he appeared less violent and at his own request with promises of good behaviour had the waistcoat taken off.

4 month 19. Has been loose since and no repetitions of mischiefs have occurred – NB he is noisy in a morning and calmer towards night pretty regularly.

6 month 3. In order to try if by any means he might be made calm by kind treatment and not suffer from cold, he was suffered to spend the days in the upper gallery where he was tried a long time but got no better. At last we deemed it prudent to try what seculsion from society would effect and the weather being warm he was for about a week shut up in the back room and let out for

Appendix

an hour or two each day to walk, and now is become calm and sensible. This paroxysm has held him nearly nine weeks.

1810 6 month 27. Having with unremitted attention to his state of body and mind been pretty well since the last paroxysm, and behaved with more humility than in any former interval, he set off to see his relations at Godalming, Alton etc. and this morning was with great difficulty brought back quite a maniac by Chas. and John Wansborough nearly having bruised and wounded them and damaged five or six chaises on the journey. Samuel W. has also got several bruises in their contests.

6 month 29. He kicked his attendants, got one of the common strait waistcoats off and broke some windows so that we are under the necessity of confining him in one covered on the sleeves with calf leather and sometimes fastening his legs with straps. Is rather quieter this morning.

7 month 26. After being pretty much confined in the back room preaching, using abusive language kicking and otherwise abusing his attendant he became about the 21st inst. more calm and has now been several days in the upper dining room and today dined in the Committee room, but he is still high-spirited and at times evidently not quite himself.

7 month 31. Has been calm and sometimes a little low.

1811 7 month 21. Has been very active and healthy for some months; today he went to see his sister Mary* at the Appendage. Spent from half an hour to an hour with her, she talking with him much about her property, her communications, etc. He confessed in the evening that it was more than he could well bear.

7 month 25. Symptoms of flightiness having taken place soon after the interview with his sister, they gradually increased. Yesterday morning he was up by 5 and this morning before 3. Is now confined to the gallery, talking and ordering almost perpetually. In the evening he absolutely refused to go to bed unless he was compelled. We were therefore under the necessity of putting on the strait waistcoat and having him conveyed by force.

7 month 26. Has been noisy all night. Has been in a cold bath today.

7 month 27. Noisy all night, as usual has torn his bedclothes.

8 month 23. Has been somewhat more himself 2 or 3 days past

---

* Case 110, and in the Retreat from 1806 to 1819.

and this evening walked a little in the garden and returned quietly, with the keeper, to his room.

9 month 1.   Worse today – preaching loudly.

9 month 16.   After a quiet of 2 or 3 days he came out to dinner today and behaved well. – Spirits brisk.

9 month 18.   Went to Meeting but rather too full of projects and talkative.

1813 2 month 9.   Since the last report 9 month 18, 1811, he has continued mostly pretty well in the mind and willing to take advice but has had frequent bodily complaints, principally of the nervous kind, and several times appeared nearly on the verge of a paroxysm which appeared to have been warded off by medical means and attention in keeping him quiet and guarding him against such things as were likely to elevate his spirits. Last 7th day, the 6th of February, he went to Charlott R.'s about a poem she had written on the Bible Society which he copied and read in the Committee room and ere he had proceeded far, raised his voice in a singing tone – the first manifest symptom of a beginning paroxysm. On first day very flighty, second day worse. Of necessity tied in bed at night – got loose and broke 11 panes in the window of his lodging room. This morning taken into the back low room.

3 month 9.   Yesterday was rather calm and good-natured. Was out in the lower sitting room when he behaved pretty well but was talkative. He has mostly been fastened in the strait waistcoat this time for, when at any time he was loose through a wish to render him more comfortable, he was sure to do some mischief. Loose all night, rather wild in the morning.

3 month 26.   After the last report he soon became high, noisy and mischievous so long as he had the use of his hands. He was then confined in the strait waistcoat and has continued very turbulent till the night before last, had a quiet night, was quiet yesterday, and at liberty this morning he appears to be recovered. This paroxysm has been of about 7 weeks duration.

11 month 13.   He has continued pretty steady till within 2 or 3 weeks back – since he has become gradually more talkative, suspicious, irritable and full of projects. This morning he arose about 2 and became sick and with the assistance of camomile tea, vomited freely; after which he was prevailed with to return to bed but was soon up again and began his usual practice of preaching etc.

Appendix

In the evening he had become quite outrageous and was by 3 men jacketed by force.

12 month 28. He had the strait waistcoat only a few days after which he was most days several hours in the lower dining room when a little approaching to calmness, he has not done much mischief but frequently noisy and very censorious. On the 25th Inst. H. Tuke came up and as we thought S. W. getting better, H. T. went into the room to see him when he began to exhibit many complaints and produced a paper of his own writing fraught with some falsity and many exaggerations of a spiteful tendency* and upon my contradicting one of his false assertions, he struck several times apparently with all his force at my legs and one stroke took effect and broke my shin. To avoid the blow I suppose I held up my leg and he continuing his efforts, struck his leg I suppose against my foot which broke his shin and raised a lump on his leg. When returned to his room he told the men I had kicked his leg which H. T., who was by all the time and pushed him from me down the gallery, knows to be false. This circumstance I note in order that if at any future time S. W. should renew the subject to my disadvantage the real state of the case may not be forgot. This evening he appears pretty calm but not well.

1814 1 month 2. He came this morning into the parlour pretty much himself after being in confinement near 7 weeks, but nearly all the time had his hands at liberty, having a man to attend particularly to him which rendered close confinement less necessary.

2 month 11. On account of some complaint in his head he was cupped and scarified this evening and relieved.

10 month 6. The 4th, he began to talk perpetually having been a few days before earnestly and anxiously employed about copying some papers respecting the Emperor of Russia. This evening he was become so ungovernable as to render close confinement indispensable.

10 month 11. In the evening after the patients had gone to bed, W. B. liberated him and brought him his supper to the fireside in the east sitting room and at his request W. B. left him to fetch an egg in addition to a good supper and whilst he was gone, S. W. took the candle which was left standing by him and set fire to two

---

* See Chap. 7, 'Performance' where this letter is reproduced.

heaps of straw which he had put close to the boarded ceiling on the north side of the low room – he then shut the double doors, and sat down to his supper where W. B. found him sitting as if nothing was the matter and the fire had made considerable progress in the room before it was discovered. It was however extinguished in time to prevent its extending beyond the room where it began.

11 month 24. He has been getting gradually calmer for about a week, was yesterday in his usual dress, dined with the parlour party, slept loose and tonight goes to his own bed. W. B. is dismissed from his attendance. The paroxysm has been of 7 weeks duration.

1817 4 month 29. This has been the longest interval he has had since he came to the Retreat and probably might have continued had not an occurrence occasioned a relapse. On the 20 Inst. his son came to see him and stayed 5 days. They went to Castle Howard on 24th Inst. The father seemed much pleased with the son's company, but the interview proved too much for the former who very soon after the son's departure discovered symptoms of disorder. On the 27th he arose about 1 in the morning with great hurry about his spirits – went early to the city, made some unnecessary purchases and was during the day exceedingly loquacious. 28th – rose early again and would probably have gone had we not pre vented him by the precaution of locking the gallery door. This forenoon the disorder prevailed so much as to render it necessary to put him under close restraint.

5 month 12. He was very disturbing to the patients last night and the night before after having been without any fastening several days and nights before. Yesterday he struck Samuel L[ay] twice with his fist and kicked him with his foot on the thigh. In consequence of this outrage he had the strait waistcoat put on since which he has been frequently very noisy. He also kicked up his foot, threw down and broke a number of plates and dishes.

6 month 7. He has frequently been very noisy and abusive since the last report but after a good night's rest 2 or 3 nights ago became rather suddenly calm and this day returned to his usual room; but at his own request has his servant to attend him another week. – This paroxysm has been about 6 weeks in duration.

11 month 1. After having been more than a week in an unsettled state of mind in consequence of an advance of his terms, a

proposal for his going to sleep in the new building, and two letters from his son and brother on interesting subjects, he got up at 3 this morning, came down, made a great noise, and rambled about most of the day earnestly engaged in various projects and manifested great irritability with some malignity of temper.

11 month 2.   Rose again about 3 this morning. In the evening gave us the slip and after considerable search and much anxiety on our part was found at W. Tuke's (after having rambled about in the lanes a considerable time in the dark) and was brought home in a chaise.

11 month 3.   He ranted about in his own sitting room, pulled off his breeches and ran about in the yard quite frantic, then we got him into his usual lodging room. Samuel Bottomley came to take care of him.

11 month 4.   He has passed a very disturbed and disturbing night, being put loose in his usual bed and S. B. lodging in the room with him.

11 month 5.   Another turbulent night fastened in bed.

11 month 6.   To the composing draught at night.

11 month 7.   Has had a better night.

11 month 8.   Draught omitted last night – had a very bad night – got loose and struck his attendant several blows with pewter chamberpot. About 10 oz. of blood was taken from his shoulders by cupping on the 5th and on the 6th he took a strong cathartic, but neither proved any apparent relief.

12 month 1.   Had a complete quiet night.

12 month 2.   Another quiet night. Has had his usual clothes on yesterday and today and behaved pretty well.

12 month 3 and 4.   Two noisy nights and two bad days.

12 month 7.   Last night and today quiet.

12 month 11.   He continued pretty orderly and yesterday was permitted to be in his sitting room. – This morning went down with S. Bottomley to the barber's in Walmgate and came back very quietly. This paroxysm has been of about or near 7 weeks duration.

1818 4 month 20.   Having been some weeks much agitated about his son's marriage, H. P.'s poetry, the distress of the Greenlanders on the 18th he got all afloat and this day we got S. Bottomley to take care of him and tonight I got his key. Has been up several mornings very early, this morning at 3, but the precaution of taking all the keys of the out doors away at nights having been attended to by us, he has not got out to range about in the city etc.

4 month 21. This morning he was up ranting about in his room by one o'clock, pounding at the door, swearing etc.

4 month 25. He still continues mischievous so as to render it necessary to keep him pretty close confined.

4 month 26. This morning after a quiet night he was pretty steady, was dressed and walked in the garden with S. B.

4 month 27. Has been extremely noisy and mischievous last night and is under confinement this morning.

4 month 30. Has dressed and walked out with the men yesterday – behaved tolerably tho' very talkative. – During the last night as bad as ever – swearing, ranting, threatening. N.B. Indulgence seems to make him worse.

5 month 25. He has been extremely raving mostly since – rather quieter this evening.

5 month 26. Has had quiet night without disturbing anyone and is quiet this morning.

5 month 28. Yesterday, pretty quiet. Had a good night's sleep, this morning arose calm and appears today much himself.

1819 2 month 16. Having been several weeks verging towards a paroxysm within this few days he has been very flighty, buying pictures, promoting a new publication, getting pieces in verse printed and making presents of them to various of his friends. Going to different friends' houses and others and talking incessantly till it has now become necessary to keep him in and last night he was put under the care of Samuel Smith at the Lodge. He was got to bed last night with some difficulty about 12 and was up again between 1 and 2. Remained up till morning. I got his keys, knives and watch from him this morning.

5 month 6. He went to Doncaster in company with G. J[epson] to meet his brother Edward, his son and his son's wife. The company stopped at Doncaster 2 nights and then all went to Ackworth on the 8th. The brother and son and daughter parted with him there the same day after which his spirits soon got afloat.

S. W. and G. J. got home on the 11th and S. W. grew gradually worse till the 13th night when it became absolutely necessary to put him under close restraint.

6 month 17. Was dressed and permitted to walk in the front garden.

6 month 18. Dined with family in the Lodge.

6 month 19. Appears quite recovered – drank tea in the Committee room. This paroxysm has been of about 6 weeks duration.

1820 1 month 2. At a sitting of the Q[ua]r[terly] Meeting in York 2 appeals depend. He got up wishing to address the meeting and was brought home in a chaise by W. Maud and H. Ponsonby.

1 month 3. Got up at 2 this morning, has been kept quiet in a room this day in his usual dress.

2 month 22. Having been kept much to himself with an attendant, he has got over this paroxysm without doing any material mischief. Restored to liberty this day.

1821 1 month 26. Has been talkative and full of remarks, today rather more so.

1 month 29. His disorder has increased but he is still at liberty.

1 month 31. Yesterday he was restless, noisy, full of projects, in an humour to give away and buy everything that came in his way. At night he was put under restraint in the small parlour at the Lodge.

5 month 20. He got over this paroxysm better than usual in about 4 weeks.

7 month 16. Has continued generally well since May 20 and this morning set off for Scarborough taking a servant (William Ellis) along with him.

8 month 13. Returned a little improved in his health.

11 month 16. After being manifestly growing more and more flighty and talkative and fond of buying etc. as formerly, he was this evening secluded from company in a comfortable room at the Lodge.

12 month 16. Had gone on pretty quietly till last night when he was vociferous and mischievous which rendered more close confinement necessary.

1822 2 month 28. About this time he got pretty calm.

7 month 7. About a week or more ago, having been at Scarborough a week, he became more and more flighty and unsettled, saying many unnecessary things, getting up by 2 in the morning, and disturbing the family at his lodgings – he was brought him this evening, confined.

8 month 3. He is now parts of the day pretty calm; but is frequently noisy and vociferous at other times. Upon the whole getting rather better.

8 month 12. About this time he became calm and was liberated.

1823 6 month 2. Has had for several weeks marked symptoms of an approaching paroxysm, which he appears himself more conscious and more to guard against than formerly.

6 month 6. He was indulged in all his eccentricities till this morning he became quarrelsome and intolerable. He was put into room under the care of W. Hart.

CASE 651: LUCY F.

Lucy F., aged 17, single, daughter of a banker's clerk at Southampton, born at Newington Green, W. London, was admitted into the Retreat, July 14th 1842. Her father has been married twice, but has had no other offspring; her mother was not a Friend, consequently she was not born in membership; but was received into the Society in her infancy. Soon after her birth (a few weeks), her mother began to be troubled with symptoms of cancer of the womb, and died of that disease within nine months. (The disease had therefore been probably in existence during the pregnancy.) Her father married again within two or three years.

L. F. did not evince any peculiarity bodily or mental – unless some obstinacy of temper be so regarded – up to about three years of age when she had a very severe attack of whooping cough, and this was followed by water on the head; for which leeches, blistering etc. were used, but, as appeared to the parents with prejudicial effect. The disorder was followed by squinting and defective vision, which have continued up to the present time.

There was no hereditary tendency to insanity and the friends are no doubt correct in attributing the strange perversity of the moral feelings, which had more or less been ever since noticed to the defective development arising from this disease. The parents state that the disposition and character of the patient have always been marked by the following characteristics and peculiarities. Her perception is very quick, and when a stranger would suppose from the defect in her sight, that she was almost unconscious of what was going on, she is really noticing everything very closely. She is gifted with a good memory, and an ability to acquire knowledge of some kinds, she is nevertheless defective in those mental qualities which would enable her to attain to proficiency in any eventual pursuit; for no description of which has her mind ever indicated any predilection. The moral feelings have always been

Appendix

marked by remarkable want of power; and though abstractedly she knows right from wrong; yet she never appeared able to follow the former, like other children, from the motive of the love of approbation, and similar motives. On the contrary there appeared to be an innate love of mischief, theft and falsehood, and great artfulness, which could never be counteracted by any ordinary methods of education. She was sent to a boarding school for three years, and would have continued much longer, but for the foregoing peculiarities of her disposition. Her parents then procured her admission into Croydon School, but the managers would not keep her on these accounts and recommended her being placed under proper care. Whilst there, she exhibited her artfulness and ingenuity by feigning blindness, and requiring to be led about, with the view of exciting commiseration, and to be discharged [from] the school.

After leaving Croydon she was placed out to board under the care of an elderly female, in a village near Southampton, with whom she has since continued. As a child she was always observed to prefer boys as her companions, but this did not attract any particular attention, until the period of puberty, which took place very early, the catamenia* appearing at 13 1/2 years. Ever since this the sexual appetite has been very prominent and has led her into numerous improprieties, and has given her parents great anxiety.

For about 7 years past, she has resided with an elderly female in the neighbourhood of Southampton, and whilst under her care, has several times eluded her vigilance and got into the company of men of low habits and with whom she has been found in the fields and lanes: – indeed the premature and excessive 'desire for the male sex' is regarded by her friends as the peculiar feature of her disorder. It was determined to place her under care in consequence of her having escaped a considerable distance about a month ago, being found in a field by the roadside in the company of a man; and being only taken by the guard of the coach and another person, after considerable resistance. Upon her return she stated that her design had been to get a situation as a laundry maid, that she might earn some money, to buy clothes, when she would get married, and go to Australia.

The disorder is considered to be gradually increasing. Her bod-

---

* Menstrual periods.

ily health is stated to be good. She has shown no disposition to refuse food or to injure herself, nor to acts of destruction or violence of any kind; but she is stated to require 'a little care' as regards habits of cleanliness.

State on admission

Is of short stature but stout to corpulency; shoulders broad, bosoms large, arms short, lower extremities imperfectly developed; has a singular waddling walk, and altogether a very peculiar appearance, her whole manner etc. exhibiting a decided preponderance of the physical and animal over the intellectual and moral. The bulk of the body resembles that of a stout woman but the head and limbs are those of a girl, a little girl. The head is of a round, flattened form, wide in the centre and full behind; the neck very short and thick, the forehead is low and shallow, but wide and above the eyes is moderately full.

The axes of the eyes do not correspond and the lid of the right is almost constantly dropped from loss of power over the levator palpebrae muscle; the left pupil is dilated, but it is difficult to ascertain the exact state of either eye from her unwillingness to submit to any close examination. The cheeks are plump, the expression when pleased childish but cunning and amorous, and she will often hide herself behind the door-post and pass out in a half-laughing playful mood, with the eyes but half-opened and [?] in a peculiar way. When displeased by anything which passes around her, which she is very readily and on the most trifling occasions, the impress of anger, disdain and of the other angry passions on the countenance is very marked, and the change from one to the other is as sudden as it is marked.

In bodily health there does not appear to be anything requiring notice, except that she is subject to great constipation of the bowels, and has been often two weeks without an evacuation. The catamenia are regular. The circulation in the hands is feeble and they are often blue and cold.

Mental state

L. F. is characterised by a shrewdness of observation and rapidity of perception which are exquisitely feminine. The memory too is strong and ready, so that she readily commits to memory considerable portions both of poetry and prose composition. In solidarity of judgement however she appears entirely wanting. She manifests strong attachments and aversions and her love to her father appears particularly strong. She is however very wayward, her will obstinate and capricious; and the faults of temper coupled with the early development and force of the amative propensity perhaps justify the conclusion that there is a degree of 'moral insanity' as certified by Dr. Williams of Southampton, who was consulted previous to her being sent here. The case would perhaps better be regarded as one of congenital moral imbecility, the 'brutality' of Dr. Mayo.

She writes a poor crabbed hand, without regard to capital letters or punctuation, but spells and reads tolerably. For a copy of one of her letters see Dec. 2nd 1842.

She was placed under the watchful care of her nurse, and as strict separation of the opposite sex, as the construction of the Retreat permits, was enjoined. Employment in domestic affairs and in needlework, with frequent exercise in the open air were also enjoined.

[From July to November of 1842 Lucy F.'s case-notes deal entirely with the treatment of various physical complaints that culminated in a serious illness in November in which the patient became delirious.]

Dec 2nd appears quite well and looks better and stouter than I have before seen her. She only complains of a little pain occasionally in the right side (hypochondriacal). The enema last ordered was not required and the bowels and kidneys perform their functions healthily. She takes the electuary* daily or on alternate days. She may now omit the quinine.

The following letter to her parents was written today:

Dear Father and Mother,

I hope these few lines will find you quite well. I am sorry to inform you I have been very ill but I am now quite well. John Thurnam was very kind to me during my illness, he was like a father to me. I think father you have certainly forgotton me, the only child you have but father I don't forget you. I think it unkind

---

* A medicine mixed with jam or honey.

as you did not answer my letter but out of sight out of mind. I often think of what you said before I left home. I do not forget if you do, dear father. Give my love to [?] and [?] and tell them I have signed the pledge to teetotalism. Give my love to Albert and to Aunt and Uncle Hodges. Give my respects to young Mr. Cray. Give my kind love to Mother, accept some for yourself. I remain your affectionate daughter,

L. F.

[Left the Retreat on 5 May 1846 and was stated to have 'recovered': no case-notes were apparently made between 2 December 1842 and her discharge.]

CASE 754: LUCY F.

Readmitted 1846 10 month 26. The apparent recovery on her discharge proved fallacious, and both at Northampton and Castle Donnington where she has been residing with her uncles and aunts since she left the Retreat she has been a constant source of anxiety and trouble by her morbid perversity and disposition of excitement. It may however be questioned whether if she had been received at home by her parents and not sent to those who though relatives were still strangers to her the result might not have been different. It was at least a grievous disappointment to her when she left the Retreat, which she did with great forebodings, as to the future. Within a month of her discharge there were applications of a very urgent kind for her readmission, but at that time had we been disposed to them, they could not procure medical certificates.

Her friends state that since her discharge the disease has manifested itself by an almost constant desire for change and rambling abroad often labouring under great excitement of mind producing high and low spirits and frequently fits of illness of short duration. The latter pretty plainly having their origin in the preceding mental excitement. The disposition to falsehood and deceit had continued very strong, so that she often told diametrically opposite stories of the same events to her uncle and to her aunt, who have been quite unable to rely on her word. It is not thought that there has been any improper familiarity with the opposite sex since her discharge. The medical men state that she has the particular delusion of addressing absent persons, that she manifests unconnected emotions and exhibits acts of extravagance and condition of morbid excitement, in addition to her disposition to wander about without any determined object. At one time she expressed a great desire to change her religious profession and even took what she regarded as some little steps towards doing so. This disposition has of late not been seen. About a fortnight ago (and this determined her friends to place her under care) she left her uncle's house and proceeded to Derby and procured a ticket for London [by] Rail. On the way however she lost the ticket, was obliged to return to Derby and being found by her uncle at the Station was brought home. Her object in going to London was *probably* that of going to her father's [home] at Southampton. How she had procured the necessary money was not discussed. She has refused food at times, and what was a source of anxiety to her friends, a little Laudanum was found in her workbox. Has suffered at times of late from pain in head and hysteria with other symptoms brought on apparently by mental excitement.

On admission

Appears in good bodily health. The seton was removed from her right side about a month after leaving and she continued free from pain for a long time; though she has of late had an occasional return of pain, and also of headache. The bowels are still subject to constipation and she has frequently to take pills which were prescribed at Castle Donnington. Her aunt reports that the catamenia were absent at the last period.

Morally and mentally

There seems little to report, appears rather subdued and more reserved in manner than she used to be but not more so than may be regarded under her circumstances, at present.

10 month 31. Conducts herself quite properly, and is generally employed in needlework [and] housework when I go into the gallery.

1850 1 month 30. A few days ago, she acquainted me that she had for some time suffered pain in the vaginal region and loins, had fluor ablus and felt out of health* . . .

11 month 12. Has lately suffered much from spinal irritation. The pain is acute in the back and side, chiefly the right* . . . In mind, she is quarrelsome, dissatisified and cunning.

1853 2 month 14. During the last 12 months an imperceptible improvement appears to have been going on in this case. She is more orderly, and altogether better regulated in herself so that I have thought it right to recommend that she have a trial at home, her family are now arranging for her return. She still suffers from spinal irritation and occasional leucorrhoea.

[On 19 April 1853 she was discharged 'recovered'.]

CASE 911: LUCY F.

Readmitted 6 month 16, 1855. On leaving the Retreat in 1853 she went to her parents at Southampton. Before she left the Superintendent took every opportunity of advising L. F. to avoid those follies and imprudences which had led her into so many troubles before and it was strongly pointed out to her that the consequence of pursuing the same line of conduct must either be the entire loss of character as a virtuous woman, or the conviction that she was permanently insane. There was at that time a male patient in the Retreat towards whom L. F. had [been] cultivating a foolish attachment, and with whom there was not the least prospect of ever forming an honourable union. She made the most solemn promises that she would never again attempt to renew any intercourse with this person. She left the Retreat with apparently the best intentions and became the governess of some young children at home. Not long after her discharge she attempted by letters to open an intercourse with the patient referred to, and fearing the letters would be intercepted by the handwriting being recognised, she directed them to the postmaster at York, with a request that he would hand them to the person intended. Becoming at last dissatisfied with her situation at home she was committed to the care of a female friend at Winchester, who unfortunately failed in maintaining the degree of oversight necessary in L. F.'s case. Her father thus gives her history: 'For a considerable time she con-

* Details of medical therapy for these physical symptoms are omitted.

ducted herself as well as we could expect under her circumstances but she gradually became dissatisfied with being at home, until at last we were obliged to remove her to Winchester, to reside with a person we have known many years, and whom we considered very suitable to the care of Lucy, and there she conducted herself satisfactorily, for some months, but again became dissatisfied and we now learn to our grief that she has with the assistance of the servant become acquainted with several young men, one of whom she has induced to promise to marry her, for she states she is determined to get married.'

The young man who had promised to marry L. F. is said to be a person of decidedly weak mind; he regards Lucy as a sane person. His opinion however is opposed to that of many who know L. F. at Winchester. The attendant who fetched her from that place states that everybody considered [her] insane at Winchester, and his impression was deepened by her conduct at the railway station, when she took a public and affectionate leave of Hayward, to whom after kissing him she continued waving her handkerchief from the carriage window 'till out of sight.

The certificates on which she was received into the Retreat state as facts 'imperfect intellectual development evinced in her conversation and behaviour, want of common discretion and judgement, and determination to gratify her inclinations without regard to the consequences – general impropriety of conduct, want of female delicacy etc.'

The first night of her return she talked in a wild, extravagant and abandoned manner, relating unlikely stories and lascivious adventures. The next day she was calm, and has remained so ever since.

1855 8 month. Her general conduct has been orderly, her manners obliging, and her variations of spirits much less than on the former occasions. She has acted with so much caution, and displayed so little manifestation of disorder that the propriety of retaining her as a patient can only be determined by the experience of what she is when out of an asylum.

1855 9 month. The Superintendent informed her father that her conduct here was unexceptionable [sic], that her detention much longer would be of questionable propriety, and it would therefore be advisable to procure some situation for her, where judicious care might be extended without the restraint of an asylum.

The whole history of this case shows a mind defective in intellectual power, dominated by animal passions and perverted in all the moral faculties to such an extent as to constitute a real case of insanity. Notwithstanding, the small amount of aberration evinced during her present sojourn here, which has been owing to the withdrawal of exciting causes and the possession of a powerful motive for self-control in the hope of accomplishing her liberation and marriage, of the propriety of her confinement, there can be no reasonable doubt. The only question is whether she can be considered convalescent. There is too much reason to apprehend that her present state, however much it may resemble convalescence, is simply a suspension by the wholesome restraints of an asylum, of a morbid condition ready on the first liberation, to declare itself with all the force of former times.

1856 5 month 20. Left the Retreat 'recovered'. George Hayward, the person alluded to, appealed to the Commissioners [in Lunacy] (some time after the letter was written to [the] patient's father by the Superintendent suggesting her removal) and they in consequence wrote for information respecting the case. The following reply was sent to them, embodying also the facts of the case as stated in this case book.

To the Secretary

Respected Friend,

I am very glad of the opportunity of laying before the Commissioners in Lunacy a statement of the case of L. F. I was informed by a person named George Hayward that he intended appealing to the Commissioners of Lunacy for L. F.'s liberation and believing him to be a person of weak mind, quite ignorant of the sad consequences that would be entailed upon himself if he succeeded in forming a matrimonial alliance with her, I thought it incumbent upon me to represent strongly to him the danger he was incurring. These representations have not convinced him; and there can be no surprise at his believing Lucy to be of sound mind. It is one of those subtle cases, when self-control is possessed to a great extent, and this coupled with the art of making plausible representations is calculated to impose upon persons, ignorant of the nature of insanity. It requires an acquaintance with L. F. when she has no strong controlling motive at work, to feel satisfied that she is insane, and it is in this and similar cases that the assistance of the

Appendix

Commissioners may be very valuable both to society, and to the superintendents of asylums, in assisting the latter with their judgement upon the propriety of retaining certain persons in confinement and thus giving to the former an assurance that a calm judgement free from every disinterested bias may be secured in all cases of obscurity or doubtfulness.

With these few remarks I enclose a full report of L. F.'s case. I am respectfully theirs,

John Kitching.

CASE 1437: THOMAS HOYLE W.

Admitted 12 May 1881. Not connected with the Society of Friends. Male. Age, 7 3/4 years. Single. No occupation – son of a manufacturer.
Previous place of abode – Holly Mount, Rawtenstall.
Birthplace —.

History

This patient has been an idiot ever since birth; he has always hitherto been looked after at home. No cause can be assigned for his defective condition. He has had convulsions (one or more) each time he has cut a tooth. Some time before his birth his mother was startled by hearing of the illness or the death of a friend.

His father's sister has been insane for 12 years. An elder sister has epileptic fits almost every night.

Mental state on admission

He is evidently an idiot. He is almost entirely unable to speak, but when asked his name occasionally says something which sounds like 'little Tom'; can also say, 'mamma' and 'papa'. He pays attention when spoken to, but only makes unmeaning (or rather unintelligible) sounds in reply. When thwarted he is very passionate, and stamps on the floor or throws himself about the room; when in a good humour he is very affectionate, and is fond of jumping about and standing almost on his head. He is fond of music and plays with a little musical box: he can hum several tunes. He is pleased with picture-books; the pictures which he picks out are those of a horse and of a cart-wheel. He likes playing with a ball, and trundling a hoop.

He appears to have no idea of *number;* but of *locality* there seems to be some idea, for after going in a given direction several times he appears to recognize familiar landmarks. As regards *form,* he always prefers rounded figures to such as are irregular. He seems to have very little colour sense.

Physical condition

Height: 3 feet 10 inches; *Weight:* —.
Expression of face vacant, often mischievous.
Head measurements: Circumference 18 3/4 inches. From root of nose to spine of occiput* – 11 3/4 inches. From ear to ear 11 inches. Hair is fair with brownish tinge. There is slight right external strabismus.

Palate slightly arched. Teeth irregular and rather crowded, three or four decaying incisors notched. Ears illformed and rather pointed. Complexion often dusky.

On account of his struggling and noise it was impossible to examine the chest satisfactorily; but the examination so far as it was carried [out] detected nothing morbid.

Progress

13-5-81. Did not sleep well last night; he jumped and tumbled about in his bed for an hour after being undressed. Will not drink milk, and has a habit of smelling food before he eats it. Has a little diarrhoea.

18-5-81. Has taken some of the Cordial Mixture which has almost stopped the diarrhoea. He is not sleeping well, but always tumbles about for some time after going to bed. Is taking a fair quantity of food, but will not drink tea or coffee, or milk. When offered some milk and water he smelt it, and then refused to taste it. He takes his food very slowly, and has a habit of holding it in his mouth for a long time without swallowing it.

25-5-81. Is usually very affectionate, but when displeased is very cross and wilful.

---

* The occiput is the back part of the head.

27-5-81. Was visited today by his mother and sister, whom he recognised and seemed very much pleased to see. After their visit he was rather excited, jumping and capering about. He will now drink milk and water with a little reluctance. There is still a little occasional diarrhoea, but not more than he has always been subject to.

2-6-81. No change. Goes out every fine day.

8-6-81. Is taking food better than on admission, but is still very slow in masticating and swallowing it. He went to church last Saturday and Sunday and behaved very well being much attracted by the music.

When a box of coloured cards is placed before him, he always picks out the blue cards; and he chooses rings and circles in preference to angular forms.

15-6-81. No change. Goes out everyday, frequently into the city, and behaves well.

13-8-81. . . . it is worth mentioning that he has learnt his letters, and can pick each one out as it is named.

16-10-81. Has gone home today on leave for 2 weeks.

3-10-81. Has returned to the 'Cottage'.* There is little change of recent occurrence; but his family consider him much improved in many respects since his admission. He is more tractable and takes his food better.

22-12-81. . . . At 2 pm today he had an (epileptic?) fit, slight and short duration (about 2 minutes): there was no cry, not much convulsive movement, except of the eyes; convulsions bilateral . . .

28-10-82. Since the admission of this patient a fair amount of improvement has occurred, at least as great as could be expected in the time. He is cleaner and more regular in his habits, and more obedient. He has learnt several letters, and can identify the pictures of animals, toys etc. Is very affectionate, and recognises many people. His memory is on the whole good; he recognizes his relations and others after an absence of many months. He is now and then rather excited and apt to strike. Is usually in good bodily health.

12-7-83. Had an epileptic fit this morning at 5 o'clock, the third since admission. It only lasted half a minute, but he was quite

---

* The Cottage Hospital – a separate building in the grounds used on rare occasions for infectious cases.

unconscious; no marked convulsions, but twitching all over. There was no cry before the fit. He was very dull and heavy all day yesterday.

15-2-84. . . . He is somewhat improved mentally, taking more notice of what is passing, paying more attention to directions given him, and being able to recognize a number of letters and pictures. He cannot speak, only making unintelligible sounds . . .

27-10-84. . . . There is no change in his mental condition: he appears to be about at a standstill. His memory for people is good; and he is also able to recognize many tunes when sung or played.

28-2-85. Was at home for three weeks, during which time he behaved very well on the whole. There is no change in his general condition. He takes plenty of out-door exercise, and enjoys riding on a tricycle, playing ball etc. Makes various articulate sounds, but cannot speak so as to make himself understood.

26-5-85. Remains in the same idiotic condition . . .

24-11-86. . . . He was at home at Christmas for 3 weeks during which time he spoke two words distinctly . . .

2-4-86. This patient remains in the same condition more or less. About 3 weeks ago he spoke one word 'tired' when going to bed. The sense of colour has developed since he came here and now he can match colours together. He has a good ear for music. Lately he has slept very badly. Appears to know what is spoken to him. . . .

30-3-89. This young patient is mentally as demented as ever. There is no improvement whatever. He is boisterous, unintelligible, offers no articulate sound. Physically he seems in very good health . . .

1-8-91. On June 6th this patient's nurse was withdrawn and a male attendant was placed in charge of him. He was too animal and too manly for a nurse any longer . . .

2-11-91. He was on leave of absence at Scarbro' for a change with his attendant for four weeks from the 29th September. He has returned in good bodily health. Mentally unchanged.

1-2-92. Is an imbecile . . .

31-8-93. Is just as usual.

11-10-93. . . . Shows no mental improvement, remains as imbecile as ever. . . .

17-4-95. He remains in the same imbecile state, unable to speak. He has to be attended like a child. He is in fairly good health.

15-7-95. There is no change in his condition. He was away with his attendant, visiting his parents for three weeks at the English Lakes. . . .

29-9-98. No change.

30-12-98. He is ill suffering apparently from pneumonia . . .

2-1-99. He refused all nourishment and got rapidly worse and died rather suddenly at 8.30 pm. on Dec. 31st 1898 in presence of A. G. Jarvis and Isaac Hodgson. A P[ost] M[ortem] was held. Cause of death Pneumonia.

CASE 1653: ROBERT H.

Admitted December 18 1888 from Hurlington Middlesex.
Male, aged 24, single. Religion, Friend.
This is the first attack and has lasted about one week but from what I can learn he has evidently been very eccentric for some months. Supposed cause religious excitement. Suicidal and dangerous to others.
Extract from certificates:
'He sits in a dejected attitude constantly moaning to himself and frequently muttering 'too late, too late'. He either does not answer questions addressed to him or begins to talk about something quite irrelevant. He had tried to murder Dr. Fox.'

On admission

I append a photograph of how he appeared [see Plate 27]. He has adopted this strange garb for some time and has allowed his hair to grow quite long. His height is 5 ft. 2 in. Sallow, ruddy complexion. Black hair, grey eyes. Strongly built.

Mental condition

When addressed he stares fixedly at you for several minutes and then either turns away without answering or begins talking some rigmarole about the light of Christ having entered into him. About the only question I got him to answer sensibly was as to where he came from.

[*Dec.*] *21.* Still appears to be in this wrapt [*sic*] ecstatic condition. Last night he had an attack almost like a hysterical attack. He refused to stand up but bent his head right back and arched his body backwards and screamed terribly.

[*Dec.*] *24.* Mr. H. has now got his hair cut and a suit of ordinary clothes on and consequently looks more rational but he, though quieter, is still very deluded. He hears voices he tells me.

Dec. 28. This patient employs himself usefully about the gallery but when he has nothing to do he is a great nuisance as he is always annoying the other patients by stroking their hair and holding their hands.

1889 Jan. 1. Mr. H. has improved in bodily health since admission and eats and sleeps well. He tore up a paper one day because it had 'football notes' in it.

Jan. 2. This patient has been constantly trying to undress himself today and this afternoon he managed to get into a bucket of water and began scrubbing himself.

Jan. 8. Mr. H. has been fairly quiet lately. He has an idea that the patients here are in need of some ministration or consolation and is often going up to them and holding out his hand to them. He will stand in front of of a demented patient for an hour or more (if allowed) holding out his hand and saying 'Friend, wilt thou not shake hands with me?'

Feb. 1. This patient has improved considerably lately and is more rational in his behaviour.

Feb. 21. Mr. H. [incorrect name inserted at first] has since last entry gone back considerably. He talks great nonsense from time to time to my dog calling it 'The lion of the tribe of Judah'. He sometimes lies on his belly and kicks about making a curious animal noise.

March 29. Mr. H. has markedly improved since the last entry. He looks well and is very active. Mentally he is more capable. His appetite is good and his general health is satisfactory. He is however still addicted to self-abuse and has to be watched.

May 10. Robert H. appears dazed today. He is dull, listless, talks nonsense when spoken to. Appears to desire to be left to himself. These symptoms appear to be due to extreme self-abuse. He was ordered a cold shower bath today to rouse him.

May 11. Mr. H. appears better today, and takes more interest in his surroundings.

July 10. This patient appears to be dull, listless and stupid today. He stands in one position and on one spot and gazes on the ground; alternately he laughs immoderately, next he draws long sighs. When he is in this mood he does no work and will not occupy himself in any way. His face appears bloated, the eyes look dull and as if a haze were over them. He inanely repeats everything one says to him. He confesses that he abuses himself immoderately just now.

July 15. Robert H. is still in the above described state. He was shouting last night – this has been reported to me by the night watch.

July 20. Robert H. is slowly emerging from his melancholic state. He was given last night a draught containing Pot[assium] Brom[ide] gr[ains] XV, Chloral Hydrate gr[ains] XX for insomnia.

July 29. This patient is cheerful and well-behaved now. He is industrious and goes about his work as before his last relapse. His face is losing the dull, vacant expression. His eyes are clearer and less dazed-looking. He confesses to having abused himself to an extreme state, in spite of being watched.

Nov. 20. He has at last been quite industrious and intelligent for the last few days. He has been allowed walks in the country and seems just now pretty well. He takes his food well and sleeps well.

Dec. 6. Mr. H. is this morning in a dazed condition. He looks dull, heavy and listless. He has numbers of trivial complaints to make and during the recital of these he flew into a passion and used the terms 'and if you will allow a person to be submitted to these things, I can only say damn you'. He knows that the trifles complained of are in no way attributable to me personally and yet he is abusive to *me*.

Dec. 10. This patient is somewhat quieter, more cheerful and better behaved.

1890 March 4. This patient has relapsed into a dazed, incoherent condition. He does nothing, mutters to himself, laughs aloud at his own mutterings, when spoken to he answers quite wide of the mark. His sexual self-abuse is largely responsible for his relapses. They are always at any rate ushered in by his indulging in this manner. His health is not particularly good, as these attacks reduce him.

March 8. He is quite delusional today and states that a 'Mrs Holloway' has been to see him and that she struck him and scratched his eye.

May 1. This patient's condition appears to have settled down into one of recurrent mania. He gets periodic attacks of mania, associated with excitement, self-abuse, violence, incoherence, etc. His foreskin and fren[ul]um have been painted with liq[uid] epispasticus* to prevent his abusing himself.

June 4. This man is now in a maniacal condition. He uses obscene language, shouts, quotes scripture, stands in the middle of the grounds and preaches, gesticulates and is regardless of what he does. His nights are much disturbed and sleepless. He has been given a nightly draught of Pot[assium] Brom[ide] gr. XV and Chloral Hydrate gr. XX, for the present.

July 15. The night draught was this day discontinued for the present. The patient is on the whole quieter and less excited.

Aug. 1. Just now, this patient is extremely well and natural in manner. He knits and is industrious and good tempered. His physical health is very satisfactory.

Nov. 3. This patient keeps well and rational. He was away on leave of absence from Sept. 13–20th at Gainsbro' House, Scarborough,† and enjoyed the change exceedingly.

Dec. 24. This patient, continuing well, was this day discharged 'recovered' by order [i.e. at the request] of his father, John H.

---

* A blistering agent, also used in other asylums (e.g. Ticehurst) for this purpose.
† The Retreat's convalescent home.

Notes

The place of publication is London unless otherwise stated. The Retreat's archives are deposited at the Borthwick Institute of Historical Research, York, referred to here as BIHR.

1. THE BIRTH OF THE ASYLUM

1. M. MacDonald, *Mystical Bedlam: Madness, Anxiety, and Healing in Seventeenth-Century England* (Cambridge, 1981), pp. 168–9; M. V. Deporte, *Nightmares and Hobbyhorses: Swift, Sterne and Augustan Ideas of Madness* (San Marino, 1974), pp. 3, 14; M. Byrd, *Visits to Bedlam: Madness and Literature in the Eighteenth Century* (Columbia, S.C., 1974), pp. 17–18, 38.
2. G. Rosen, 'Social Attitudes to Irrationality and Madness in Seventeenth and Eighteenth Century Europe', *Journal of History of Medicine*, XVIII (1963), p. 233; M. Foucault, *Madness and Civilization: A History of Insanity in the Age of Reason* (1967), pp. 115–16.
3. Deporte, *Nightmares*, pp. 28–9, 37–9; Byrd, *Bedlam*, pp. 46–9; M. MacDonald, 'Insanity and the Realities of History in Early Modern England; *Psychological Medicine*, 11 (1981), p. 14; R. Porter, 'Being Mad in Georgian England', *History Today*, 31 (1981), p. 48; R. Porter, 'The Rage of Party: A Glorious Revolution in English Psychiatry?' *Medical History*, 27 (1983), pp. 35–50.
4. A. O. Lovejoy, *The Great Chain of Being*, 2d ed. (Cambridge, Mass., 1961), pp. 190, 195–6, 234.
5. Foucault, *Madness*, pp. 46–8, 64; Byrd, *Bedlam*, pp. 22–30.
6. A. Fessler, 'The Management of Lunacy in Seventeenth Century England, An Investigation of Quarter-Sessions Records', *Proceedings of the Royal Society of Medicine*, 49 (1956), pp. 903–5; W. L. Parry-Jones, *The Trade in Lunacy* (1972), p. 282.
7. W. Battie, *A Treatise on Madness*, 2d ed. (1963), p. 93.
8. *Liverpool Advertiser*, 15 Oct. 1789.
9. D. Leigh, *The Historical Development of British Psychiatry* (Oxford, 1961), p. 78.
10. M. G. Hay, 'Understanding Madness: Some Approaches to Mental Illness c 1650–1800' (Ph.D. thesis, University of York, 1979), pp. 15, 192.
11. Battie, *Treatise*, p. 94.
12. J. M. Cox, *Practical Observations on Insanity*, 2d ed. (1806), p. 100.
13. W. F. Bynum, 'The Great Chain of Being after Forty Years: An Appraisal', *History of Science*, 13 (1975), pp. 12–13; Byrd, *Bedlam*, pp. 145, 175.
14. J. Locke, *An Essay Concerning Human Understanding*, Everyman ed. 2 vols. (1965), I, p. 127.
15. J. Haslam, *Observations on Insanity* (1798), p. 10.
16. W. Pargeter, *Observations on Maniacal Disorders* (Reading, 1792), p. 49.
17. Haslam, *Observations*, p. 128.
18. J. Ferriar, *Medical Histories and Recollections*, 3 vols. (Manchester, 1792–8), II, pp. 107, 110.

19. Foucault, *Madness*, pp. 182–3. See also Chap. 4 for a fuller discussion of this point.
20. Cox, *Insanity*, p. 137.
21. *First Lines of the Practice of Physic*, 4 vols. (Edinburgh, 1789), IV, p. 153.
22. V. Skultans, *English Madness: Ideas on Insanity, 1580–1890* (1979), pp. 26–8.
23. N. Roberts, *Cheadle Royal Hospital: A Bicentenary History* (Altrincham, 1967), p. 7; *York Courant*, 5 Sept. 1772.
24. G. McLoughlin, *A Short History of the First Liverpool Infirmary, 1749–1824* (1978), p. 108.
25. Foucault, *Madness*, pp. 46–53, 64; K. Doerner, *Madmen and the Bourgeoisie: A Social History of Insanity and Psychiatry* (Oxford, 1981), pp. 69–72; A. T. Scull, *Museums of Madness: The Social Organisation of Insanity in Nineteenth-Century England* (1979), pp. 30, 34.
26. A. Masters, *Bedlam* (1977), p. 47; C. N. French, *The Story of St. Luke's Hospital* (1951), p. 35; Roberts, *Cheadle Royal*, pp. 27–9; *York Courant* August 1800; McLoughlin, *Liverpool Infirmary*, p. 53.
27. Parry-Jones, *Lunacy*, pp. 29, 46.
28. Masters, *Bedlam*, pp. 47–57.
29. French, *St. Luke's*, pp. 37–8; D. H. Tuke, *Chapters in the History of the Insane in the British Isles* (1882), p. 114.
30. M. Fears, 'The "Moral Treatment" of Insanity: a Study in the Social Construction of Human Nature' (Ph.D. thesis, University of Edinburgh, 1978), pp. 79–80.
31. *Liverpool Advertiser*, 29 Aug. 1789; Roberts, *Cheadle Royal*, p. 6.
32. Roberts, *Cheadle Royal*, p. 16.
33. Ferriar, *Medical Histories*, II, p. 112.
34. Roberts, *Cheadle Royal*, pp. 22–4.
35. *York Courant*, 11 Aug., 5 Sept. 1772.
36. [A. Hunter], *A Letter from a Subscriber to the York Lunatic Asylum to the Governors of that Charity* (York, 1788), p. 13.
37. *York Courant*, 5 Sept. 1772.
38. *York Courant*, 22 March 1774; J. Gray, *A History of the York Lunatic Asylum* (York, 1815), App. 3.
39. Bootham Park Hospital, York, Admissions Book, 1777–86.
40. Bootham Park Hospital, *A Charity Sermon at Church of St. Michael Le Belfrey by Rev. Dr. Marsden*.
41. [A. Hunter], *The History of the Rise and Progress of the York Lunatic Asylum* (York, 1792), p. 1.
42. A. Digby, 'Changes in the Asylum: The Case of York, 1777–1815', *Economic History Review*, 2d ser., XXXVI (1983), pp. 218–39.

2. THE RETREAT: A DISTINCTIVE CONCEPT

1. S. Tuke, *Review of the Early History of the Retreat* (York, 1846), p. 10.
2. R. M. Jones, *The Later Periods of Quakerism*, 2 vols. (1921), I, chap. X.
3. BIHR E/2, S. Birchall to W. Tuke, 1 April 1793; W. Tuke to W. Alexander, 22 July 1793; W. Birkbeck to W. Tuke, 19 Dec. 1793; S. Tuke, *Description of the Retreat*, 2d ed. (1964), pp. 34–5.
4. Quoted in W. K. Sessions and E. M. Sessions, *The Tukes of York* (1971), p. 55.
5. *A Memorial of York Monthly Meeting Concerning William Tuke* (York, 1823), p. 8.
6. Bootham Park Hospital, York, Admissions Book, 1787–1802, case 610; Tuke, *Description*, p. 22; York Public Library, Y362.2, W. Burgh to W. Wilberforce, 10 Nov. 1791.
7. Quoted in Sessions and Sessions, *Tukes*, p. 58.
8. Sessions and Sessions, *Tukes*, p. 93.
9. Sessions and Sessions, *Tukes*, p. 58.
10. Tuke, *Description*, p. 27.

Notes to pages 17–27   297

11. BIHR A/1/1, Directors Minutes 1792–1841, Circulars and Minutes 1793–5; Tuke, *Description*, pp. 30–41. Twenty acres of land were bought originally and eight acres sold as likely to be surplus to the requirements of the Retreat.
12. BIHR A/1/1, circular of 28 June 1792, article 7, and minute of 5 April 1793.
13. Tuke, *Description*, p. 33; Retreat *Report* (1851).
14. BIHR A/1/1, 5 April 1793.
15. C. L. Cherry, 'The Southern Retreat, Thomas Hodgkin, and Achille-Louis Foville', *Medical History*, 23 (1979), p. 315.
16. BIHR H/1, J. Bevans to W. Tuke, 2 Dec. 1793, 20 Jan. 1794, and 26 Feb. 1794; H. Tuke to W. Alexander, 22 Oct. 1793; D. H. Tuke, *Reform in the Treatment of the Insane: Early History of the Retreat* (1892), p. 14.
17. BIHR H/1. Two letters from W. Tuke to J. Bevans undated but probably November and December 1793; J. Bevans to W. Tuke, 31 Jan. 1794.
18. BIHR H/1, W. Tuke to J. Bevans n.d., probably Nov. 1793; J. Bevans to W. Tuke, 20 Jan. and 26 Feb. 1794.
19. Sessions and Sessions, *Tukes*, p. 26.
20. Retreat's *Reports* 1797–1821; S. Tuke, *A Sketch of the Origin, Progress, and Present State of the Retreat* (York, 1828), pp. 40–2.
21. *Description*, pp. 69–70.
22. Retreat *Report* (1821).
23. Retreat *Rules*, item 3. A revision of the rules in 1876 raised the qualifying donation to £50 and also added that legacies of £100 or more conferred the same privilege.
24. *Rules*; E. Isichei, *Victorian Quakers* (Oxford, 1970), pp. 70–2.
25. BIHR A/1/1, 1 Jan. 1796.
26. Sessions and Sessions, *Tukes*, p. 62.
27. BIHR H/2, W. Tuke to W. Maud, 13 Feb. 1797.
28. Ibid.
29. BIHR A/3/1, Committee Minute Book, 1796–1825, 12 Jan. 1797; BIHR C/1, R. Dearman to W. Tuke, 21 Jan. 1797.
30. BIHR A/3/1, J. Cordingley (April 1796–Jan. 1797), R. Driver (May 1797–Jan. 1798), J. Taylor (April–June 1798), J. Duxbury (Jan. 1799–Sept. 1800), T. Ventriss (Feb. 1799–Feb. 1803) and J. Beale (Dec. 1799–July 1801).
31. BIHR A/3/1, 3 May, 23 May, 29 Aug. 1796.
32. BIHR C/1, W. Tuke to W. Maud, 14 April 1797; BIHR A/3/1, 14 April 1797. Jane King was treated for mania and melancholy for three months in 1808 and then almost continuously from 1811 to 1828 (cases 123, 582, 584, 224).
33. Parry-Jones, *Trade in Lunacy*, p. 112; BIHR C/1, Dr Fox (brother of Edward Long Fox) to W. Tuke, 9 Aug. 1796, and undated note from John Hipsley.
34. Tuke, *Description*, pp. 46, 60–2; B. Pierce, 'Psychiatry a Hundred Years Ago', *Journal of Mental Science*, Oct. 1919; T. Fowler, *Medical Reports of the Effects of Tobacco* (1785); and *Medical Reports of the Effects of Arsenic* (1786).
35. BIHR C/1, W. Tuke to W. Maud, 24 July 1801.
36. The Cappe Bequest included specialist works on insanity by W. Battie, J. M. Cox, W. Cullen, W. Falconer, A. Harper and J. Monro.
37. BIHR L/1, L. Murray to Henry Tuke and other members of Retreat Committee, Aug. 1802.
38. BIHR C/1, J. Morris to T. Allis, 4 Feb. 1800.
39. BIHR A/1/1, 28 June 1797.
40. H. C. Hunt, *A Retired Habitation* (1932), p. 16.
41. S. Tuke, *Memoirs*, 2 vols. (1860), I, p. 230.
42. BIHR C/I, letter dated 19 Jan. 1802.
43. BIHR C/I, D. Harris to George Jepson, 17 June 1806.
44. BIHR C/I, S. Hodgson and W. Beavington to G. Jepson, 7 June 1802.
45. *Memoirs*, II, pp. 224–5.
46. Introduction by S. Tuke to M. Jacobi, *On the Construction and Management of Hospitals for the Insane* (1841), p. xx.

47. Tuke, *Review*, p. 37.
48. Tuke, *Description*, p. 138.
49. Ibid., pp. 131–2.
50. M. J. Clark, 'The Rejection of Psychological Approaches to Mental Disorder in Late Nineteenth Century British Psychiatry', in A. Scull, ed. *Madhouses, Mad-Doctors, and Madmen* (1981), p. 271; M. J. Clark, ' "A Plastic Power Ministering to Organisation": Interpretations of the Third Body Relation in Late Nineteenth-Century British Psychiatry', *Psychological Medicine*, 13 (1983), p. 490.
51. Retreat *Report* (1871).
52. *J. S. Rowntree; His Life and Work* (1908), p. 107.
53. Quoted in J. S. Rowntree, *Quakerism Past and Present* (1895), p. 17.
54. Tuke, *Review*, p. 10.
55. See chap. 5.
56. R. Hunter and I. MacAlpine, 'Samuel Tuke's First Publication on the Treatment of Patients at the Retreat, 1811', *British Journal of Psychiatry*, 111 (1965), p. 771.
57. Tuke, *Sketch*, p. 11; *Review*, p. 16.
58. Tuke, *Description*, pp. 133–4.
59. BIHR C/1, letter to W. Maud of 1 Dec. 1796.
60. BIHR D/3/1, Visitors Book, 1798–1822.
61. J. Griscom, *A Year in Europe in 1818 and 1819*, 2 vols. (New York, 1823), II, p. 302; Griscom had earlier visited the asylum at Geneva.
62. G. Zilboorg, *A History of Medical Psychology*, 2d ed. (New York, 1967), p. 317.
63. G. Mora, 'Vincenzo Chiarugi (1759–1820) and his Psychiatric Reform in Florence in the Late 18th Century', *Journal of History of Medicine and Allied Sciences*, XIV (1959), p. 431.
64. K. M. Grange, 'Pinel or Chiarugi?' *Medical History*, 7 (1963), p. 371.
65. Quoted in Mora, 'Chiarugi', p. 432.
66. The ensuing paragraphs are heavily indebted to E. A. Woods and E. T. Coulson, 'Psychiatry of Phillipe Pinel', *Bulletin of the History of Medicine*, XXXV (1961), and K. M. Grange, 'Pinel and Eighteenth Century Psychiatry', *Bulletin of the History of Medicine*, XXXV (1961).
67. P. Pinel, *A Treatise on Insanity*, trans. D. Davis (Sheffield, 1806), p. 221.
68. For the repressive side of Pinel's moral treatment see C. Jones, 'The "New Treatment" of the Insane in Paris', *History Today*, 30 (1980), p. 10.
69. E. H. Ackerknecht, *A Short History of Psychiatry*, 2d ed. (New York, 1968), p. 45.
70. *Memoirs*, I, p. 171.

3. MORAL TREATMENT

1. J. G. Kohl, *Travels in England and Wales*, 2d ed. (1968), p. 97.
2. A. Walk, 'Some Aspects of the "Moral Treatment" of the Insane Up to 1854', *Journal of Mental Science*, 100 (1954), pp. 808–9.
3. See chap. 1.
4. *Sketch of the Retreat*, p. 36.
5. *Book of Christian Discipline of the Religious Society of Friends* (1883), chap. IX.
6. Deporte, *Nightmares and Hobbyhorses*, pp. 144–7; Haslam, *Observations* (1798), p. 130.
7. E. T. Carlson and N. Dain, 'The Psychotherapy that was Moral Treatment', *American Journal of Psychiatry*, 117 (1960), pp. 519–24.
8. Tuke, *Description*, p. 178.
9. Quoted by G. Newman, 'The Application of Quaker Principles in Medical Practice', *Friends' Quarterly Examiner*, 64 (1930), p. 62.
10. N. Penney, ed., *The Journal of George Fox*, 2 vols. (Cambridge, 1911), I, pp. 420–1; R. A. Clark and J. R. Elkington, *The Quaker Heritage in Medicine* (Pacific Grove, Calif. 1978), p. 31.
11. W. C. Braithwaite, *The Beginnings of Quakerism* (1923), pp. 131, 140, 499, 524.

12. M. MacDonald, 'Religion, Social Change and Psychological Healing in England, 1600–1800', in W. J. Sheils, ed., *The Church and Healing* (Oxford, 1982), pp. 110–12.
13. D. H. Tuke, *Reform in the Treatment of the Insane: Early History of the Retreat* (1892), p. 23.
14. Tuke, *Review*, p. 37.
15. BIHR C/1, letter from T. Richardson to G. and C. Jepson, 28 June 1822.
16. *Retreat Report* (1859).
17. See M. Donnelly, *Managing the Mind* (1983), chap. 4, for an interesting discussion on architecture as a therapeutic tool.
18. BIHR L/3/2, State of an Institution (1797).
19. BIHR H/1, J. Bevans to W. Tuke, 20 Jan. 1794. John Bevans (1743–1809) began in a small way in the building industry and became quite a notable builder. He was an Elder of the Peel (Quaker) Meeting in London and also took an active part in the Yearly Meetings of the Society of Friends. There he was sometimes mentioned as being involved in the same activities as William Tuke.
20. French, *St. Luke's*, pp. 37–8.
21. D. H. Tuke, *Chapters in the History of the Insane in the British Isles* (1882), p. 114.
22. BIHR H/1, J. Bevans to W. Tuke, 26 Feb. 1794.
23. Brislington House seems to have been the first purpose-built private establishment; its new buildings were started in 1804 and opened in 1806.
24. *Retreat Report* (1824).
25. BIHR H/1, W. Tuke to J. Bevans, n. d., but probably Nov. 1793.
26. BIHR H/1, correspondence between Tuke and Bevans, autumn to spring 1793–4 and Tuke, *Description*, for early plans of the Retreat facing pp. 94, 100.
27. BIHR H/1, bills of the joiner, W. Farkinson; S. Tuke, *Practical Hints on the Construction and Economy of Pauper Lunatic Asylums*, 2d ed. (Wakefield, 1819), p. 11.
28. Tuke, *Review*, pp. 32–3.
29. Quoted in Tuke, *Description*, p. 225.
30. Tuke, *Memoirs*, I, p. 231.
31. *Retreat Report* (1852).
32. *Retreat Report* (1874), 'Retrospect', by J. Kitching.
33. *Retreat Report* (1855).
34. 'Retrospect', by J. Kitching.
35. The elevation of the Retreat, the finite capacity of York Waterworks Company and the huge amount of water used in this Institution (10,000 gallons daily by 1895) led to recurrent problems and the periodic installation of new steam pumps, as in 1865 and 1872.
36. BIHR L/3/2, State of an Institution (1797).
37. Tuke, *Description*, pp. 152, 158, 186.
38. Unless otherwise stated, generalisations here are based on details given in patients' case-books (the K/2 series at the Borthwick Institute) and in the annual printed *Reports* of the Retreat.
39. BIHR L/1, E. Pumphery, 'Recollections of the Retreat of 50 Years Ago', p. 94. Elizabeth Pumphery, daughter of Superintendent T. Allis, married an assistant keeper at the Retreat – William Pumphery.
40. *Retreat Report* (1839).
41. See chap. 8, 'The Changing Social Character of Patients'.
42. For example, BIHR K/2/1, case 2; K/2/2, case 19.
43. BIHR A/3/1, Committee Minute Book (1796–1825), 29 Aug. 1796.
44. Pumphery, 'Recollections', pp. 92, 94–5.
45. For example, BIHR K/2/2, case 25; K/2/3, cases 408, 420.
46. BIHR A/1/1, Directors Minutes, 27 Dec. 1821; Tuke, *Sketch*, p. 25.
47. For example, BIHR K/2/8, cases 848, 883, 905.
48. Tuke, *Memoirs*, II, p. 450.
49. For example, BIHR K/2/8–10, cases 808, 848, 883, 922, 1030.
50. See chap. 9, 'Outcome of Treatment,' for a discussion of the convalescent state.

51. Retreat *Report* (1894).
52. For example, K/2/2, case 80; K/2/3, case 390; K/2/6, cases 676, 709; K/2/7, case 725.
53. BIHR K/2/2, case 80; K/2/4, case 144; K/2/3, cases 438, 465; K/2/10, case 1010; K/2/16, case 1702.
54. BIHR, Unclassified, Matron's Report Books, 1897, 1902, 1907, 1909.
55. BIHR K/2/4, case 70; K/2/1, case 183; K/2/3, case 548.
56. BIHR K/2/10, case 1050.
57. BIHR K/2/1, case 183, comment dated 29 March 1815.
58. Retreat *Report* (1870).
59. Pumphery 'Recollections', p. 75.
60. BIHR C/1, letter from W. J., 21 Jan. 1803, concerning case 54, who had entered the institution in 1800 and was to remain there for sixty years.
61. BIHR C/1, letter from J. S., 11 Feb. 1803. He had been in the Retreat from Aug. to Dec. 1802.
62. BIHR C/1, letter from J. P., 7 Feb. 1819. He had been a patient from Dec. 1814 to March 1815 and again from Nov. 1818 to Jan. 1819.
63. C/1, letter from H. B. to T. Allis, 1 Nov. 1833, concerning his wife who had been a patient for six months earlier in that year.
64. Tuke, *Description*, p. 136.
65. BIHR K/2/4, case 122; Pumphery, 'Recollections', pp. 83–4.
66. BIHR K/2/7, case 776; K/2/10, case 987; Pumphery, 'Recollections', p. 84.
67. BIHR K/2/8, case 838.
68. BIHR K/2/3, case 446.
69. *Report* (1874).
70. See chap. 6, 'From Lay Therapist to Medical Practitioner', for a fuller discussion of medical personnel and their policies.
71. BIHR K/2/4, case 544.
72. J. Thurnam, *The Statistics of the Retreat, 1796 to 1840* (York, 1841), table 44.
73. BIHR C/1, undated letter probably written in Nov. 1793.
74. Tuke, *Description*, pp. 99–103.
75. Tuke, *Sketch*, p. 73.
76. BIHR K/2/9, case 977, letter of 30 April 1860 to Commissioners in Lunacy.
77. See chap. 10.
78. Pumphery, 'Recollections', p. 43.
79. E. N. C., 'Letter written to a Friend in 1878 by a Former Patient in the Retreat'.

4. MORAL MANAGEMENT

1. J. Conolly, *Treatment of the Insane without Mechanical Restraint*, 2d ed. (1973), p. 17.
2. K. Jones, *Lunacy, Law and Conscience, 1744–1845* (1955), p. 65.
3. M. Foucault, *Madness and Civilization: A History of Insanity in the Age of Reason* (1967), pp. 244–5.
4. Quoted in Tuke, *Description*, p. 223.
5. Foucault, *Madness*, pp. 252–3.
6. *Description*, p. 178; *Review*, p. 34.
7. Pumphery, 'Recollections', p. 82.
8. BIHR C/1, J. Harvey to W. Tuke, 14 March 1811.
9. BIHR K/2/8, case 824; K/2/7, case 778.
10. Tuke, *Description*, p. 159.
11. BIHR K/2/8, case 843; K/2/8, cases 828, 883.
12. *Description*, p. 150.
13. *A Letter from J. Fothergill Relative to the Intended School at Ackworth* (1778), p. 17.
14. J. J. Gurney, *Thoughts on Habit and Discipline* (1844), p. 75.
15. BIHR K/2/10, case 1149, observation of 18 April 1864.
16. J. C. Bucknill and D. H. Tuke, *A Manual of Psychological Medicine* (1858), p. 509.
17. *Sketch*, p. 36.

18. *Book of Christian Discipline of the Religious Society of Friends*, preface (1883).
19. BIHR C/1, W. Whitehead to W. Tuke, 6 April 1809, concerning case 134, and J. Thwaite to T. Allis, 14 May 1836, concerning case 549.
20. BIHR C/1, H. Jermyn to G. Jepson, 4 Jan. 1808, concerning case 115, and L. Sutton to G. Jepson, 23 June 1806.
21. S. Tuke, *A Letter on Pauper Lunatic Asylums* (New York, 1815); BIHR L/3/2, *State of an Institution* (1797).
22. Gurney, *Thoughts*, pp. 216, 218.
23. BIHR C/1, J. Brunton to T. Allis, 29 April 1839, concerning his brother, case 432, a patient from 1829 to 1849.
24. BIHR K/2/10, case 1053; K/2/8, case 883; K/2/4, case 559.
25. Foucault, *Madness*, p. 247.
26. Letter from W. Finch, 19 Feb. 1838.
27. Contrast the enthusiasm shown by Tuke in 1813 with the cautious advocacy of 1841 and 1850 (*Description*, pp. 180–6; Introduction to M. Jacobi, *On the Construction and Management of Hospitals for the Insane*, p. xxx; *Memoirs*, II, pp. 450–2.)
28. For example, BIHR K/2/4, case 544; K/2/5, case 632; K/2/8, case 864; K/2/9, cases 889, 897.
29. Foucault, *Madness*, pp. 244, 247–8, 252–3, 274.
30. Retreat *Report* (1854); BIHR D/1/1, Male Vistors Book (1815–67), 21 Nov. 1855.
31. Tuke, *Practical Hints*, p. 13.
32. K. Doerner, *Madmen and the Bourgeoisie* (Oxford, 1981), p. 66.
33. BIHR C/1, J. Brunton to T. Allis, 29 April 1839.
34. Quoted in Walk, 'Moral Treatment', pp. 816–7.
35. E. Goffman, *Asylums* (1961), p. 361.
36. Scull, *Museums of Madness*, p. 121.
37. Ferriar, *Medical Histories*, III, pp. 17–19; Haslam, *Observations* (1798), p. 127.
38. Principal sources for the section on classification are annual *Reports*; plans of the Retreat, mainly those in category H/1/6 at the Borthwick Institute; together with Tuke, *Description*, pp. 96–103; *Sketch*, pp. 44–6; J. Thurnam, *The Statistics of the Retreat* (York, 1841), pp. 19–22.
39. In the *Sketch* of 1828 (p. 45) these two subgroups are divided so that women are said to have five classes.
40. *Description*, p. 102; Thurnam, *Statistics*, p. 21.
41. *Practical Hints*, pp. 6–7.
42. *Description*, p. 141.
43. BIHR K/2/9, case 909.
44. BIHR K/2/9, observation of 10 Jan. 1859.
45. BIHR K/2/9, case 894.
46. BIHR E/2; Retreat *Report* (1896).
47. Tuke, *Description*, p. 146; BIHR K/2/10, case 1156.
48. BIHR K/2/4, case 470, observation of 28 March 1839.
49. S. Tuke, *Hints on the Treatment of Insane Persons* (1811).
50. BIHR K/2/9, case 979.
51. BIHR K/2/12, case 1416.
52. Retreat *Report* (1866).
53. BIHR K/2/2, case 85.
54. Foucault, *Madness*, p. 247.
55. BIHR K/2/, case 19.
56. BIHR K/2/8, case 847, observation dated 5 Nov. 1851. This patient was diagnosed as suffering from a monomania of anger or self-will.
57. BIHR K/2/9, case 897, observation dated 10 May 1855.
58. BIHR K/2/11, case 1135, observation of 12 Jan. 1874.
59. BIHR K/2/9, case 1191, observation of 1 April 1872. See A. Scull, 'The Domestication of Madness', *Medical History*, 27 (1983), pp. 233–48, for an interesting discussion on the domestication of the lunatic from the seventeenth to the early nineteenth centuries.

60. BIHR K/2/11, case 1205.
61. BIHR K/2/16, case 1753, observation of 10 July 1892.
62. BIHR K/2/9, case 967.
63. BIHR K/2/7, case 864, later readmitted as case 892, observation of 28 Jan. 1854.
64. Tuke, *Description*, p. 141.
65. Tuke, *Description*, pp. 141–3, 148.
66. *Description*, p. 149; *Sketch*, pp. 10–11.
67. M. Fears, 'Therapeutic Optimism and the Treatment of the Insane' in R. Dingwall, C. Heath, M. Reid, M. Stacey, eds., *Health Care and Health Knowledge* (1977), p. 68.
68. BIHR K/2/2, case 85, observation of 13 Nov. 1813.
69. Tuke, *Description*, p. 144; *Review*, p. 24.
70. BIHR L/3/1, G. Jepson to G. Higgins, undated but probably written in 1814.
71. BIHR C/1, Mr Reid to G. Jepson, 13 June 1813. C/1, miscellaneous bills for manufacture and repair of jackets in 1799.
72. BIHR K/2/2, case 15, observation of 19 Jan. 1816.
73. BIHR K/2/3, case 380, observation of 5 Sept. 1828, and case 389, 25 July 1828.
74. For example, BIHR K/2/2, case 15, observations of 24 Aug. 1813, 18 Jan. 1816.
75. BIHR C/1, bills of the joiners W. Farkinson and T. Fox for 1799 and 1801.
76. Delarive noted this during his visit in 1798 and his observations are quoted in Walk, 'Moral Treatment', p. 816.
77. BIHR D/1/1, 30 Sept. 1815.
78. See chap. 10.
79. *Description*, pp. 165–6.
80. *Description*, p. 67; BIHR D/1/1, Male Visitors Book, 1815–67; *Review*, p. 26; *Sketch*, p. 30.
81. *Description*, p. 164.
82. BIHR D/1/1, Male Visitors Book.
83. See chap. 10.
84. *Eighth Report of the Commissioners in Lunacy*, Parliamentary Papers, 1854, XXIX, p. 157.
85. *Review*, p. 28.
86. D. H. Tuke, *Prize Essay on the Moral Management of the Insane* (1854), p. 97; Retreat *Reports* 1851 and 1854.
87. *Review*, p. 29.
88. See chap. 6, 'Medical Treatment'.
89. BIHR K/3/1–9, Medical Journals and Weekly Reports.
90. BIHR G/1/1, Report of Visiting Commissioners in Lunacy, 12 April 1893.
91. Retreat *Report* (1854).
92. BIHR K/2/8, case 835.
93. BIHR K/2/9, case 912.
94. BIHR K/2/8, case 848.
95. *Description*, p. 142.
96. BIHR K/2/7, case 758.
97. BIHR K/2/3, case 380, 5 Sept. 1828; D/1/1, 2 Feb. 1836; C/1, letter of 18 Jan. 1835 concerning case 491.
98. BIHR G/1/1, 26 July 1862, 4 Nov. 1886.
99. *Description*, p. 157.
100. E. N. C., 'Letter Written to a Friend in 1878 by a Former Patient in the Retreat'.
101. BIHR K/2/6, case 886, 5 Feb. 1855.
102. BIHR L/3/2, S. Tuke to S. W. Nicholl, 12 July 1814.
103. Quoted in Walk, 'Moral Treatment', p. 816.

5. A QUAKER INSTITUTION

1. BIHR A/1/1, Director's Minute Book, 5 April 1793.
2. J. S. Rowntree, *Quakerism, Past and Present* (1859), p. 120.
3. Rowntree, *Quakerism*, p. 122.

Notes to pages 88–96

4. Ibid., p. 137; Isichei, *Victorian Quakers* (Oxford, 1970), pp. 144–6.
5. *Observations on the Religious Pecularities of the Society of Friends*, 5th ed. (1825), pp. 313–4.
6. *Observations*, p. 312.
7. Ibid., pp. 277–8.
8. H. Tuke, *The Principles of Religion as Professed by the Quakers* (1805), p. 158.
9. T. Clarkson, *A Portraiture of Quakerism*, 3 vols. (1806), I, p. 187.
10. BIHR K/2/4, case 541.
11. BIHR K/2/8, case 879.
12. L. J. Ray, 'Priests of the Body: Professionalisation and Medical Ideas about Insanity in Nineteenth-Century England' (Ph.D. diss., University of Sussex, 1981), p. 232.
13. BIHR K/2/11, case 1,327.
14. E. H. Hare, 'Masturbatory Insanity: the History of an Idea', *Journal of Mental Science*, 108 (1962), pp. 10–11.
15. BIHR K/2/14–15, cases 1526, 1561, 1563.
16. BIHR K/2/4, case 470.
17. BIHR K/2/10, case 1083.
18. J. J. Gurney, *Thoughts on Habit and Discipline*, 2d ed. (1844), pp. 98, 155.
19. BIHR K/2/1, case 208.
20. BIHR C/1, declaration dated 22 Feb. 1829.
21. BIHR C/1, J. Fryer to T. Allis, 28 June 1832.
22. *Observations on several clauses of the Bill 'For the regulation of the care and treatment of Lunatics in England and Wales' so far as it relates to Charitable Hospitals* (July 1845).
23. Gurney, *Observations on Religious Peculiarities*, p. 272; BIHR K/2/13, Case 1446, letter dated 11 April 1882.
24. BIHR K/2/1, case 129.
25. BIHR K/2/12, case 1440, observation of 23 June 1881.
26. BIHR K/2/1, case 117.
27. BIHR K/2/3, case 400.
28. E. T. Carlson and N. Dain, 'The Meaning of Moral Insanity', *Bulletin of the History of Medicine*, 36 (1962), pp. 132–4; R. Smith, *Trial by Medicine: Insanity and Responsibility in Victorian Trials* (Edinburgh, 1981), pp. 36–40, 102.
29. D. Leigh, 'James Cowles Prichard, M.D., 1786–1848', *Proceedings of the Royal Society of Medicine*, 48 (1955), pp. 586–7.
30. *A Treatise on Insanity* (1835), p. 4.
31. *On the Different Forms of Insanity in Relation to Jurisprudence* (1847), p. 31.
32. J. Kitching, *The Principles of Moral Insanity* (York, 1857), Introduction, pp. 23–4, 28–9.
33. J. C. Bucknill, *Unsoundness of Mind in Relation to Criminal Insanity* (1854), p. 17.
34. Cases 107, 158, 199, 282, 465, 543, 651 (readmitted as 754 and 911), 671 (readmitted as 753), 675, 676, 711, 716, 722, 724, 737, 739 (readmitted as 766), 748 (readmitted as 1012), 764, 766, 776, 912, 1052, 1399 (readmitted as 1447). Cases 465, 764, 912 and 1052 were those of non-Quakers. Details of the cases are to be found at BIHR, in J/1/1, Admissions Register and the K/2 series of case-books. Dr Thurnam's rediagnoses are not included as cases of moral insanity in Table 5.1.
35. BIHR K/2/7, fos. 147–155:
36. BIHR K/2/6, fos. 258–64.
37. BIHR K/2/6, entry of 7 Feb. 1844.
38. See also the discussion of the nature of moral management in chap. 4, sec. 2.
39. BIHR K/2/7, fos. 35–40, 348, entries for 5 and 7 July 1845.
40. BIHR K/2/6, fos. 41–50.
41. *Retreat Report* (1855).
42. BIHR K/2/7, foe. 283.
43. BIHR K/2/7, fos. 255–6.
44. E. Showalter, 'Victorian Women and Insanity', in A. Scull, ed., *Madhouses, Mad-Doctors, and Madness* (1981), p. 330.

45. BIHR J/1/1, K/2/1.
46. BIHR K/2/7, fos. 69–73, 75–7, 165, 213.
47. W. R. Huggard, 'The Standard of Sanity', *British Medical Journal* (1885), p. 1,013.
48. *Quakerism*, III, p. 150.
49. Quakerism, III, p. 402.
50. Retreat *Report* (1858).
51. Carlson and Dain, 'Moral Insanity', pp. 138–9.
52. J. Thurnam, *The Statistics of the Retreat* (York, 1841), pp. 18–19, and Table 11.
53. Retreat *Report* (1872).
54. Isichei, *Quakers*, p. 168.
55. BIHR K/2/3, foe. 27.
56. Retreat *Report* (1872).
57. Retreat *Report* (1875). Table 8.3 gives rather lower proportions of the celibate among *admissions*, but the single tended to stay in the Retreat for longer periods than the married and hence formed a higher proportion of the *inmates* at any one time. See A. Digby, 'The Changing Profile of a Nineteenth-Century Asylum: The York Retreat', *Psychological Medicine*, 14 (1984), for a fuller discussion of inmate composition.
58. Retreat *Report* (1906). Figures for the Retreat were 54.3 per cent compared to the national estimate of 22.4 per cent made by the Commissioners in Lunacy.
59. BIHR A/1/1, Directors' Minutes, circular of 25 Sept. 1794.
60. BIHR C/1, letter from T. B. Lowe, 14 July 1845.
61. S. Tuke, *Memoirs*, II, pp. 224–5.
62. Retreat *Report* (1827).
63. Clifford Street deposit, Brotherton Library University of Leeds, K.2.1., Applications for Membership, etc., of York Monthly Meeting, and K.4.1., Records of Members for York Monthly Meeting.
64. BIHR A/1/1, Directors Minutes, 28 June 1827.
65. William Waller MSS, Diary.
66. Waller MSS, poem 'Our Table', written Feb. 1856.
67. S. Tuke, *Review* (1846), p. 10.
68. BIHR K/2/3, case 178, entry of 31 Oct 1838.
69. BIHR K/1/1, case 258.
70. BIHR G/1/1, Vistors' Book of Commissioners in Lunacy, 29 Nov. 1848, and 9 Dec. 1858.
71. Tuke, *Practical Hints*, p. 13.
72. J. Travis Mills, *John Bright and the Quakers*, 2 vols. (1935), I, p. 233.
73. For example, BIHR K/2/8, case 846, and K/2/7, case 748.
74. For example, J. Griscom, *A Year in Europe in 1818 and 1819*, 2 vols. (New York, 1823), II, p. 307.
75. H. W. Sturge and T. Clark, *The Mount School* (York, 1931), p. 73.
76. Royal Bethlem Archives, *Report on the Expediency of Appointing a Chaplain to Bethlem Hospital* (1817).
77. One-third of the Retreat's income from 1796 to 1840 came from subscriptions, legacies and donations (Thurnam, *Statistics*, p. 5.).
78. BIHR C/1, letter to S. Tuke, 6 Dec. 1844.
79. BIHR A/1/1, Directors' Minutes, 31 Jan. 1889.
80. Isichei, *Quakers*, pp. 10–11, 158–9.
81. Ibid., pp. 156, 164.
82. Ibid., p. 75.
83. BIHR A/1/1, 31 Jan. 1889.
84. BIHR A/1/1, Annual Report for 1824.

6. THE ASCENDANCY OF MEDICINE

1. BIHR A/1/1, circular dated 28 June 1792; cover of ninety-ninth *Report* (1895).
2. A. T. Scull, 'Mad-Doctors and Magistrates: English Psychiatry's Struggle for Professional Autonomy in the Nineteenth Century', *Archives Européenes de So-*

Notes to pages 105–112   305

     ciologie, XVII (1976), pp. 279–305; A. T. Scull, 'From Madness to Mental Illness: Medical Men as Moral Entrepreneurs', *Archives Européenes de Sociologie*, XVI (1975), pp. 218–51.
3. S. Tuke's introduction to Jacobi, *Construction and Management*, p. xix, and Tuke, *Memoirs*, II, p. 45.
4. *Review of the Retreat* (1846), p. 37.
5. BIHR L/1, T. Allis to S. Tuke, Sept. 1822.
6. *Review* (1846), p. 16.
7. *Retreat Report* (1822).
8. BIHR L/1, letter of September 1822. By *materia medica* Allis meant the remedial substances employed in medicine.
9. *Description*, p. 112.
10. *Plarr's Lives of the Fellows of the Royal College of Surgeons*, 2 vols. (1930); H. Hutchinson, *Jonathan Hutchinson. Life and Letters* (1946), p. 20.
11. C. Williams, *Observations on the Criminal Responsibility of the Insane Founded on the Trials of James Hill and William Dove* (York, 1856).
12. He took his M.D. at Aberdeen in 1855 and became a member of the Royal College of Physicians in 1859.
13. Pumphery, 'Recollections', p. 81; *Retreat Report* (1849); Friends Library, Biographical Catalogue.
14. J. H. Wetherill, 'The York Medical School', *Medical History*, V (1961), p. 257; W. Hargrove and J. Hargrove, *A New Guide for Strangers and Residents in the City of York*, 2d ed. (1971), pp. 103, 106.
15. Scull, *Madness*, pp. 158–63.
16. BIHR C/1, S. Tuke to P. D. Tuckett, 27 July 1841.
17. Thomas Allis (1788–1875) was the son of a Burford hosier, who was engaged at various times in hosiery in Bristol and Tewkesbury, as well as in other more agricultural pursuits. He became increasingly interested in ornithological osteology, was appointed Curator of the Department of Comparative Anatomy in the Yorkshire Museum (1839–75) and also became a member of the Council of Yorkshire Philosophical Society (1852–4). His collections went ultimately to the society. He also became a member of the British Association and a Fellow of the Linnaean Society – a tribute to his numerous scientific papers. See S. Melmore. 'Thomas Allis, Osteologist', (Yorkshire Philosophical Society, 1930); and Friends Library, Biographical Catalogue.
18. BIHR L/1, T. Allis to S. Tuke, Sept. 1822.
19. *Retreat Report* (1823).
20. Pumphery, 'Recollections', p. 81.
21. BIHR C/1, letter to P. D. Tuckett, 27 July 1841.
22. Friends Library, Biographical Catalogue.
23. BIHR A/1/1, 6 June 1841. In this context it is interesting that it was not until 1848, when he became a director, that it appears Allis could bear to have a direct contact with the Retreat.
24. Cases 487, 535, 632 (BIHR K/2/4–5).
25. BIHR C/1, P. D. Tuckett to S. Tuke, 25 July 1841, and Tuke's reply of 27 July.
26. BIHR C/1, J. Proctor to T. Allis, 21 Nov. 1841.
27. BIHR C/1, C. Cathcart to S. Tuke, 20 Nov. 1841.
28. Quoted in *Osbaldwick, the History of a Suburban Village* (Osbaldwick History Group, 1980), p. 93.
29. *Osbaldwick*, p. 92. In 1853 Pumphery became the joint licensee of Hollytree House.
30. BIHR L/1, Joseph Rowntree, 'Memories of the Retreat', dated 24 July 1924.
31. BIHR A/3/1; the Petition from Committee of 'The Friends Retreat' to the Commons of the United Kingdom, July 1845, had asked that 'the precise position and style of the Medical Officer be left to the Managers of the Institution', but the Lunatics Act of 1845 (8 and 9 V.c.100.s.57), ruled that for asylums with over 100 patients the superintendent should possess medical qualifications. By the third quarter of that year there were over 100 patients at York.
32. *Sketch of the Retreat* (1828), p. 57.

Notes to pages 112–120

33. Advertisement dated 30 June 1841.
34. BIHR C/1, J. Candler to S. Tuke, 11 Oct. 1841.
35. Quoted in Scull, 'Mad-Doctors and Magistrates', p. 295.
36. Scull, *Madness*, pp. 141–2, 158–63, 170–1.
37. R. J. Cooter, 'Phrenology and British Alienists. Part II: Doctrine and Practice', *Medical History*, 20 (1976), pp. 135–6, 143.
38. BIHR K/2/3. The Retreat library contains a copy of G. Combe, *A System of Phrenology*, 4th ed., 2 vols. (Edinburgh, 1836).
39. BIHR K/2/4, fol. 517.
40. K/2/5, case 617.
41. *Dictionary of National Biography*.
42. Friends Library, Biographical Catalogue; Retreat *Report* (1874); Pumphery 'Recollections', p. 81. Kitching also translated Jacobi's *On the Construction and Management of Hospitals for the Insane* (1841). He wrote *A Lecture Addressed to Working Men on the Opportunities which They Have for Improving their Minds* (York, 1860), and *The Principles of Moral Insanity* (1857). After retiring as Retreat superintendent he was appointed visiting physician, a post he retained until his death in 1878.
43. Retreat *Report* (1861).
44. Kitching, *Moral Insanity*, p. 24.
45. M. J. Clark, 'The Rejection of Psychological Approaches to Mental Disorder in Late Nineteenth-Century British Psychiatry', in A. Scull, ed., *Madhouses, Mad-Doctors and Madmen* (1981), p. 271.
46. Scull, *Madness*, p. 185.
47. Retreat *Report* (1910); Pumphery, 'Recollections', p. 35. Robert Baker (1843–1910) had qualified as a doctor at Edinburgh in 1864 and had also studied in Paris. He practised in Thirsk, North Yorkshire, after 1867, and from 1872 he was the licensee of a private asylum – Lawrence House – in York, previously run by William and Elizabeth Pumphery – the son-in-law and daughter of Thomas Allis. He published *Notes on Some Asylum Specialities in Use at the Retreat* (1890) and papers on the benefits of Turkish baths, and the hospital villa system, in the *Journal of Mental Science* in 1889 and 1891. After his retirement as superintendent in 1892, he was appointed consulting physician to the Retreat, an office he held until his death in 1910.
48. P. McCandless, ' "Build! Build!" The Controversy over the Care of the Chronically Insane in England 1855–1870', *Bulletin of the History of Medicine*, 53 (1979), pp. 553–74, discusses the large-scale asylum-building programme for incurables and the mainly unsuccessful attempts by more progressive psychiatrists to get smaller buildings, rather than huge asylum blocks, created.
49. The Belle Vue estate of house and three acres of land was sold to the Retreat by Jonathan Burtt, who was its treasurer (1865–88) and was also Baker's uncle.
50. R. Baker, *Our Hospitals for the Insane: Their Position and Influence* (York 1892), p. 4. This first appeared in the *Journal of Mental Science* in 1891.
51. *Review of the Retreat* (1846), p. 10.
52. BIHR G/1/1, Minute 29 July 1892; M. Garrod, 'The Retreat was my Home' (typescript in the Retreat Library), pp. 10–12; Dr Garrod was Pierce's daughter.
53. See chap. 7, 'From Attendant to Mental Nurse'.
54. Garrod typescript, pp. 8–13; H. C. Hunt, *A Retired Habitation* (1932), p. 109.
55. Garrod typescript, pp. 10–11; B. Pierce, 'Some of our Difficulties in Practice' (Address to the York Medical Society, 14 Sept. 1901).
56. His seven case-books in the Retreat library indicated the size of his private practice: he was permitted to attend two afternoons a week at consulting rooms in Leeds. At first fees went to the Retreat but later Pierce bore the cost himself and took the fees (A/1/1 27 July 1892; Retreat *Report* [1903]).
57. L. J. Ray, 'Models of Madness in Victorian Asylum Practice', *Archives Européenes de Sociologie*, XXII (1981), p. 259.
58. *Our Hospitals for the Insane*, p. 4.

Notes to pages 120–132

59. Retreat *Report* (1906).
60. B. Pierce, *Psychiatry a Hundred Years Ago: With Comments on the Problems of Today* (1919), p. 16.
61. Hunt, *Habitation*, p. 109.
62. *Description*, p. 108, Retreat *Report* (1896).
63. A French Traveller [L. Simond], *Journal of a Tour and Residence in Great Britain During the Years 1810 and 1811*, 2 vols. (Edinburgh, 1815), II, p. 69.
64. See C. MacKenzie, 'Women and Psychiatric Professionalization, 1780–1914' (Paper presented at the History of Psychiatry conference at the Wellcome Institute, London, Sept. 1980). At the Retreat in 1893 ladies were formally associated with the Committee of Management and in 1898 the first female director was selected – a belated recognition of women's work as Female Visitors to the Retreat during the previous century.
65. Retreat *Report* (1912), and 'Address to the staff of the Retreat' given by Dr Kemp on 14 Dec. 1926. Dr Kemp left the Retreat in 1912 to take up general practice.
66. Tuke, *Description*, p. 111.
67. Thurnam, *Statistics of Insanity*, pp. 36–7.
68. Tuke, *Description*, pp. 110–116; *Sketch of the Retreat*, pp. 11–12.
69. *Statistics*, p. 28.
70. J. C. Bucknill and D. H. Tuke, *A Manual of Psychological Medicine* (1858), p. 472.
71. D. H. Tuke, *Prize on the Moral Management of the Insane* (1854), p. 68.
72. D. J. Mellett, *The Prerogative of Asylumdom* (1982), p. 41; M. Finnane, *Insanity and the Insane in Post-Famine Ireland* (1981), p. 208.
73. At Colney Hatch, e.g., only 6 per cent of patients were under medication in 1859 (R. Hunter and I. MacAlpine, *Psychiatry for the Poor* [1974], p. 18).
74. Generalisations on the Retreat's medical treatment are based on detailed examination of the Retreat's seventeen surviving medical case-books (BIHR K/2/1–17), which provide a superb record of the asylum's medical practice until the early 1890s.
75. *Description*, p. 118; Bucknill and Tuke, *Psychological Medicine*, p. 477.
76. BIHR C/1, bill from Thomas Surr, Sept. 1798.
77. BIHR unclassified, Journal (1792–1804), item July 1798.
78. Bucknill and Tuke, *Psychological Medicine* p. 474.
79. *Select Committee on Lunacy Law*, Parliamentary Papers 1877, XIII, Q8896 (evidence of Dr J. M. Granville).
80. E. B. C., 'Letter written to a Friend in 1878' (typescript in Retreat Library). Cases of excitement were minuted in the Retreat's medical journals (K/3/1–9).
81. For example, BIHR K/2/5, case 630; K/2/7, case 725; and K/2/9, case 917 were cases where medicine was refused. Edwin R. was in the Retreat as case 233 (April to July 1820), as case 497 (from Dec. 1834 to April 1835) and as case 627 (from Jan. to June 1841). Later, he was readmitted as case 713 (from April 1845 to June 1846) and as case 851 (from Dec. 1851 to June 1852).
82. *Madness*, p. 221.
83. BIHR K/2/5, case 627, observation of 28 June 1841.
84. E. N. C., 'Letter Written to a Friend in 1878': K/2/11, case 1279, fos. 299–300.
85. BIHR K/2/11, case 1303, observation of 21 May 1877; K/2/12, case 1366, observation of 8 April 1879.
86. *Description*, p. 124.
87. BIHR C/1, J. Brunton to J. Candler, 2 Nov. 1842.
88. See chap. 5.
89. *Statistics of Insanity*, pp. 32–3.
90. For Dr Belcombe see BIHR K/2/3, cases 466 and 473, and for Dr. Thurnam, K/2/6, case 671.
91. This is particularly evident in cases 601–50 in K/2/5–6.
92. B. S. Turner, 'The Government of the Body: Medical Regimens and the Rationalisation of Diet', *British Journal of Sociology*, XXXIII (1982), pp. 259–65.
93. BIHR K/2/3, case 446; K/2/6, case 666.

94. BIHR C/1, G. Jepson to W. Alexander, 1 Sept. 1820.
95. BIHR C/1, A. Mackintosh to T. Allis, 9 June 1830.
96. BIHR K/2/11, case 1232.
97. BIHR K/2/13, case 1508, observation of 21 Sept. 1883.
98. BIHR K/2/1, case 75.
99. BIHR C/1, Jepson to Alexander, 1 Sept. 1820; K/2/13, case 1464, observation of 1 Jan. 1883.
100. Tuke, *Description,* pp. 112–3; Thurnam, *Statistics,* p. 36.
101. BIHR K/2/2, case 91; K/2/6, case 658; K/2/8, case 850; K/2/9, case 935.
102. BIHR K/2/9, case 955; K/2/11, case 1134.
103. BIHR K/2/2, cases 68, 85; *Description,* p. 114.
104. Thurnam, *Statistics,* p. 36; BIHR K/2/6, case 671; K/2/7, case 716; K/2/12, case 1375.
105. BIHR K/2/8, case 866.
106. BIHR K/2/9, case 924.
107. BIHR J/1/1–3, Returns of Admissions.
108. BIHR K/2/4, fol. 330.
109. BIHR J/1/1, cases 160, 470.
110. BIHR K/2/6, fol. 409.
111. Retreat *Report* (1904).
112. 'The Treatment of the Insane: A Survey of the Work of Friends in England and America', *Friends Quarterly Examiner* (1902).
113. B. Clarke, *Mental Disorder in Earlier Britain* (Cardiff, 1975), pp. 99, 105; J. C. Bucknell and D. H. Tuke, *A Dictionary of Psychological Medicine,* 2 vols. (1892), II, p. 813.
114. For example, in cases of mania, BIHR K/2/4, case 271, and K/2/5, case 615; for melancholia, K/2/2, cases 91, 101.
115. For example, BIHR K/2/4, cases 470, 541, and K/2/8, cases 853, 877, 941.
116. BIHR J/1/1, cases 171, 309, 542, 603, 701.
117. Retreat *Report* (1885).
118. BIHR K/2/3, cases 393, 399, 404.
119. BIHR K/2/8–9, case 866, observation of 7 March 1854.
120. D. Pierce, 'The Undermind' (Paper given to the Quaker Medical Society on 11 Feb. 1918).

7. THE ASYLUM ATTENDANT

1. *Ninth Report of Commissioners in Lunacy,* Parliamentary Papers 1854–5, XVII, p. 576.
2. J. T. Arlidge, *On the State of Lunacy and the Legal Provision for the Insane* (1859), pp. 105–6.
3. *Thirteenth Report of Commissioners in Lunacy,* Parliamentary Papers 1859, sess. 2, XIV, p. 597.
4. For example, in 1869, 122 attendants were dismissed from asylums of whom 46, or nearly one-third, had been violent or rough with their patients. This included the two attendants from Lancaster Asylum who were convicted of the manslaughter of their patient and given seven years' penal servitude. (*Twenty-fourth Report of Commissioners in Lunacy,* Parliamentary Papers 1870, XXXIV, p. 80).
5. BIHR C/1, S. Tuke to T. Stordy, 22 Nov. 1826.
6. See chap. 5.
7. See chap. 2 and chap. 2, n. 30.
8. BIHR A/3/1, Committee of Management Minutes; the 'Clifford Street deposit' at Brotherton Library, University of Leeds, K.4.1., Record of Members and Account of Families, 1790–1841 in York Monthly Meeting.
9. BIHR, Unclassified, Retreat Journal 1842–53; and 'Clifford Street deposit', K.4.1, and M.3.1., York Monthly Meeting List of Members, 1837–1907.

Notes to pages 142–152   309

10. BIHR F/1/1, Appointment testimonials, 1841; C/1, E. Penty to T. Allis, 27 Jan. 1841.
11. BIHR, Journal 1842–53; J. Walton, 'The Treatment of Pauper Lunatics in Victorian England: the Case of the Lancaster Asylum, 1816–70', in A. Scull, ed., *Madhouses, Mad-Doctors, and Madmen* (1981), p. 180.
12. BIHR A/3/1, 17 July 1801.
13. BIHR C/1, letter to T. Stordy, 22 Nov. 1826.
14. S. Tuke, *A Letter on Pauper Lunatic Asylums* (New York, 1815), p. 27.
15. *An Enquiry into the Present State of Visitation, in Asylums* (1828), p. 3.
16. A New Governor [S. W. Nicoll], *A Vindication of Mr. Higgins from the Charges of Corrector Addressed to the Earl Fitzwilliam* (York, 1814), p. 37.
17. *Retreat Report* (1900).
18. Sources for Table 7.1 are BIHR A/1/1 for patient numbers; for attendants: (1797) A/3/1; (1813) Tuke, *Description*, p. 108; (1823) C/1, Notes on back of letter from W. Percy, 5 Dec. 1823; (1828) *Sketch of the Retreat*, p. 48; (1840) Thurnam, *Statistics*, table 44; (1847) G/1/1; (1863–77) Retreat Journals, 1853–70, 1870–8.
19. Parry-Jones, *Trade in Lunacy*, p. 186; Walton, 'Pauper Lunatics', p. 180; Tuke, Introduction to Jacobi, *Hospitals for the Insane*, p. xxi; J. Conolly, *The Construction and Government of Lunatic Asylums and Hospitals for the Insane* (1847), p. 83.
20. Tuke, *Practical Hints*, p. 3.
21. Tuke, Introduction to Jacobi, *Hospitals for the Insane*, p. xxi.
22. *Sketch of the Retreat*, pp. 58–9.
23. *Rules for the Government of Attendants and Servants, at the Retreat near York; with Instructions as to the Management of Patients* etc. (York, 1842, 1847).
24. Conolly's views had been printed in the *Lancet* in 1846 before publication in *The Construction and Government of Lunatic Asylums and Hospitals* in the following year. Rule books of many asylums apparently followed the same model (Public Record Office MH51/44B, Collection of rule books).
25. The *Rules* of 1897 specified a weekly warm bath. Already in the 1840s, Hanwell was providing a weekly bath for its inmates. (Conolly, *Construction and Government*, p. 109.)
26. Parry-Jones, *Trade in Lunacy*, p. 189.
27. Walton, 'Pauper Lunatics', p. 180. I am grateful to Nicholas Hervey for the information on attendants in Kent and Surrey.
28. Tuke, *Description*, p. 151.
29. See chap. 4, 'Rewards and Punishments'.
30. Tuke, *Description*, p. 172.
31. Colney Hatch, for example, employed them in 1858 (R. Hunter and I. MacAlpine, *Psychiatry for the Poor* [1974], p. 96).
32. Walton, 'Pauper Lunatics', p. 180.
33. *Retreat Report* (1850) and (1854).
34. BIHR K/2/10, case 1010.
35. *Retreat Report* (1861).
36. BIHR K/2/10, case 1143, 15 April 1873.
37. BIHR K/2/8, case 866.
38. BIHR K/2/9, case 889, 1 Feb. 1855.
39. BIHR K/2/9, case 891, 12 Aug. 1854.
40. BIHR K/2/9, case 955, 10 June 1858.
41. BIHR K/2/10, case 1036, 28 May 1863.
42. BIHR K/2/8, case 878, 18 Jan. 1854.
43. S. W. to the Retreat Committee, 27 Dec. 1813. For details of this letter see Appendix on Samuel W., and entry for 12 month 28 in 1813.
44. Samuel W. had come to the Retreat at his own request in Dec. 1803 (after experiencing several attacks of remittent mania in the preceding dozen years), and stayed there until his death in 1824. Waring got to know members of York Monthly Meeting well, amongst them the respected American grammarian, Lindley Murray. The keepers he mentioned, Samuel Smith and John Binns (both

appointed in 1801) and Isaac Stansfield (appointed in 1807), could, from the point of chronology, have played the roles he assigned them. This was also true of the patients: Joseph G. (at the Retreat from 1803 to 1804 and again from 1826); James B. (1798–1843); J. C. (1804–5 and 1805–14); and J. W. (1801–9).
45. BIHR A/3/1, 23 March 1812.
46. BIHR C/1, T. Crowley to W. Tuke, 26 Sept. 1803.
47. BIHR K/2/2, case 171.
48. Tuke, *Description*, p. 172; Conolly, *Construction and Government*, p. 115.
49. BIHR K/2/11, case 1222, 5 Dec. 1873.
50. Care and Treatment of Lunatics Act and Lunatic Asylums Act of 1853 (16 and 17 Victoria c. 96 and 97).
51. A/3/5, 3 Aug. and 21 Aug. 1894; *Yorkshire Herald*, 10 Aug. 1894.
52. For example, the Rules of 1847 specified that attendants were 'expected to set a good example to the patients in habits of cleanliness, regularity and order, and in neatness and propriety of dress and manners'.
53. Rule 13 (1842).
54. BIHR K/2/10, case 1044.
55. BIHR K/2/9, case 967.
56. BIHR K/2/8, case 821.
57. I am most grateful to Mr Brian Walster for allowing me to consult the private papers of William Waller while his own work on Waller's biography was in progress.
58. Journal of religious experiences, 1839–95.
59. Journal, 16 Feb. 1843.
60. Fragment of diary, undated.
61. BIHR A/4/6, Rough Committee Minutes, 1 Dec. 1843.
62. Diary, n.d.
63. Diary.
64. Diary.
65. BIHR K/2/6, case 669; J/2, Returns of Admissions; J/1/2, Admissions record; K/1/4 certification.
66. BIHR A/3/3, 17 Feb. 1845; 22 Sept. 1845; 21 Oct. 1846; 18 Sept. 1848; 24 June 1851; 15 Nov. 1852; 17 April 1854.
67. Letter to Mr. Isaac Wood, 17 Dec. 1849.
68. Journal, 11 Dec. 1843.
69. Ibid.
70. Journal, 6 July 1847.
71. Journal, 15 June 1851.
72. 'Our Table', written Feb. 1856; verses 7 and 10.
73. Journal, 6 Jan. 1856.
74. BIHR A/3/3, 18 July 1856.
75. Elizabeth Slee had worked as a nurse at the Retreat since 1843 and was considered to be good at her job. The patient 'has been under the care of a much more efficient attendant (Elizabeth Slee)' recorded the case-notes on patient 877 in K/2/8, on 2 Oct. 1853. She left her employment when she married Waller.
76. Journal, 15 March 1857.
77. Journal, 23 Nov. 1842.
78. Conolly, *Construction and Government*, p. 83.
79. *Report on the Training of Nurses* (1890), p. 4.
80. Retreat *Report* (1894).
81. Retreat *Report* (1902).
82. Retreat *Report* (1907).
83. Retreat *Report* (1908).
84. Retreat *Report* (1902, 1908).
85. B. Pierce, 'On the Training of Nurses in Institutions for the Insane', *Journal of Mental Science* (Jan. 1903).
86. Retreat *Report* (1874, 1875).

87. I am indebted to Mrs. W. K. Sessions, the daughter of Ethelwyn Rowntree, for this information.
88. Retreat *Reports*, 1894–1911; *Rules and Instructions for the Guidance of the Attendants, Nurses, Artisans and other Servants Employed at the Retreat, York* (York, 1897).
89. M. Finnane, *Insanity and the Insane in Post-Famine Ireland* (1981), p. 182.
90. BIHR A/3/5, 21 March 1893; Retreat *Report* (1901).
91. Retreat *Report* (1905).
92. I am grateful to Charlotte MacAlpine for this information on Ticehurst; BIHR F/3, Notes on Female Nurses; F/4, Notes on Male Attendants.
93. *Rules* (1847).
94. Intemperance was cited quite frequently in BIHR F/4 as a cause of notice being given to attendants.
95. BIHR A/3/1, 12 Jan. 1897.
96. See chap. 2, n. 29.
97. Hunter and MacAlpine, *Psychiatry for the Poor*, p. 112; Walton, 'Pauper Lunatics', pp. 186–7; Finnane, *Insanity*, pp. 210–11; Scull, *Madness*, p. 204.
98. Quoted in D. H. Tuke, *On the Moral Management of the Insane* (1854), p. 100.

8. PATIENTS

1. BIHR K/1/1–20, admissions certificates; J/1/1–2, admissions registers; K/2/1–17, medical case-books; J/2, tabulated return of admissions.
2. See chap. 6, 'From Lay Therapist to Medical Practitioner'.
3. Cases 2090, 2278.
4. E. Showalter, 'Victorian Women and Insanity', in A. Scull, ed., *Madhouses, Mad-doctors, and Madmen* (London, 1981), pp. 315–16. Overall, 44.1 per cent of patients at the Retreat were male and 55.9 per cent female (1796–1910).
5. B. Mitchell and P. Deane, *Abstract of British Historical Statistics* (Cambridge, 1962), p. 7.
6. Isichei, *Victorian Quakers*, p. 167. It is interesting that in the York Monthly Meeting between 1822 and 1844, 43 per cent of members were men and 57 per cent women (Brotherton Special Collection, University of Leeds, M6, Statistical Notes on York Monthly Meeting by S. Tuke).
7. See Showalter, 'Women and Insanity', pp. 322–4, and V. Skultans, *Madness and Morals: Ideas on Insanity in the Nineteenth Century* (1975), chap. VIII for fascinating discussions on the predisposition of the female to insanity as revealed in late Victorian psychiatric literature.
8. Some other mental institutions, notably Witney (1828–56) and Bowhill House (1801–69), had a greater proportion of single than married patients although the disparity was not so great as that at the Retreat.
9. Retreat *Report* (1872).
10. In 1861, 3.6 per cent of the male population of England and Wales and 7.4 per cent of the female were widowed, whereas under Dr Kitching (1849–74) 3.3 per cent of male patients and 6.0 of the females were in this category. In 1881, 3.4 per cent of the male population and 7.5 per cent of the female were widowed, whereas under Dr Baker (1874–92), 3.2 per cent of male patients and 7.0 per cent of females were in this category.
11. There were 317 married men and the same number of married women, whereas there were 485 single men in contrast to 645 single women, and 64 widowers in contrast to 113 widows. Married men outnumbered women in four of our sub-periods, but there were slightly more women under Kitching and substantially more under Pierce.
12. BIHR K/2/2, case 366. See also, e.g. K/2/3, cases 401, 409.
13. Showalter, 'Women and Insanity', p. 325.
14. Thurnam, *Statistics*, table C and table 9; Parry-Jones, *Trade in Lunacy*, p. 163; and information on Bowhill House kindly supplied by Nicholas Hervey.
15. The census of 1851 showed 45.2 per cent of the population of England and Wales

to be under twenty, and that of 1881 revealed a comparable figure of 46.2 per cent (Mitchell and Deane, *Historical Statistics*, p. 12).
16. *The Facilities and Services of Mental Illness and Mental Handicap Hospitals in England* (DHSS Statistical and Research Report Series 21, 1980), table A1.1.
17. BIHR G/1/1, 3 July 1883.
18. Isichei, *Victorian Quakers*, pp. 168–70.
19. BIHR C/1, W. Tuke to Dr Fox, 14 Aug. 1796.
20. BIHR C/1, W. Jackson to W. Tuke, 4 Nov. 1804.
21. Retreat *Report* (1844). This examination of patients' fees had been prompted by the worsening financial predicament of the asylum since the late thirties.
22. BIHR C/1, S. Tuke to J. Barnes, 25 Nov. 1841.
23. Figures for non-economic fee payers were given in the Retreat's *Reports* for 1862, 1883, 1889, 1890 and 1898.
24. Retreat *Report* (1893).
25. BIHR C/1, F. Fox to W. Tuke, 27 Sept. 1800.
26. BIHR K/2/15, case 1,741.
27. Retreat *Report* (1894).
28. BIHR G/1/1, 29 July 1870.
29. See, e.g., C/1, T. Allis to F. Nicoll, 27 March 1824.
30. BIHR G/1/1, 5 March 1881.
31. E. Isichei, *Victorian Quakers* pp. 288–91. Isichei followed the work of Charlotte Erikson in *British Industrialists: Steel and Hosiery 1850–1950* (Cambridge, 1959), pp. 230–2.
32. Retreat *Reports* (1905, 1910).
33. Reproduced in D. Peterson, ed., *A Mad People's History of Madness* (Pittsburgh, 1982), pp. 94, 106–7.
34. BIHR K/2/4, case 597.
35. BIHR K/2/10, cases 1104, 1057.
36. BIHR L/1, Pumphery, 'Recollections', pp. 87–8.
37. BIHR K/2/6, case 657.
38. By the 1870s fifty-four keys were needed to go round the asylum (BIHR E/13).
39. James W. [case 719] to J. Candler, 16 Nov. 1845. The patient was in the Retreat from 6 Aug. to 1 Oct. 1845.
40. BIHR K/2/15, cases 1653, 1725.
41. BIHR K/2/5, case 611; K/2/6, case 697.
42. BIHR K/2/5, case 608.
43. BIHR K/2/6, case 1737.
44. Showalter comments that textbook cases of female insanity usually described disobedient or rebellious women ('Women and Insanity', p. 324).
45. E. N. C., 'Letter to a friend M. R. in 1878'.
46. BIHR K/2/12, case 1,443.
47. S. Tuke, *Practical Hints*, p. 3.
48. Waller, MSS, poem, 'Our Table' (1856), verse 5.
49. *Madness or the Maniac's Hall,* p. 219. Edwin R. had been in the Retreat as case 233 (1820–2), case 497 (1834–5) and was at this time undergoing further treatment as case 627.
50. See chap. 7, 'Performance'.
51. BIHR C/1, letter of 19 Sept. 1819.
52. BIHR K/2/9, cases 917, 978.
53. BIHR K/2/11, case 1261; K/2/13, cases 1484, 1512.
54. See the occasional entries in K/3/1, Medical Journal and Weekly Reports.
55. BIHR G/1/1, comment of 31 July 1883; K/2/3, cases 442, 280; K/2/1, case 314 describing case 318.
56. Annual statement in the appendix to printed *Reports* of the Retreat.
57. H. Thompson, *A History of Ackworth School* (1879), pp. 139, 178–9, 255.
58. For example, BIHR C/1, E. Lambert to G. Jepson, 8 Oct. 1805.
59. BIHR C/1, Jane P. to T. Allis, 7 March 1841.

60. E. N. C., 'Letter to a friend M. R. in 1878'. It is interesting that until the mid-nineteenth century, pupils at Quaker schools also had their outgoing letters read (W. A. Campbell Stewart, *Quakers and Education* [1953], p. 212).
61. BIHR C/1, W. H. to G. Jepson, 21 Feb. 1803, about his wife, who was the first patient at the Retreat.
62. Retreat *Report* (1899).
63. Bootham Park Hospital, Visitors Reports (1814–28), 7 July 1817.
64. BIHR A/3/1, 29 Aug. 1796, and 31 Aug. 1814.
65. BIHR C/1, J. Ellis to G. Jepson, 18 Nov. and 4 Dec. 1821.
66. BIHR K/2/13, case 1,460, letter dated 23 Feb. 1882.
67. BIHR K/2/13, case 1,446, letter dated 11 April 1882.
68. BIHR C/1, T. G. to T. Allis, 19 Feb. 1830.
69. BIHR C/1, T. Crowley to W. Tuke, 26 Sept. 1803.
70. *Madness or the Maniac's Hall*, pp. 252–3.
71. BIHR K/2/13, case 1,501; K/2/6, case 710.
72. BIHR K/2/13, case 1,483. Charles Reade's *Hard Cash*, published in 1863, was a somewhat sensational compilation of previous, isolated cases of abuse in mental institutions that was recast in fictional form. Given comtemporary concern over wrongful confinement in lunatic asylums it attracted a wide readership.
73. BIHR G/1/1, 3 May 1895.
74. BIHR K/2/5, case 601.
75. BIHR K/2/4, case 454.
76. Retreat *Report* (1897).
77. BIHR K/2/3, case 471; Retreat *Report* (1875).
78. BIHR K/2/9, case 896.
79. BIHR C/1, J. Burtt to T. Allis, 18 and 22 Nov. 1836.
80. BIHR C/1, W. Pickford to T. Allis, 16 Sept. 1836.
81. BIHR K/2/10, case 1153.
82. BIHR K/2/2, case 78.
83. BIHR K/2/12, case 1368.
84. BIHR K/2/8, case 879.
85. BIHR K/2/9, case 967. See also chap. 4, 'Internal Restraint'.
86. BIHR K/2/12, case 1375, Dr Baker to Commissioners in Lunacy, 3 Jan. 1881. The patient had been in the Retreat from 25 March to 31 Dec. 1880.
87. E. Goffman, *Asylums* (New York, 1981), pp. 41, 63–4.
88. Scull, *Museums of Madness*, p. 198; Hunter and McAlpine, *Psychiatry for the Poor*, pp. 11, 79–80.
89. At Colney Hatch, for example, four to six doctors were responsible for 2,250 patients from the 1860s to the early twentieth century. (*Psychiatry for the Poor*, pp. 79–80).
90. BIHR K/2/6, case 710.
91. Case 1795. Unfortunately, this patient's case-notes have not been found, but some information on his illness is given on his admission certificate (BIHR K/1/11).

9. THE RETREAT'S RECORDS

1. In 1827 the average asylum had 116 patients and in 1890, 802 (Scull, *Museums of Madness*, p. 198).
2. BIHR A/3/1, 4 April 1816; J/1/1, case 194.
3. Retreat *Report* (1799).
4. Retreat *Report* (1800).
5. Lunatics Act, 1828, (9 George IV c.41), Lunatics Act, 1845 (8 and 9 Victoria c.100).
6. P. McCandless, 'Liberty and Lunacy: the Victorians and Wrongful Confinement', in A. Scull, ed., *Madhouses, Mad-Doctors and Madmen*, pp. 339–62.
7. K. Jones, *Mental Health and Social Policy* (1960), p. 110; B. Pierce, 'Treatment of

Mental Disorders in their Early Stages', *Friends Quarterly Examiner*, April 1920; Retreat *Report* (1905).
8. Retreat *Report* (1880).
9. BIHR K/2/13. Bryan S. was first admitted as case 1,419, and this extract came from his medical record between this first stay as a certificated patient, and his next formal admission as case 1,458. He had treatment as a certificated patient on eight occasions between 1880 and 1902.
10. BIHR J/2, Returns of Admissions, 1796–1910; Retreat *Reports*, 1901–8.
11. B. Pierce, *The Hospital Treatment of Incipient Insanity* 1908. (Address to the British Medical Association.)
12. J. Thurnam, *The Statistics of the Retreat, 1796–1840* (York, 1841), tables 13–14.
13. Tuke, *Description*, p. 208.
14. BIHR J/1/1, cases 514, 600.
15. L. J. Ray, 'Models of Madness in Victorian Asylum Practice', *Archives Européenes de Sociologie*, XXII (1981), p. 264.
16. BIHR K/1/16, Admissions Certificates (1903–4), case 2,141.
17. See chap. 5.
18. *Description*, pp. 211–12; Thurnam, *Statistics*, pp. 18–19; Ray, 'Models of Madness', p. 264.
19. BIHR K/1/18, Admissions Certificates (1906–7), cases 2344, 2353.
20. BIHR K/1/17, Admissions Certificates (1904–6); case 2289 was admitted in Nov. 1906.
21. BIHR K/1/6, Admissions Certificates (1861–75), case 1063.
22. Information on admissions certificates during Jepson's time was very patchy, partly because relatively few certificates have survived and also because in the early days relatives were not prompted to give information by formal questionnaires. However, this lack was more than compensated for by information obtained from relatives through correspondence or visits to the Retreat, which was then inserted into the admissions registers.
23. Mellett, *Prerogative of Asylumdom*, pp. 76–7.
24. Returns given in Parliamentary Papers in appendices to the annual *Reports of the Commissioners in Lunacy*
25. BIHR G/1/3, Returns to Commissioners in Lunacy; Scull, *Museums of Madness*, pp. 190, 192.
26. Retreat *Report* (1900).
27. Retreat *Report* (1899, 1896).
28. BIHR K/2/4, case 15.
29. Retreat *Report* (1902).
30. Retreat *Report* (1903).
31. Scull, *Museums of Madness*, p. 190.
32. Retreat *Report* (1903). Modern therapists might see such an incident as an embarrassing failure to perceive, and give therapy to, a treatable case.
33. Quoted by G. D. Knight in 'The Quaker Contribution to Psychiatric Thought', in *Addresses on the Occasion of the Retreat's 150th Anniversary* (York, 1946), p. 35.
34. Tuke, *Description*, p. 212; Thurnam, *Statistics*, pp. 25–6; Retreat *Report* (1912).
35. *Yorkshire Express*, 5 Dec. 1868.
36. BIHR K/2/12–13, case 1437. In 1895 the visiting Commissioners in Lunacy considered "the idiot boy . . . to be well looked after" (Retreat *Report* [1896]).
37. BIHR K/2/12, case 1,359.
38. Tuke, *Description*, p. 211; Thurnam, *Statistics*, table 36.
39. Bucknill and Tuke, *Psychological Medicine*, pp. 736–43; BIHR K/2/10, case 1062, was treated with a bismuth mixture, and K/2/12, case 1395, indicates a borax mixture was used.
40. BIHR G/1/1, 24 July 1880; Retreat *Report* (1897).
41. Ray, 'Models of Madness', pp. 262–3; Parry-Jones, *Trade in Lunacy*, pp. 207, 210; A. Digby, 'The Changing Profile of a Nineteenth-Century Asylum: The York Retreat', *Psychological Medicine* 14 (1984).

42. Thurnam, *Statistics*, table 19.
43. Tuke, *Description*, p. 216.
44. Thurnam, *Statistics*, p. 29.
45. Retreat *Report* (1910).
46. Ray, 'Models of Madness', p. 256; Parry-Jones, *Trade in Lunacy*, p. 202.
47. BIHR K/2/2, case 708.
48. BIHR C/1, S. Thorpe to George Jepson, 5 March 1814.
49. Thurnam, *Statistics*, p. 29.
50. BIHR K/2/8, case 862.
51. BIHR K/2/9, case 963, observation of 9 Feb. 1863.
52. BIHR K/2/3, case 395.
53. BIHR K/2/3, case 408.
54. He was readmitted as case 772 and then 830.
55. Retreat *Report* (1905).
56. Tuke, *Description*, p. 202; Thurnam, *Statistics*, p. 30.
57. Retreat *Report* (1904).
58. For example, case 150 (BIHR J/1/1).
59. Thurnam, *Statistics*, table 36.
60. Ibid., tables 32, 36.
61. BIHR K/2/8, case 347.
62. Thurnam, *Statistics*, appendix.
63. J. Conolly, *The Construction and Government of Lunatic Asylums* (1847), p. 151.
64. Returns given in Parliamentary Papers in appendices to the annual *Reports of the Commissioners in Lunacy*.
65. B. R. Mitchell and P. Deane, *Abstract of British Historical Statistics* (Cambridge, 1962), pp. 36–7.
66. Retreat *Report* (1924).
67. Thurnam, *Statistics*, appendix; Conolly, *Lunatic Asylums*, p. 151.
68. Thurnam, *Statistics*, p. 33.
69. Tuke, *Description*, p. 202.
70. BIHR L/3/2, Thurnam's return of 1844; Retreat *Report* (1845); Thurnam, *Statistics*, pp. 33–4.
71. BIHR C/1, J. Nevill to S. Tuke, 26 April 1824. Ann B. was first admitted as case 94 and readmitted as case 293.
72. Samuel W. was admitted as case 85 and Margaret B. as case 116.
73. Sarah G. was first admitted as case 178, Elizabeth G. as case 285 and Elizabeth W. as case 1722.
74. Tuke, *Description*, p. 216.
75. Parry-Jones, *Trade in Lunacy*, p. 160.
76. I am grateful to Nicholas Hervey for kindly supplying me with further details on the patients' record than was contained in his *Bowhill House* (Exeter, 1980).

10. THE RETREAT'S INFLUENCE

1. M. A. Crowther, 'A Grand Tour of Total Institutions: From Dickens to Goffman', *Social History Society Newsletter*, 8 (1983). (A Summary of a paper given to the Social History Society Conference, Jan. 1983.)
2. Tuke, *Memoirs*, I, chap. V.
3. Ibid., entries 3 Jan. 1811, 25 Oct. 1810.
4. Ibid., I, chap. V.
5. *Description*, pp. 146–7, 198.
6. BIHR L/3/2, S. Tuke to G. Higgins, 23 Dec. 1815.
7. Ibid.
8. *York Chronicle*, 22 Sept. 1813. For a fuller discussion see A. Digby, 'Changes in the Asylum: The Case of York, 1777–1815', *Economic History Review*, 2d ser., XXVI (1983), pp. 218–39.
9. *York Chronicle*, 29 Sept. 1813.

10. *York Chronicle*, 7 Oct. 1813 and (as 'Observator') 14 Oct. 1813.
11. 'Civis' (J. Wemyss) in *York Herald*, 16 Oct. 1813.
12. S. W. Nicoll, Recorder of Doncaster, advised S. Tuke to stay in the background lest projected reform should appear that of a Retreat party (BIHR L/3/2, S. Tuke to G. Higgins, 7 Dec. 1813).
13. 'Non-Irrisor', in *York Herald*, 23 Oct. 1813; 'Monitor', in *York Chronicle*, 18 Nov. 1813.
14. 'Monitor', *York Chronicle*, 27 Nov. 1813.
15. G. Higgins, *A Letter to the Earl Fitzwilliam* (Doncaster, 1814), pp. 10–11; J. Gray, *A History of the York Lunatic Asylum* (York, 1815), pp. 22–3, 38–41; BIHR L/3/2, correspondence between S. Tuke and G. Higgins, Dec. 1813–April 1814.
16. BIHR L/3/1, Introduction to Papers Respecting the York Lunatic Asylum.
17. BIHR L/3/2, S. Tuke to G. Higgins, 22 Jan. 1814.
18. BIHR L/3/1, *Reports of Governors of York Lunatic Asylum* (1814–39); Bootham Park Hospital, Proceedings of Committee (1821–34).
19. Tuke, *Memoirs*, I, p. 258.
20. BIHR L/3/2, S. Tuke to G. Higgins, 23 Dec. 1815.
21. Digby, 'Changes in the Asylum', pp. 218–39.
22. See, e.g., the pamphlet by the apothecary C. Atkinson, *Retaliation; or Hints, to some of the Governors of the York Lunatic Asylum* (York, 1814) and that by Corrector, *A Few Free Remarks on Mr. Higgins' Publications* (York, 1814).
23. *Evidence taken before a committee of the House of Commons respecting the asylums at York* (Doncaster, 1816), p. 2.
24. *Second Report from the Committee on Madhouses in England*, Parliamentary Papers 1814–15, IV (Evidence, 26 May 1815).
25. Parry-Jones, *Trade in Lunacy*, pp. 173, 187.
26. Ibid. appendix B and index of private madhouses; J. A. R. Bickford and M. E. Bickford, *The Private Lunatic Asylums of the East Riding* (E. Riding Local History Society, 1976).
27. *York Chronicle*, 29 Sept. 1813.
28. *Osbaldwick* (Osbaldwick History Group, 1980), pp. 91–2.
29. Bickford and Bickford, pp. 23–5, 29–34.
30. Ibid., p. 27.
31. Ibid., p. 14.
32. William Charles Ellis became the first superintendent of Hanwell in 1831 and was later the first psychiatrist to be honoured with a knighthood. In 1815 he had published *Letter to Thomas Thompson, M. P.* in which he welcomed the treatment developed at the York Retreat.
33. BIHR D/3/1, Visitors Book (1798–1822). Caleb Crowther, visiting physician to the asylum, also visited in Dec. 1817.
34. D. H. Tuke, *The Past and Present Provision for the Insane Poor in Yorkshire* (1889), p. 8.
35. BIHR L/3/2, G. Higgins to S. Tuke, 24 Oct. 1814; *Letter to Earl Fitzwilliam*, p. 16.
36. Stanley Royd Hospital, Wakefield; Order Book, Pauper Lunatic Asylum, 30 Nov. 1814, 5 April 1815. (The Stanley Royd Hospital is the successor of the West Riding Asylum.) I am grateful to Mr. A. L. Ashworth for his expert guidance on the hospital's records.
37. BIHR L/3/2, S. Tuke to G. Higgins, 4 Nov. 1814, and G. Higgins to S. Tuke, 18 June 1815.
38. Order Book, Pauper Lunatic Asylum, 2 Nov. 1815.
39. *Plans, Elevations, Sections and Description of the Pauper Lunatic Asylum by Watson and Pritchett* (York, 1819).
40. A. L. Ashworth, *Stanley Royd Hospital Wakefield: One Hundred and Fifty Years, A History* (Wakefield, 1975), p. 15.
41. See chap. 3, 'A Therapeutic Environment'.
42. *Practical Hints*, p. 8.

Notes to pages 245–251   317

43. Ibid., p. 5.
44. BIHR D/3/1–3, Visitors Books, 1798–1860.
45. A. P. Williamson, 'The Origins of the Irish Mental Hospital Service' (M. Litt. thesis, 1970. Trinity College, University of Dublin), pp. 11, 68–71, 94, 99, 108, 113; M. Finnane, *Insanity and the Insane in Poet-Famine Ireland* (1981), pp. 23, 32, 227.
46. *Memoirs*, I, p. 166.
47. BIHR C/1, T. Morris to G. Jepson, 6 Dec. 1811; L/3/2, Dr. Pennington to S. Tuke, 16 July 1814.
48. BIHR C/1, T. Morris to G. Jepson, 10 July 1814.
49. In this context it is interesting that the architect of Hanwell, William Anderson, consulted Samuel Tuke over his design. (C. Tylor, *Samuel Tuke: His Life, Work and Thoughts* [1900] p. 165).
50. Order Book, Pauper Lunatic Asylum, 11 Dec. 1817; BIHR L/3/2, S. Tuke to G. Higgins, Sept. (?) 1815.
51. BIHR C/1, J. Ewen to G. Jepson, 18 Sept. 1813; W. Griffiths to G. Jepson, 2 Feb. 1813.
52. BIHR C/1, A. Cruikshank to G. Jepson, 16 Feb. 1813, 10 April 1813; Quoted in Tuke, *Description*, p. 226.
53. W. Stark, *Remarks on the Construction and Management of Public Hospitals for the cure of mental derangement* (Glasgow, 1810), pp. 11–13; E. O. Checkland, *Philanthropy in Victorian Scotland: Social Welfare and the Voluntary Principle* (Edinburgh, 1980), p. 170.
54. BIHR C/1, F. Nicoll to T. Allis, 4 March 1834.
55. BIHR C/1, Memorandum of Mr Reid, 1813.
56. BIHR C/1, W. Drury to G. Jepson, 12 June 1817.
57. BIHR C/1, A. Macintosh to T. Allis, 9 June 1830.
58. For example, M. Ellis of Wakefield Asylum to G. Jepson, 2 Sept. 1819.
59. BIHR C/1, C. Cresson to G. Jepson, 4 March 1817, 24 May 1817.
60. See F. B. Tolles, *Quakers and the Atlantic Culture* (New York, 1960), chaps. 1 and 2 for the origins of this community, and G. N. Grob, *Mental Institutions in America: Social Policy to 1875* (New York, 1973), pp. 19, 26, 30–1, 48, for an account of early American provision.
61. *Memoirs*, I, p. 158, entry for 9 March 1811.
62. R. Hunter and I. MacAlpine, 'Samuel Tuke's First Publication on the Treatment of Patients at the Retreat', *British Journal of Psychiatry*, 111 (1965), p. 770.
63. J. Griscom, *A Year in Europe in 1818 and 1819*, 2 vols. (New York, 1823), II, p. 302.
64. *Friends Asylum for the Insane 1813–1913* (Philadelphia, 1913), pp. 14–16, 63.
65. A. Scull, 'The Discovery of the Asylum Revisited: Lunacy Reform in the New American Republic', in Scull, ed., *Madhouses, Mad-Doctors, and Madmen* (London, 1981), p. 147.
66. S. Tuke, *A Letter to Thomas Eddy of New York on Pauper Lunatic Asylums* (New York, 1815).
67. T. Eddy, *Hints for Introducing an Improved Mode of Treating the Insane in the Asylum: Read before the Governors of New York Hospital on 4 April 1815* (New York, 1815), p. 5.
68. Grob, *Mental Institutions*, p. 63.
69. *A Psychiatric Milestone: Bloomingdale Hospital Centenary, 1821–1921* (Society of the New York Hospital, 1921), p. 212.
70. BIHR L/3/2, S. Tuke to G. Higgins, 9 Dec. 1815.
71. Quoted in D. H. Tuke, *Chapters in the History of the Insane in the British Isles* (1882), p. 134; Scull, 'Asylum Revisited', pp. 148–51.
72. L. K. Eaton, 'Eli Todd and the Hartford Retreat', *New England Quarterly*, XXVI (1953), pp. 435–6, 441; F. J. Braceland, *The Institute of Living: The Hartford Retreat, 1822–1972* (Hartford, Conn. 1972), p. 13.
73. Scull, 'Asylum Revisited', p. 151.

74. Ibid., p. 149; Eaton, 'Eli Todd', p. 452.
75. Eaton, 'Eli Todd', p. 453.
76. BIHR D/3/3, entry of 2 June 1856.
77. Eaton, 'Eli Todd', p. 452.
78. Scull, 'Asylum Revisited', pp. 156–7.
79. Grob, *Mental Institutions*, p. 104; BIHR D/3/3, entry for 16 Aug. 1845. Other visitors included Luther V. Bell of the McLean, Dr. H. A. Buttolph of Utica, Rufus Woodward of Worcester State Hospital and W. Porter of the Hartwell Retreat.
80. N. Dain, *Concepts of Insanity in the United States, 1789–1865* (New Brunswick, N. J., 1964), pp. 21–2; Scull, 'Asylum Revisited', pp. 151–3; N. Dain and E. T. Carlson, 'Milieu Therapy in the Nineteenth Century: Patient Care at the Friends Asylum, Frankford, Pennsylvania 1817–61', *Journal of Nervous and Mental Diseases*, 131 (1960), pp. 277–90.
81. Grob, *Mental Institutions*, p. 169.
82. J. S. Bockhoven, *Moral Treatment in American Psychiatry* (New York, 1963), p. 70.
83. G. Zilboorg, *A History of Medical Psychology*, 2d ed. (New York, 1967), p. 409.
84. Tylor, *Samuel Tuke*, p. 81.
85. See chap. 4, 'Patients as children' and 'Moral Management and Moral Treatment'.
86. Quoted in D. Palliser and M. Palliser, eds, *York as They Saw It* (York, 1979), p. 57.
87. Quoted in Hunt, *Retired Habitation*, p. 56.
88. K. Doerner, *Madmen and the Bourgeoisie: A Social History of Insanity and Psychiatry* (Oxford, 1981), pp. 260–3, 339; D. H. Tuke, *Reform in the Treatment of the Insane: Early History of the Retreat, York* (1892), p. 51.
89. J. G. Kohl, *Travels in Ireland, Scotland and England*, 2d ed. (1968), p. 97.
90. *Memoirs*, I, p. 198, entry for 8 May 1813.
91. 'An Account of the York Retreat', *Edinburgh Review*, 23 (1814), p. 190.
92. BIHR H/2, S. Tuke to A. R. Barclay.
93. *Select Committee on State of Pauper Lunatics*, Parliamentary Papers 1826–7, VI, Q.37.
94. D. H. Tuke, *Prize Essay on the Moral Management of the Insane* (1854), p. 83.
95. R. G. Hill, *The Non-Restraint System* (London, 1857), p. 12.
96. D. H. Tuke, *Reform in Treatment*, p. 51; J. Conolly, *Treatment of the Insane without Mechanical Restraint* (London, 1856), p. x.
97. Conolly, *Treatment*, p. 18.
98. G. E. Bryant and G. P. Baker, eds., *A Quaker Journal being the Diary and Reminiscences of William Lucas of Hitchin*, 2 vols. (1933), II, p. 400.
99. Tuke, *Memoirs*, I, pp. 281–2. Nicholas was on a Grand Tour of Western Europe (H. Seton Watson, *The Russian Empire* [Oxford, 1967], p. 199).
100. Retreat *Report* (1892).

Index

In this index f refers to a figure, p to a plate, t to a table, and n to an endnote.

Ackworth School, 15, 16, 18–19, 21, 60, 114, 193, 246
Acts of Parliament, Lunatics (1845), 112, 126, 205, 223, 305 n31; Lunacy (1862) 205, 223; Lunacy (1890), 205, 223; Mental Deficiency (1913), 217
Adams, Thomas, 1
Admissions, 187, 203–4, 204f, 314 n22
Alexander, R. D., 101
Allen, Catherine *see* Jepson, Catherine
Allis, Mary, 109p
Allis, Thomas, appearance, 109p, 112; career, 106, 173, 305 n17; as lay therapist, 42, 50–2, 55–6, 63, 80; and medicine, 106, 124–6, 138; runs private madhouse, 111–12, 243; and religious healing, 25, 35; resignation, 111
Arlidge, J. T. 140
Arnold, Thomas, 5, 9, 11, 93, 236
Asylums (*see also* Private madhouses)
ENGLAND:
  County and Borough: Bedfordshire, 246; Cornwall, 246; Derby, 248; Lancashire, 144, 150, 208–9, 218, 246; Middlesex, Colney Hatch, 200, 313 n89; Middlesex, Hanwell, 82, 146, 309 n25; Nottingham, 246, 247; Surrey, Brookwood, 208, 209, 218; Wiltshire, 114; West Riding of Yorkshire (Wakefield), 146, 225, 244–6, 248
  Idiot: Bath, 217
  Public Subscription or Registered Hospitals: Bethlem, 2, 3, 6, 37, 66, 100, 119, 242, 246; Bowhill House, Exeter, 176, 177, 200, 235; Leicester, 4, 9; Lincoln, 197, 255; Liverpool, 4, 8, 9, 10, 246; Manchester, 4, 7, 8, 9, 10, 11, 66, 246; Newcastle, 4, 11; St. Luke's, London, 4–5, 9, 18, 21, 37, 140; York, 4, 8, 9, 10–12, 21, 37, 43, 130, 145, 146, 176, 213, 225, 239–42, 245, 246
FRANCE: Bicêtre, 31, 253; Salpetrière, 31
GERMANY: Siegburg, 254
IRELAND: Richmond, 246–7
SCOTLAND: Aberdeen, 248; Dundee, 249; Edinburgh, 119, 248, 249; Glasgow, 248–9
UNITED STATES OF AMERICA: Bloomingdale, New York, 250–1; Brattleborough, Vermont, 252; Frankford Retreat, 250, 251, 252; Hartford Retreat, 251, 252; McLean, Boston, 251–2; Utica, New York, 252; Worcester State Hospital, 252–3
Attendants, attitudes of, 99, 159–60; dismissal, 145, 153–4, 170; duties, 143, 144, 147–50, 169; hours, 149, 150, 151, 168; length of service, 100, 142–3, 166; ratio to patients, 145, 146; recruitment, 99, 141–2 156–8; relationship with patients, 66, 74, 79, 150–6, 161, 308 n4; training, 158, 165–7; viewed by others, 140–1, 148, 150, 155, 162, 165, 169; wages, 143–4, 158, 165, 167, 168; *see also* Waller, William

Baker, Robert, 86, 98, 116p, 167; career, 56, 115, 173, 306 n47; use of hydrotherapy, 134, 306 n47; emphasis on medical treatment, 115–16, 120, 124–7, 129; and moral treatment, 46; interest in mental handicap, 261, 287–90
Battie, William, 4–5, 11
Belcombe, H. S., 52, 107–8, 113, 127, 132
Belcombe, W. 24, 52, 101, 107–8, 127, 239, 243

319

Best, Charles, 239–41
Bevans, John, 18, 37–8, 54, 299 n19
Blanqui, Jerome, 253
Board of Control, 120; *see also* commissioners in Lunacy
Bompas, George, 246
Brigham, Amariah, 252, 253
Bright, John, 100
Bucknill, J. C., 61
Buildings of the Retreat, amenities, 40, 55, 209 n35; appearance, 37, 44p; the Appendage, 20, 23, 44p, 45, 69, 101, 141, 222, 271; cost, 18–20; Cottage Hospital, 115, 289; furnishings, 39–40; Gainsborough House, 69, 121, 124; grounds, 33, 37, 43; the Lodge, 23, 47p, 54, 115, 158, 276; and other asylums' buildings, 30–2; plans, 18, 38–40, 53, 68–9, 68p; security of, 39–40, 188, 312 n38; site, 33, 37, 43; Throxenby Hall, 69, 70p; villas, 54, 67, 115–19, 118p, 119p, 121
Burtt, Jonathan, 52, 306 n49

Candler, John, 112
Candler, Maria, 112
Cappe, Catherine, 267
Cappe, Dr, 24, 32, 127
Charlesworth, E. P., 197, 256
Cheyne, George, 8, 132
Chiarugi, Vincenzo, 30–1, 253
Clark, Michael, 28
Clarkson, Thomas, 89
Combe, George, 93
Commissioners in Lunacy, 84, 115, 117, 134, 140, 165, 182, 196, 212, 214, 215; *see also* Board of Control
Conolly, John, 57, 146, 147, 165, 225, 233, 255
Convalescence, 46, 69, 222–3
Cooter, R. J., 113
Cox, J. M., 5, 7–8
Cresson, Caleb, 249

Daquin, Joseph, 30–1, 253
Deaths, 28, 221, 224–6, 226f, 227t, 228t, 229t; *see also* Suicide
Delarive, Dr, 32, 58, 66, 87, 253
Description of the Retreat, 59, 61, 69, 78, 85, 106, 122, 131, 186; nature and influence of, xiii, 36, 237–55; *see also* Tuke, Samuel
Diet, 29, 51, 52, 101, 131–3
Dix, Dorothea, 252
Doerner, K., 8, 65
Duncan, Andrew, senior, 248

Eddy, Thomas, 250, 251
Education of patients, 58–61, 96–7
Ellis, Sir, W. C., 244, 316 n32
Employment of patients, 62–4
Epilepsy, 204, 217–18, 225, 260, 287–91
Escapes, 73, 188, 196–8
Esquirol, Jean, 93, 137, 170, 253
Evangelicalism, 6, 12, 23

Fears, Michael, 79
Ferriar, John, 5, 7, 10–11, 66–7, 236
Foucault, M., 7, 8, 57–58, 63–64, 75, 77
Fowler, Thomas, 23, 106, 122, 127
Fox, E. L., 23, 101, 186
Fox, George, 28, 35, 216
Fry, Elizabeth, 256
Freud, Sigmund, 139

Galen, 4
Goffman, E., 66
Griscom, John, 30, 250
Gurney, J. J., 88, 256

Hard Cash, 196, 313 n72
Haslam, John, 5, 6, 7, 66, 237
Higgins, Godfrey, 240–2, 244
Hill, R. Gardiner, 236
Hippocrates, 4
Hipsley, John, 21
Hogarth, William, 2
Howard, John, 18
Hunter, Alexander, 11–12, 241

Imbeciles, *see* Mental handicap
Insanity, *see* Mental illness
Isichei, E., 183, 185

Jacobi, Maximilian, 256
Jepson, Catherine (née Allen), 22p, 22–3, 50, 52–3, 108, 121
Jepson, George, 22p, 138, 173, 238, 241, 256, 259; appointment, 22–3; as lay therapist, 27, 35, 42, 72, 74, 79, 81, 101, 124–6, 132–3, 152–3, 261–78; and Retreat family, 26, 50–1, 53, 58, 121

Keepers *see* Attendants
Kemp, Norah, 117p, 121–2
Kitching, John, 56, 98, 116p, 254, 306 n42; early life, 53, 107, 108; sees insanity as disease, 28, 93–4, 114–15; treatment of mental illness, 35, 40, 46, 49, 74, 93–4, 97, 124–7, 134, 216–17; and patients, 61, 190, 260, 283–7; and attendants, 150, 162, 164, 169

Index

Kitching, W., 52
Kohl, J. G., 254

Lay therapy, 25–30, 106–13, 232
Lee, T. G., 252
Locke, John, 6, 10, 29, 34, 60, 81
Lunatics *see* Patients, Social character of patients, and Medical character of patients

McCandless, P., 306 n48
McKenzie, Dr, 117p
Madness *see* Mental illness
Maud, Timothy, 21
Maud, William, 24
Maudsley, Henry, 208
Medical character of patients, chronic, 42, 213–15, 219; curable, 213, 314 n32; deluded, 192–3, 200–1; violent, 67, 69, 74, 78–80, 149–51, 161, 193, 204, 263, 264, 268, 271, 274; *see also* Convalescence, Epilepsy, Mental handicap, Recoveries
Medical treatment, 218; bleeding, 5, 127, 129, 263, 264, 266, 267, 273, 275; case records, 36, 46, 61, 111, 113, 115, 189; counter-irritants, 5, 128, 262, 264, 266, 273; doctors and patients, 189–91, 200, 313 n89; force feeding, 132–3; postmortems, 225; villa system, 54, 67, 115–19, 118p, 119p, 121; *see also* Diet, Treatment
Medicine, aloes, 128; aperients, 5, 11, 128–9, 263, 264, 275; asafetida, 264; bismuth, 218; borax, 218; calomel, 128, 263; castor oil, 128; cephalic essence, 263; chloral hydrate, 129–30, 293, 294; cost of, 124–6, 125f, 126t; emetics, 5, 11, 128–9, 264; epasticus liquid, 294; hyoscyamine, 130; mercurials, 128; opiates, 127–8, 151; potassium bromide, 128–9, 218, 293, 294; saline mixtures, 128; tartrate of antimony, 128, 263; use made of, 122–7; *see also* Restraint
Medico-Psychological Association, 117, 120, 165, 206, 256
Mental handicap, 67, 188p, 209, 210, 211f, 212, 216–17, 220, 259, 261, 287–91
Mental illness, 37–8, 94; causes, 90–2, 97–8, 137–8, 207–13, 209t, 211f, 261, 292; classification of, 78, 135–7, 136t (*see also*, Epilepsy, Mental handicap, Mental illness); duration of, 213–21, 219t, 226–7, 227t, 228t; outcome of, 221–3; *see also*, Deaths, Readmissions, Recoveries
Mental nurses, *see* Attendants
Methodism, 35, 157
Moral insanity, 93–7, 95t, 259, 278–87
Moral management, 34, 61; and attendants, 155–6; classification of patients, 66–72; code of honour, 73–4, 189; discipline of patients, 62, 73, 76, 96–7; and moral treatment, 85–7, 115, 189, 199; *see also* Education of patients, Employment of patients, Patients, Restraint
Moral treatment, 33–4, 36, 115; and moral management, 85–7, 115, 189, 199; and Quaker values in 34–5, 40–1, 60; and religion, 34–6, 99–101; and Retreat family, 49–55, 57, 61, 147, 182, 191–3; and a therapeutic environment, 33–4, 37–42; *see also* Employment of patients, Lay therapy, Treatment, Spiritual healing
Murray, Lindley, 24, 152, 250

Newington, Hayes, 169
Newington, Samuel 246
Nicholas, Grand Duke of Russia, 256
Nicoll, S. W., 145, 241
Non-restraint movement, 82, 84, 178, 256
Nurses, *see* Attendants

Occupational therapy, *see* Treatment
Owen, Robert, 256

Pargeter, W., 6
Pascal, Blaise, 2
Patients, certificated, 205–6; as children, 52, 57–9, 64, 86; clothing of, 92, 189, 261, 291–2; and families, 26, 71, 193–4, 207, 212, 281–2; letters, 193–4; views on treatment, 36, 56, 63, 77, 129–30, 195, 196, 238, 281; views on visitors, 59, 194; voluntary, 206–7, 223–4; *see also* Medical character of patients, Social character of patients
Pecchio, Count, 253–4
Perceval, John, 186–7
Phrenology, 93–4, 113–14, 115
Pierce, Dr Bedford, 72, 117p, 121, 139; career, 117–20, 306 n56; and moral treatment, 46, 55–6, 72, 83; and mental illness, 137, 214, 216, 221; and mental nurses, 166–9
Pinel, Philippe, 30–2, 93, 237, 251, 252, 256
Ponsonby, Harriet, 50, 52, 108, 110p, 121

Pope, Alexander, 2
Prichard, James Cowles, 93
Private madhouses (*see also* Asylums)
ENGLAND: Brislington House, Bristol, 23, 146, 186, 246; Cleeve Hill, Bristol, 243; Cottingham Retreat, Yorks, 243; Darnall House, Yorks, 114; Duddeston Hall, Birmingham, 129; Fishponds, Bristol, 5, 246; Hessle Retreat, Yorks, 243; Hook Norton, Oxon, 177, 219, 235; Hollytree House, York, 243; Laverstock House, Salisbury, 242; Lawrence House, York, 306 n47; Painthorpe, Yorks, 114; The Poplars, York, 217; Sculcoates Refuge, Yorks, 243–4; Southcoates Retreat, Yorks, 243; Ticehurst, Sussex, 146, 169, 246, 294; Witney, Oxon, 177, 219, 235, 311 n8
IRELAND: Donnybrook, Dublin, 246: Loughall, Armagh, 246
Pumphery, Elizabeth, 58, 299 n39
Pumphery, William, 112, 306 n47

Quakers, *see* Society of Friends

Ray, Isaac, 252
Readmissions, 233–6, 236t
Recoveries, 221–2, 224, 226–33, 227t, 228t, 230t, 231t, 232f, 235
Reid, Robert, 248
Restraint, chemical, 128–9, 151, 261; internal, 72–8, 87, 260; mechanical, 78–84, 80p, 85, 260–1, 264, 268, 269, 274, 276
Retreat, The, constitution, 20–1, 101; finances, 17–20, 101–2, 104, 180–2, 184, 205, 220; influence of, 237–9, 247–56; origins, 12, 14–16; rules, 147–8; size, 53, 107, 108, 120–1, 199–200, 203, 203f; staffing, 22–4, 53, 104, 107–8, 120–1, 199–200, 203, 203f; visitors to, 43, 55, 59, 74, 121, 184–5, 237, 246f, 256, 257p; *see also* Admissions, Attendants, Buildings of the Retreat, *Description of the Retreat*, Patients, Society of Friends, Superintendents of the Retreat, Treatment
Richardson, Charlotte, 267, 269, 272
Rowntree, E., 167, 167p
Rush, Benjamin, 252

Scattergood, Thomas, 250
Scull, A. T., 8, 9, 66, 113, 215, 301 n59
Slee, Elizabeth, 162, 163p, 310 n75
Smith, Sydney, 254
Social character of patients, age, 176–7, 177t, 220, 225; gender differentiation, 42–3, 45, 48, 67–8, 96–7, 122, 174–5, 174t, 183, 186, 189–91, 209, 210, 212, 220; geographical origins, 177–80, 179t, 186; marital status, 175–6, 175t, 219–20, 311 n11; occupational background, 54, 183–4, 183t; Quaker and non-Quaker inmates, differentiation of, 42, 54, 102–4 103f, 173, 174–5, 178–80, 180t, 181, 186, 220t, 225, 236
Southern Retreat, 18
Society of Friends, discipline of, 34, 60, 88–93, 102, 175–6; disownments from, 88–9, 95–6, 175; and mental illness, 26–7, 35–6, 64–5, 89–101, 208; and the Retreat, 12–13, 16–17, 20–1, 25, 43, 45, 101–4, 175, social character of members, 14, 175, 178, 183, 185–6; *see also* Ackworth School, Fox, George
Spiritual healing, 27–8, 35–6
Stark, William, 39, 248
Suicide, 77, 79–80, 198–9
Superintendents of the Retreat, 21–3, 112–13; *see also* Allis, Thomas; Baker, Robert; Jepson, George; Kitching, John; Pierce, Bedford; Thurnam, John

Thurnam, John, 69, 110p; career, 107–8, 112; diagnoses, 136, 138; organic view of mental illness, 28, 97, 122–3, 209; and outcomes of illnesses, 221, 224, 233; and patients, 72–3, 89, 129–30, 260, 278–82; *Statistics of Insanity*, 63, 111; treatment of insanity, 124–7, 129–30, 131–2, 134, 218
Todd, Eli, 251, 252
Treatment, chemotherapy, 122–30; hydrotherapy, 76, 96, 130, 133–5, 269, 271, 292, 306 n47; mesmerism, 138; occupational therapy, 42–9; psycho analysis, 138–9; seclusion, 80–4, 86, 265–6, 269, 270; *see also* Diet, Medical treatment, Medicine, Moral management, Moral treatment, Phrenology, Restraint, Spiritual healing
Tuke, Ann, 15
Tuke, Daniel Hack, 32, 52, 60–1, 83, 94, 119, 123, 244
Tuke, Esther, 15
Tuke, Henry, 18, 19, 74, 89, 238, 240, 242, 265, 267, 273
Tuke, James, 157
Tuke, Mary Maria, 25
Tuke, Samuel, 3, 19p, 20, 52, 69, 117,

Index

181, 256; on asylum staff, 27, 86, 99, 144–5, 157; and other asylums, 239–41, 244–5, 249–50, 253; attitudes to the insane, 59–60, 207; and *Description of the Retreat*, 237–9, 254; on mechanical restraint, 78–81; on medical treatment, 106, 133–4; on moral treatment, 27, 35, 58, 85, 192; views on insanity, 26, 28, 208–9, 221, 235

Tuke, William, 19p, 52, 275; building and financing the Retreat, 18–19, 54; and patients, 26, 29, 50; and origins of the Retreat, 14–16, 38, 256; and York Asylum, 239–40

Tuke, William, nursing medal, 166–7

Waller, William, xiv, 140, 163, 169; appointment, 99, 156–8; attitudes to work, 141, 159–61, 164, 192; duties and salary, 158–9; early life, 156–7, 164; marriage, 162; resignation, 162, 164

Wellington, Duke of, 256

Williams, Caleb, 53, 107–8, 113, 127

Willis, Thomas, 6

Women, as doctors, 121–2; as matrons, 23, 50, 121; as nurses, 121, 142–4, 155, 167–8; as patients, 174–6, 183, 186, 209–10, 212, 278–87; as Retreat directors and visitors, 21, 307 n64; subject to "hysteria," 122, 189–90; vulnerability to insanity, 96, 312 n44; *see also* Allen, Catherine; Kemp, Norah; Ponsonby, Harriet; Social character of Patients

Wyman, Morrill, 251

DATE DUE